Cooking for Health and Disease Prevention

Cooking for Health and Disease Prevention
From the Kitchen to the Clinic

Edited by
Nicole M. Farmer
Andres Victor Ardisson Korat

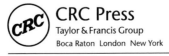

CRC Press
Taylor & Francis Group
Boca Raton London New York

CRC Press is an imprint of the
Taylor & Francis Group, an **informa** business

First edition published 2022
by CRC Press
6000 Broken Sound Parkway NW, Suite 300, Boca Raton, FL 33487-2742

and by CRC Press
2 Park Square, Milton Park, Abingdon, Oxon, OX14 4RN

© 2022 Taylor & Francis Group, LLC

CRC Press is an imprint of Taylor & Francis Group, LLC

Library of Congress Cataloging-in-Publication Data
Names: Farmer, Nicole M., editor. | Ardisson Korat, Andres V., editor.
Title: Cooking for health and disease prevention / edited by Nicole M. Farmer, Andres V. Ardisson Korat.
Description: First edition. | Boca Raton, FL : CRC Press, 2022. | Includes
bibliographical references and index. | Summary: "Chronic conditions
mainly impacted by diet and lifestyle are Alzheimer's, cancer, diabetes,
and heart disease. Numerous health benefits result from actual meal
preparation rather than the composition of the meal itself. This book
provides cooking methods and techniques to help improve nutrient
delivery and prevention or management chronic disease conditions. It
contains evidence-based information derived from food science studies
and clinical nutrition trials"—Provided by publisher.
Identifiers: LCCN 2021029908 (print) | LCCN 2021029909 (ebook) | ISBN 9781138304703 (hbk) |
ISBN 9781138304673 (pbk) | ISBN 9780203729892 (ebk)
Subjects: MESH: Diet Therapy | Cooking | Cookbooks as Topic
Classification: LCC RC271.D52 (print) | LCC RC271.D52 (ebook) | NLM WB
400 | DDC 641.5/631—dc23
LC record available at https://lccn.loc.gov/2021029908
LC ebook record available at https://lccn.loc.gov/2021029909

ISBN: 9781138304703 (hbk)
ISBN: 9781138304673 (pbk)
ISBN: 9780203729892 (ebk)

DOI: 10.1201/b22377

Typeset in Times
by codeMantra

From Nicole Farmer: To my family and friends, thank you for your support and love. Thank you for so many wonderful moments in the kitchen and around the kitchen table. In ode to some of those treasured moments are the following quotes embedded in my memories: "The greens need a little bit more time," "Don't let the plantains burn," and "You can always figure out how to make your own sauce."

From Andres Victor Ardisson Korat: To Barbara and Andrea, your love and support has been the secret ingredient for this book. I hope these pages inspire many more kitchen experiments together.

Drs. Farmer and Korat would like to acknowledge Randy Brehm and Julia Tanner of Taylor and Francis for their work and support.

Dr. Farmer would like to acknowledge that the information and contents in this book do not reflect the opinions or approved content from Health and Human Services Agency or the National Institutes of Health.

Contents

Editors

Dr. Nicole M. Farmer is currently a Staff Scientist at the NIH Clinical Center. In this intramural research position, Dr. Farmer is involved in both community-based and patient research exploring the role of cooking in chronic disease prevention and psychosocial health. Prior to joining the NIH, she was a well-established primary care clinician and routinely engaged her patients in nutrition education through cooking classes. Dr. Farmer's research focus may be categorized into three major areas: psychosocial outcomes of health behaviors, role of cooking interventions on dietary behaviors and cardiovascular outcomes, and mechanisms of health disparities. She received the 2020 William G. Coleman Minority Health and Health Disparities Research Innovation Award from the NIH's National Institute of Minority and Health Disparity for her work in exploring microbiome-related dietary metabolites in cardiovascular disease health disparities. Dr. Farmer is an alumnus of Howard University College of Medicine, received her internal medicine training from Thomas Jefferson University Hospital, and held a prior appointment at Johns Hopkins University Hospital. She has also completed fellowship-level training in Integrative Medicine from the Center for Integrative Medicine at the University of Arizona and Duke University Integrative Medicine.

Dr. Andres Victor Ardisson Korat is a nutrition researcher and a food scientist interested in investigating the role of diet in chronic disease prevention. His research draws on his expertise in the fields of nutrition, epidemiology, food processing, and culinary arts.

Dr. Ardisson Korat's training includes a doctorate in nutrition and epidemiology from the Harvard T.H. Chan School of Public Health, an M.S. in food science from Cornell University, an M.A. in gastronomy from the University of Adelaide and Le Cordon Bleu, and a B.S. in food industries engineering from Instituto Tecnológicoy de Estudios Superiores de Monterrey (ITESM) in Mexico. He also holds a certificate in culinary arts from Collin College. Prior to his studies in nutrition, he worked in research and development in the food industry creating new technologies to incorporate whole grains in food products and developing solutions to reduce sodium, eliminate trans fats, and increase fiber and whole grains in processed foods.

Andres hopes that this book can help disseminate ideas for health prevention by bringing together nutrition principles and culinary techniques.

Contributors

Andres Victor Ardisson Korat
Harvard T.H. Chan School of Public
    Health
Boston, Massachusetts

Graciela Caraballo
The George Washington University
    School of Medicine & Health
    Sciences
Washington, District of Columbia

Xonna M. Clark
Xonna Clarck, LLC
Germantown, Maryland

Kofi Essel
Children's National Hospital
Washington, District of Columbia
and
The George Washington University
    School of Medicine & Health
    Sciences
Washington, District of Columbia

Nicole M. Farmer
National Institutes of Health, Clinical
    Center
Bethesda, Maryland

Joshua Z. Goldenberg
The Goldenberg GI Center, LLC
Colorado Springs, Colorado
and
Helfgott Research Institute
Portland, Oregon

Vincent W. Li
The Angiogenesis Foundation
Cambridge, Massachusetts

Winifred Nwanety
University of Maryland Medical System
Baltimore, Maryland

Grace Rivers
Nutrition Works, Inc.
Richardson, Texas

Joel J. Schaefer
Your Allergy Chefs
Hendersonville, Nevada

Mary Schaefer
Your Allergy Chefs
Hendersonville, Nevada

Delaney K. Schurr
The Angiogenesis Foundation
Cambridge, Massachusetts

Catherine Ward
The Angiogenesis Foundation
Cambridge, Massachusetts

1 Introduction

Nicole M. Farmer
National Institutes of Health, Clinical Center

Andres Victor Ardisson Korat
Harvard T.H. Chan School of Public Health

As professionals focused on health prevention, we have witnessed the connection between our everyday food choices and our long-term health outlook in our everyday work. This is true whether directly interacting with patients or looking at dietary patterns for large groups of individuals. The idea for this book comes from the belief that what we eat and how we prepare our foods, including our selection of ingredients and cooking methods, have profound effects on our wellbeing and health. In fact, the journal *Lancet* publishes a report of the Global Burden of Disease every year, which has consistently identified poor diet and nutrition as one of the leading factors of premature death worldwide. Cardiovascular diseases, diabetes, and cancer primarily cause these deaths. With this book, we want to expand this knowledge to think about what we eat and how we select, prepare, and cook foods to present them as equally important factors. This book is about building a bridge between our kitchens and our long-term health.

Cooking is a central activity in our lives, whether we engage in food preparation ourselves or enjoy the labor of somebody else's work in the kitchen. Cooking makes our food richer by imparting complex flavors and aroma to our dishes, thus providing enjoyment to our senses. Cooking makes our food safe to eat, and it allows us to consume several foods that would otherwise remain unavailable to us, such as grains, tubers, several cuts of meats, and legumes. Cooking is an expression of our culture and traditions. French anthropologist Claude Levi-Strauss has argued that cooking makes us human: "Not only does cooking mark the transition from nature to culture, but through it and by means of it, the human state can be defined with all of its attributes." Cooking has been a central human activity throughout our history and a fundamental step in our development as a species. Cooking is so essential that anthropologist Richard Wrangham stated as follows: "We humans are the cooking apes, the creatures of the flame."

Cooking is also markedly connected to our biology. For instance, cooking starchy foods can modify our gut microbiome, which influences the presence and quantity of several microbial metabolites (chemicals made by the microbiome). Cooking can also alter antimicrobial compounds found in natural foods. On the other hand, various types of high-heat cooking can create compounds that may possess carcinogenic effects. Given the intimate role that cooking can play in our biology, it is surprising that cooking methods are not frequently queried during dietary measurements and interviews. Furthermore, cooking methods are seldom considered in dietary assessment methods, especially in large cohort studies. We suspect that one reason for this

DOI: 10.1201/b22377-1

omission is that the totality of cooking's effects on the nutritional value of food is understood in compartments but not comprehensively. Furthermore, the results from cooking are not placed within the context of how people prepare and consume foods at home. Although databases provided by the United States Department of Agriculture (USDA) offer extensive and valuable water loss tables and significant nutrient loss for commonly consumed foods, the cooking methods reflected therein do not often represent how people cook at home. In recent years, the food science literature has provided intriguing and interesting experiments focused on replicating home cooking times and traditional cooking and measurement resultant nutrients. The value of the experimental loss or retainment of nutrients stems from nutritional epidemiology and clinical trial studies that have evaluated specific nutrients and dietary patterns impacting human biology and metabolism. Cooking can also provide a vehicle for sustainability. A recent report by the EAT-*Lancet* Commission developed targets for healthy diets that met standards for sustainable food production. From a human health perspective, the report found that globally, most people consume fruits, vegetables, nuts, and legumes at levels below adequate. In contrast, red meat and sugar are consumed at levels above the current dietary recommendations, especially in North America. Conversely, consumption levels of fruits, vegetables, nuts, whole grains, and fish are currently below the recommended amounts. Choosing some foods over others influences our health. Still, it also has enormous impacts on planetary health through agricultural lands, greenhouse gas emissions, water use, and biodiversity loss, among others. Thus, the report considered that "Food is the single strongest lever to optimize human health and environmental sustainability on Earth."

This book aims to make essential connections between the foods we eat and the prevention of the most common chronic ailments in the United States and other countries. The book introduces what may at first seem common sense or appear to be widely understood (i.e., boiling of vegetables causes loss of water-soluble vitamins). But the information is subtly lost or not applied within the health and nutrition research literature on cooking. For example, which nutrients are retained when vegetables are steamed or boiled? Which traditional cooking methods or recipes can increase the bioavailability of evidence-based nutrients? And what are the possible explanations based on food science and molecular nutrition?

The book is essentially divided into three parts. Part 1 introduces the major themes of the book (Chapters 1–3). Part 2 consists of chapters focused on specific disease outcomes (Chapters 4–8). Part 3 explores the application of the knowledge in the last parts of the book (Chapters 9 and 10). Each chapter in Part 2 explores the pathophysiology of various diseases, including cardiovascular disease, diabetes, osteoarthritis, inflammatory bowel syndrome, and liver disease, as primary examples. More importantly, each chapter provides essential information regarding the connection between individual foods, cooking methods, overall dietary patterns, and the prevention of these diseases. These chapters aim at improving our collective health while offering ideas and suggestions about food choices and delicious dishes in the process. Within each chapter, there is a focus on plant-based foods. This focus is due to the emphasis on sustainability that comes from plant-based diets and the current evidence-based diets supporting the role of plant-based diets on health promotion and disease prevention. Moreover, our belief is that knowledge on how to cook vegetables is crucial to help bring evidence-based diets, such as the DASH diet, into kitchens and homes.

We hope that this book will be used as a resource in a variety of ways and settings. The information provided may be of value to not only the health-conscious home cook but also the food-focused clinician or the culinary professional interested in the capacity of food to improve health. Lastly, the fields of food science and nutrition are truly dynamic, as with time, new understandings of pathways and nutrients occur. Thus, we anticipate that as the fields continue to advance, some of the information included in this book may require updating or a renewed view.

2 Effects of Food Processing, Storage, and Cooking on Nutrients in Plant-Based Foods

Fruits, Vegetables, Cereals, and Grains

Andres Victor Ardisson Korat
Harvard T.H. Chan School of Public Health

CONTENTS

FOOD PROCESSING

The term food processing includes any method used to transform raw agricultural commodities or ingredients into food products that can be readily consumed. Food processing involves one or more steps including sorting, washing, mixing, heating, baking, freezing, packaging, and many others. The US Food and Drug Administration

DOI: 10.1201/b22377-2

definition includes a comprehensive list of transformation steps as defined in the
Code of Federal Regulations, Title 21 (21CFR1.227):

> Manufacturing/processing means making food from one or more ingredients, or syn-
> thesizing, preparing, treating, modifying or manipulating food, including food crops or
> ingredients. Examples of manufacturing/processing activities include: baking, boiling,
> bottling, canning, cooking, cooling, cutting, distilling, drying/dehydrating raw agricul-
> tural commodities to create a distinct commodity (such as drying/dehydrating grapes to
> produce raisins), evaporating, eviscerating, extracting juice, formulating, freezing, grind-
> ing, homogenizing, irradiating, labeling, milling, mixing, packaging (including modified
> atmosphere packaging), pasteurizing, peeling, rendering, treating to manipulate ripening,
> trimming, washing, or waxing. For farms and farm mixed-type facilities, manufacturing/
> processing does not include activities that are part of harvesting, packing, or holding.
>
> *US Food and Drug Administration, 2019*

Some of these processing steps, such as washing, waxing, or sorting, involve minimal food transformation, whereas other steps carry nutritional implications, including changes to the levels of vitamins, minerals, and dietary fiber, or changes to the
macronutrient composition of foods resulting from the addition of fats and sugars. Of
note, many food processes have been designed with food safety as the main objective;
however, they affect the final nutritional content of foods. For instance, pasteurization, canning, freezing, and dehydration processes are designed to slow down or stop
bacterial activity that would otherwise result in detrimental changes of the nutritional
and sensory properties of the food (spoilage) or result in pathogen growth. However,
these processes may change the levels of vitamins, minerals, and polyphenols present in these foods. Similar processing steps take place at home and in commercial
kitchens, albeit at a different scale. These include boiling, steaming, baking, frying,
grilling/griddling, and broiling to name a few. These cooking methods help transform
raw foods and ingredients into safe and ready-to-consume meals, and just like in the
case of industrial processes, the selection of cooking method carries implications not
only for the final flavor and texture of the product but also for its nutritional content.

AIMS OF FOOD PROCESSING

Industrial food processing has four primary goals: (1) extend the shelf life of foods
by slowing down the microbial and biochemical reactions that produce degradation,
(2) add nutrients required for health via supplementation or fortification, (3) provide variety to dietary choices by increasing the year-round availability of many
products, often time in markets located far from the place where the raw materials
were grown, (4) add value to the manufacturer (Park, Lamsal, & Balasubramaniam,
2014). Shelf life extension is achieved by preserving food products against physical, chemical, and biological hazards. This is accomplished through a broad range
of technologies, such as washing and sorting, to remove physical hazards including
dirt, stones and damaged product. Other steps target the mitigation of chemical and
microbial hazards by thermal inactivation of enzymes and microbial agents through
pasteurization, freezing, or drying as well as the addition of sugar, salt, or chemical
preservatives. In general, food processing is divided into primary and secondary

processing. Primary processing includes all steps from harvest or slaughter involved in the preparation raw materials for direct consumption or steps necessary to manufacture ingredients to be used in other products. Secondary processing transforms these food ingredients into ready-to-eat processed foods (Park et al., 2014). This chapter will examine the effects of various industrial processes and cooking methods (used at home and in commercial kitchens) on various nutrients and components present in fruits, vegetables, and grains.

INDUSTRIAL PROCESSING OF FRUITS AND VEGETABLES

Processing fruits and vegetables includes several primary steps occurring at the farm and at collection and distribution centers including grading, washing, and sorting as well as secondary steps including peeling, dicing, blanching, freezing, or canning.

PRIMARY PROCESSING STEPS

Grading is used to assess the quality of harvested products and to determine the price paid to the farmer. Farmers are usually paid based on the proportion of products that falls within several quality categories based on US Department of Agriculture (USDA) standards (Sumonsiri & Barringer, 2014). These quality standards are based on the degree of ripeness and other parameters such as the total solids, total sugar, color, appearance, and texture. There are separate USDA grades used for fruits and vegetables consumed fresh, dried, frozen, or canned. For instance, USDA grades for fresh vegetables in descending order of quality are U.S. Extra Fancy, U.S. Fancy, U.S. Extra No. 1, and U.S. No. 1. There are grades developed for specific vegetables when particular attributes are needed.

Washing helps eliminate dirt, microorganisms, pesticide residues, and soil and is an important step in the control of microbial residues in fruits and vegetables. Fruits and vegetables are washed either by immersing them in water tanks or water plumes with continuous water recirculation, which are used to decrease the amount of soil and dirt that come in with the harvested product (Figure 2.1).

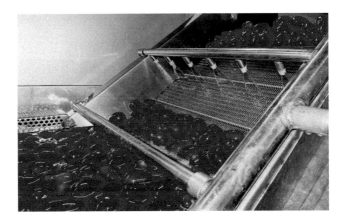

FIGURE 2.1　Tomato washing process.

Sorting is used to separate the harvested product into several streams, which may represent products of various sizes or quality standards. Sorting can be accomplished by mechanical means, especially to separate products by size, or it can be achieved manually using visual inspection to separate products of different quality standards. Mechanical sorting of several fruits and vegetables is accomplished by suspending the product between two conveyor belts onto which the product is perched, leaving a gap in the middle. As the product is conveyed forward, the gap gradually increases allowing the smallest pieces to be separated first and continuing until only the largest pieces are left. Size sorting can also be achieved by conveying products on top of a series of rollers adapted with orifices of increasing sizes. Color sorting is typically carried out by automated optical sorting units with an additional inspection step by a human operator (Figure 2.2).

Minimally processed fruits and vegetables undergo basic processing steps such as washing and sometimes peeling or cutting. Examples of these products include vegetables ready to use in salads such as lettuce, arugula, salad greens, baby carrots, and other products sold in packages ready for microwave cooking. The shelf life of these products is limited (3–7 days) and is typically extended by storage and transportation at refrigeration temperatures.

Storage and packaging technologies: The shelf life of fresh fruits and vegetables can be extended by storing them under reduced temperature conditions and/or by modifying the conditions of the packaging environment including the regulation of levels of oxygen, carbon dioxide, water vapor, and ethylene inside the packaging container (Vaclavik & Christian, 2014). Temperature-controlled storage decreases the rate of respiration, which in turn slows down fruit ripening, minimizes moisture loss, and controls microbial growth. Modification of the surrounding gases controls the respiration rate and facilitates shipping and distribution (Sumonsiri & Barringer, 2014). Fruits and vegetables continue to exchange gases with the environment after harvest. Thus, reducing the oxygen level in the environment to about 5% in a controlled-temperature environment (compared to 21% in the atmosphere) can extend the shelf life of many products. Increasing carbon dioxide levels helps prevent the growth of aerobic organisms responsible for the degradation of fruits and vegetables

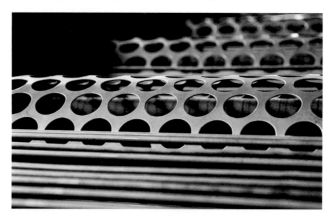

FIGURE 2.2   Perforated rolls used to sort fruit by size.

such as yeast, mold, and some types of bacteria. The two most common forms of these technologies used in the postharvest handling of fruits and vegetables are modified atmosphere packaging (MAP) and controlled atmosphere packaging (CAP).

MAP is used to introduce a mixture of gases to change the composition of the atmosphere surrounding fresh or minimally processed fruits or vegetables. MAP involves substituting the air immediately surrounding the product with an atmosphere with a gas composition different from air, usually with lower oxygen levels and higher carbon dioxide. MAP is applied to fruits and vegetables that are still undergoing respiration. Of note, the composition of the air surrounding the product is balanced for each commodity. Typically, the modified atmosphere is introduced once; thus, the composition of the atmosphere changes gradually throughout storage as a result of fruit and vegetable respiration (Vaclavik & Christian, 2014).

CAP is a system that continuously preserves the desired atmospheric composition in the packaging environment or storage containers (Vaclavik & Christian, 2014). CAP maintains the atmospheric composition constant by injecting the desired gas mixture at prescribed intervals dictated by the respiration rate of the fruit or vegetable commodity or by introducing oxygen scavenging agents into the packaging material. The former technique is compatible with large storage vessels (i.e., commercial shipping containers), whereas the latter can be applied to smaller packages.

Effects of controlled and modified atmosphere storage on selected nutrients: The use of MAP to extend the shelf life of fresh fruits and vegetables does not have apparent detrimental effects on their vitamin content when compared to storage at atmospheric conditions (Barth & Zhuang, 1996; Granado-Lorencio et al., 2008; Villanueva, Tenorio, Sagardoy, Redondo, & Saco, 2005). For instance, storage of broccoli florets at 5°C for 6 days in a modified atmosphere containing 11.2% oxygen and 7.5% carbon dioxide did not result in appreciable losses of beta-carotene and vitamin C; in contrast, the control product (without MAP) retained only about 50% of these nutrients (Barth & Zhuang, 1996). Tocopherol levels were comparable across different treatments, suggesting MAP does not have an effect on its retention (Barth & Zhuang, 1996). Two separate studies observed similar retention of beta-carotene, lutein, and tocopherols in broccoli stored in MAP conditions compared to the unpackaged product (Granado-Lorencio et al., 2008) and in sweet potatoes stored in MAP under refrigerated conditions (Erturk & Picha, 2002). These findings are consistent with a separate study that examined the effects of MAP and cold storage on beta-carotene stability in strawberries, which found similar retention profiles comparing the product stored under MAP to the product stored under normal conditions (Ekinci, Aydin, & Şeker, 2016). Of interest, this study did not find differences in the levels of these nutrients in human serum samples after randomly assigning participants to consume the products stored in MAP conditions vs. unpackaged for 4 weeks (Granado-Lorencio et al., 2008). A separate study observed differential deterioration of vitamin C during storage of asparagus samples observing higher retention rates in the product stored under MAP conditions vs. the unpackaged control (Villanueva et al., 2005). Storage of bell peppers under MAP resulted in better retention of vitamin C in mature samples (Ogawaa & Suzuki, 2016).

Storage under MAP conditions also helps retain most phenolic compounds. For instance, storage of radicchio under MAP or control conditions (both under refrigerated temperatures) did not contribute to total phenolic compound losses (Cefola, Carbone, Minasi, & Pace, 2016). In contrast, refrigerated storage of broccoli (without MAP) resulted in substantial losses (>50%) of several phenolic compounds including glucosinolates, flavonoids, and caffeoylquinic acid derivatives (Vallejo, Tomas-Barberan, & Garcia-Vigurea, 2003). In conclusion, MAP storage – especially in conjunction with refrigerated temperatures – results in better retention of most vitamins and several phenolic compounds. However, the retention profiles of each micronutrient depend greatly on the commodity, stage of maturity, and the specific settings for temperature and MAP gas composition.

SECONDARY PROCESSING STEPS

Peeling removes undesirable portions of the product and helps control microbial counts for roots and tubers, which may have higher microbial loads owing to soil residues that persist after washing. The most common methods include mechanical peeling, steam peeling, and caustic peeling (Sumonsiri & Barringer, 2014). Mechanical peeling is the physical removal of peels using blades placed in a fixed position against which fruits or vegetables rotate or with the use of an abrasive surface. Steam peeling is carried out in a pressurized vessel that breaks the cells underneath the peel of carrots, tomatoes, potatoes, and beets (Sumonsiri & Barringer, 2014). In caustic peeling, fruits or vegetables are submerged in a hot sodium hydroxide solute (10%–20%) for a few minutes to hydrolyze the pectin that keeps the skin in place. The physical removal of peels is associated with substantial decreases (10%–30%) in total crude fiber, folic acid, ascorbic acid, and moderate decreases of most minerals (<10%) (Alvi, Khan, Sheikh, & Shahid, 2003). However, no information is available regarding the nutrient retention profiles of these peeling methods (Figure 2.3).

Dicing and slicing creates even-sized product slices, cubes or shreds depending on the final product need. This operation is traditionally achieved with highly mechanized cutting blades with carefully adjusted size specifications. Whole products

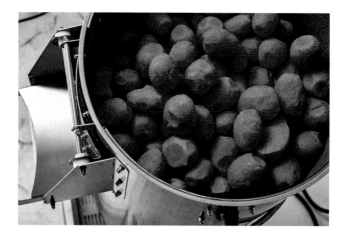

FIGURE 2.3 Machine for peeling potatoes.

traditionally rotate onto the stationary blades located in the periphery of a container. The force of the product moving against the blades forces the cut pieces through the gaps between the blades.

Blanching is mild heat treatment used in most vegetables and cut fruits prior to freezing. Its main purpose is the inactivation of enzymes that cause flavor or texture degradation during frozen storage. Examples of these enzymes include polyphenol oxidase, responsible for the development of undesirable colors through **enzymatic browning** (text box 1), and lipoxygenase that promotes the production of peroxides, which are responsible for undesirable flavors and odors. Of note, peroxidase activity is used as a proxy for lipoxygenase activity as a maker of the effectiveness of blanching because the activity of the latter is difficult to assess.

Blanching is essential to prevent food deterioration during frozen storage. Standard blanching involves submerging fruits or vegetables in boiling water for 1–3 minutes. The precise time depends on the size of the fruit piece, the type of fruit or vegetable, and the desired level of enzymatic inactivation. For instance, peas and small diced fruits and vegetables require less time, whereas longer times may be required for larger pieces. Blanching in either water or hot oil is used in french fry preparation (both, in commercial kitchens and in food manufacturing processes) to inactivate enzymes such as polyphenol oxidase and peroxidase, which produce undesirable colors trough **enzymatic browning** and to decrease levels of reducing sugars, which affect **nonenzymatic browning** reactions (text box 1) (Ngobese, Workneh, & Siwela, 2017). Blanching can also inactivate the enzyme lipoxygenase, which promotes lipid and carotenoid oxidation and degradation. After blanching, French fries are either fried for immediate consumption or frozen as a partially cooked product.

TEXT BOX 1

Enzymatic browning occurs when the phenolic compounds present in fruits and vegetables are exposed to oxygen (through bruising or cutting) and react with oxygen. Enzymatic browning produces undesirable brown colors in apples, avocados, bananas, pears and potatoes. This reaction is enhanced by the presence of enzymes such as polyphenol oxidase present in the fruit. Few control measures available, which include (1) preventing contact between phenolic compounds and atmospheric oxygen by submerging fruit and vegetable pieces in water or with the addition of an antioxidant such as ascorbic acid or citric acid, (2) inactivating the enzymes that catalyze the browning reactions through a blanching step, and (3) the use of sulfites, which reduce oxidized polyphenols into a colorless intermediate. The use of sulfites is heavily restricted in food products due to its ability to produce allergic reactions in some individuals.

Nonenzymatic browning occurs when a reducing sugar reacts with amino acids in the presence of heat. This process, called the Maillard reaction, forms molecules that provide color and flavor in a variety of food products including cooked fruits, baked goods, French fries, and roasted meats. The reaction starts when the carbonyl group in the reducing sugar interacts with the amino group in the amino acid. After several steps, it produces a large amount of color and flavor compounds. Whereas the Maillard reaction produces mostly desirable flavors and colors, it is also responsible for generating acrylamide in products such as breads, French fries, and potato chips. Acrylamide is a carcinogen; exposure in humans can occur through multiple sources (including tobacco smoke), and exposure through baked or fried carbohydrate-rich foods is relevant to human health (Tareke, Rydberg, Karlsoon, Eriksson, & Tornqvist, 2002).

Freezing relies on decreasing the temperature below the freezing point of the individual fruit or vegetable to slow down enzymatic reactions and inhibit microbial growth to extend the shelf life of the product. Many fruits and vegetables undergo a blanching step prior to freezing to inactivate enzymes that may cause flavor or texture degradation upon thawing. Industrial freezers rely on passing cooled air (−30°C) over fruits and vegetables circulated with the use of conveyor belts. A common freezing technology used for small fruits and diced vegetables is called Individual Quick Freezing (IQF). IQF works by blasting cold air through fruit or vegetable pieces as they are conveyed through a perforated belt, which enables quick freezing. One of the advantages of IQF is the prevention of large ice crystal formation, which tends to damage the product. As a result, the product pieces preserve their shape, color, and flavor upon thawing compared to processes that freeze the product in blocks.

Canning is a method of food preservation that involves heating food products in a hermetically sealed container (aluminum can, glass jars or flexible pouches) to achieve commercial sterility. A hermetic seal makes the can or container airtight so that oxygen or air does not enter and come in contact with the product during processing or storage. Commercial sterility is defined as the "degree of sterilization at which all pathogenic and toxin-forming organisms have been destroyed, as well as all other types of organisms which, if present, could grow in the product and produce spoilage under normal handling and storage conditions." Industrial canning is carried out in a large pressure cooker called retort. The time and temperature are carefully designed considering the type of product, the size of the can, and the overall rate of heat transfer to ensure that commercial sterility is achieved. Typical canning temperatures are in the range of 115°C–121°C, and the resulting time and temperature combination renders products shelf-stable for at least 6 months and up to several years.

Effects of blanching, freezing, and canning of fruits and vegetables on selected nutrients: The degree to which nutrients are preserved in frozen products compared to their fresh counterparts depends on a variety of factors including their heat sensitivity and water solubility. First, blanching involves submerging fruits and vegetables in hot water. This step may promote leaching of water-soluble components into the liquid, which depends on the size of the product and the type of fruit or vegetable. Blanching may also affect the integrity of heat-sensitive ingredients. Interestingly, blanching may promote higher retention of carotenoids due to the inactivation of enzymes such as peroxidase and lipoxygenase, which may promote oxidation of these compounds and decrease their levels (Mujumdar, 2019). Second, freezing storage may impact the content of the vitamins and minerals in the food. Evidence from studies that compared a variety of fruit and vegetable commodities as fresh or frozen shows that nutrient preservation depends on the food product and the length of frozen storage (Bouzari, Holstege, & Barrett, 2015a, 2015b; Li, Pegg, Eitenmiller, Chun, & Kerrihard, 2017). Novel technologies such as steam blanching, ohmic heating blanching, (heating through the passage of electrical current through food), microwave heating, and ultrasonic blanching may increase nutrient retention compared with conventional blanching. However, these technologies are mostly experimental, and their full effects on food composition and nutrient retention and availability are yet to be explored (Mujumdar, 2019).

Similar factors affect the ability of various nutrients to survive the canning process, including their water solubility, which determines whether they leach out into the cooking liquid, their susceptibility to degradation in thermal processes, and their ability to resist degradation during prolonged storage in an anaerobic environment (Rickman, Bruhn, & Barrett, 2007). Next is a list of several food micronutrients followed by a review of the effects that several food processes have on their stability.

Carotenoids are red, orange, and yellow fat-soluble pigments in fruits and vegetables that give tomatoes, peppers, carrots, sweet potatoes, and citrus fruits their characteristic colors. Carotenoids comprise a large number of polyisoprenoid compounds, of which about 40 are ingested by humans. Carotenoids contain several conjugated double bonds, which allows them to scavenge free radicals and absorb light in the visible spectrum, which explains the wide range of colors they can produce.

The main carotenoids found in human tissues are beta-carotene, alpha-carotene, beta-cryptoxanthin, lutein, zeaxanthin, and lycopene. Carotenes are characterized by possessing long carbon chains with unsaturated double bonds that are responsible for providing color. Beta-carotene is naturally orange in color and is one of the most common precursors of vitamin A. Alpha-carotene is found in orange vegetables (pumpkins, carrots, and squash). Alpha-carotene has one fewer double bond than beta-carotene, which makes it paler in color than beta-carotene, and lycopene has one more, thus responsible for its intense red color. Lycopene is found in tomatoes, watermelon, grapefruit, and papaya. Xanthophylls are derivatives or carotenes containing oxygen, which are naturally yellow orange in color. Xanthophylls are found in leafy greens such as spinach, kale, and Swiss chard (Figures 2.4–2.6).

Beta-carotene is substantially degraded during blanching and during frozen storage. In fact, beta-carotene levels continue decreasing during frozen storage, which suggests that several factors contribute to its degradation (Bouzari et al., 2015b). Beta-carotene is not water-soluble; thus, leaching out into an aqueous medium during blanching is likely not responsible for its decreased levels. Moreover, inactivation of lipoxygenase during blanching may contribute to better beta-carotene retention. Oxidation during storage seems to be the primary deterioration mechanism (Bouzari et al., 2015b).

Of interest, beta-carotene is minimally degraded during canning possibly because carotenoids are lipid-soluble molecules that do not leach out into the water-soluble medium that surrounds the product (Rickman, Bruhn, et al., 2007). Beta-carotene is prone to oxidation, which is minimal in the anaerobic environment of the canned product. The thermal process involved in the canning process may have a dual effect

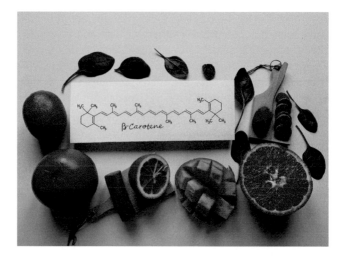

FIGURE 2.4   Molecular structure of beta-carotene and common food sources.

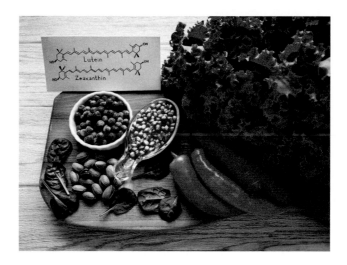

FIGURE 2.5   Molecular structure of lutein and common food sources.

on beta-carotene levels. On one hand, it may decrease its levels due to thermal degradation, while it may increase its extraction from the cellular matrix leading to increased levels compared to the fresh product (Rickman, Barrett, & Bruhn, 2007; Rickman, Bruhn, et al., 2007).

The B vitamin group includes thiamin (B1), riboflavin (B2), niacin (B3), biotin, pantothenic acid, B6, folate, and B12. Fruits and vegetables do not contain vitamin B12 and contain very little thiamin. The retention rate of this vitamins during fresh storage depends on their light and oxygen sensitivity. Among B vitamins, thiamin is considered the least stable to thermal degradation (Rickman, Barrett, et al., 2007). Reported losses of thiamin during canning of various fruits and vegetables

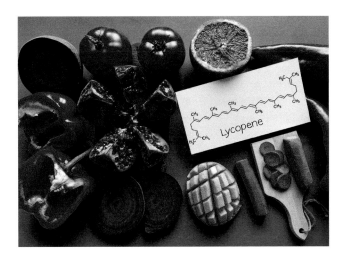

FIGURE 2.6 Molecular structure of lycopene and common food sources.

range from 25% to 66% depending on the food product (Martín-Belloso & Llanos-Barriobero, 2001; Rickman, Barrett, et al., 2007). Thiamin losses are substantial in the blanching step prior to freezing due to leaching and thermal degradation (Rickman, Barrett, et al., 2007). Overall, riboflavin is well preserved in fresh, frozen, and canned fruits and vegetables with retention ranging from 60% to 90% (Bouzari et al., 2015b; Martín-Belloso & Llanos-Barriobero, 2001; Rickman, Barrett, et al., 2007). Riboflavin is stable during frozen storage of most fruits and vegetables with some losses observed in frozen peas, possibly due to enzymatic degradation (Bouzari et al., 2015b). The retention rates of niacin, vitamin B6, and folate were moderate to good ranging from 50% to 93% depending on the food product (Martín-Belloso & Llanos-Barriobero, 2001; Rickman, Barrett, et al., 2007). Few studies have examined the stability of folate to canning, but it seems to remain constant after canning in beets and green beans (Jirantanan & Liu, 2004).

Vitamin C is sensitive to thermal degradation and oxidation, which makes it a good marker for thermal process severity (Rumm-Kreuter & Demmel, 1990). Vitamin C is water soluble, which makes it prone to leaching during washing, blanching, and canning. The average losses of vitamin C during canning are substantial (>60%) for most fruits or vegetables owing to the severity of the heat processing involved (Bouzari et al., 2015b; Rickman, Barrett, et al., 2007). However, it may also depend on the commodity as some products, such as beets, experience <10% losses (Jirantanan & Liu, 2004), and asparagus, mushrooms, lentils, and tomatoes experience moderate losses (Martín-Belloso & Llanos-Barriobero, 2001). After the thermal process, vitamin C losses during storage of canned products are actually small (<10%) possibly due to the lack of oxygen in the canned environment (Rickman, Barrett, et al., 2007).

Alpha-tocopherol (vitamin E) is the name of a group of eight different molecules that exhibit the antioxidant activity of alpha-tocopherol. The main source of vitamin E in the diet is vegetable oils, especially safflower and sunflower oils (Traber, 2006). Vitamin E is lipid-soluble and, like carotenoids, does not tend to leach out during processing, especially in those unit operations such as washing and blanching, which require the product to be immersed in water. Alpha-tocopherol levels actually increase immediately after blanching which may be explained by increased availability to the assay due to rupture of cell wall materials and remain relatively constant during frozen storage (Bouzari et al., 2015b). However, more severe heat processing, such as the conditions found in canning operations, seems to decrease levels of alpha-tocopherol to their fresh counterparts. For instance, alpha-tocopherol levels decreased by as much as 15%–20% during canning of tomato paste and asparagus compared to their fresh versions, whereas no decreases were detected in canned spinach or sweet potatoes (Rickman, Bruhn, et al., 2007). Conversely, alpha-tocopherol is well preserved in fruits and vegetables during freezing.

Water-soluble minerals (magnesium, calcium zinc, copper, and iron) are well retained in frozen commodity samples compared to their fresh counterparts (Bouzari et al., 2015a). The majority of mineral losses are the result of leaching into the blanching water irrespective of the commodity; nonetheless, 78%–91% of minerals are retained after the blanching step (Rickman, Bruhn, et al., 2007). A higher proportion of minerals is retained during canning compared to products that undergo frozen storage because there are fewer opportunities to incur into mineral losses during the process. In fact, the sodium, calcium, and iron content of several vegetable commodities is higher than in their fresh counterparts because of addition of sodium in the form of salt. Calcium levels increase as well due to the utilization of hard water and the utilization of calcium compounds to increase firmness of diced and canned vegetables (such as calcium chloride) (Martín-Belloso & Llanos-Barriobero, 2001). Canned asparagus, mushrooms, tomatoes, and lentils retained most of the potassium, iron, and magnesium after canning (65%–102%) (Martín-Belloso & Llanos-Barriobero, 2001). However, there was a 2–10-fold increase in sodium and calcium content due to addition of salt and use of hard water in the process (Martín-Belloso & Llanos-Barriobero, 2001).

Polyphenols include a vast number of phytochemicals traditionally categorized into phenolic acids, stilbenes, lignans, and flavonoids. These molecules are involved in defense mechanisms against pathogens or ultraviolet radiation (Manach, Scalbert, Morand, Rémésy, & Jiménez, 2004). Polyphenols are usually classified by their structure which is determined by the number of phenol rings and the side groups attached to them (Manach et al., 2004). The flavonoid subclass of compounds includes a large group of compounds (more than 6,000) possessing two or more aromatic rings linked by an oxygenated heterocyclic bridge possessing one oxygen and three carbon atoms (Blumberg & Milbury, 2006; Manach et al., 2004). The main classes of flavonoids include anthocyanidins, flavanols, flavanones, flavones, flavonols, and isoflavones; these compounds reflect variations of the primary backbone structure (Blumberg & Milbury, 2006)

Among specific phenolic compounds, **anthocyanins** are red, blue, and purple water-soluble pigments found in berries, in plums, in the skins of grapes and apples, and in vegetables such as beets, eggplant, red onion, and red cabbage. Anthocyanins are characterized by a structure of carbon rings including a positively charged oxygen in the central group of the molecule responsible for anthocyanins' pH sensitivity. However, there is a wide range of structural diversity, and more than 250 different structures have been identified in fruits and vegetables. In an acidic environment, anthocyanins possess a red color, but in an alkaline environment, they turn blue with

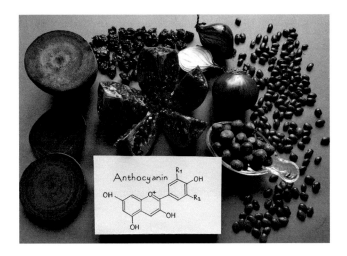

FIGURE 2.7   Molecular structure of anthocyanins and common food sources.

varying degrees of purple depending on the pH. The four forms of anthocyanins include the quinoidal base (which is blue in alkaline conditions), the red flavylium cation (which is red in acidic conditions), and the colorless chalcone and carbinol pseudo base (Sumonsiri & Barringer, 2014) (Figure 2.7).

Flavonols include quercetin, kaempferol, and myricetin and are present in fruits and vegetables such as apples, blueberries, grapes, broccoli, kale, leeks, and onions (Blumberg & Milbury, 2006). **Flavanols** are present in many fruits and seeds including apricots, apples, and grapes and are present in foods such as tea and chocolate. The primary forms of flavanols are catechin, epicatechin and epigallocatechin which tend to be relatively stable to various cooking methods. **Flavones** are found in celery, parsley, and cereals and in the rinds of citrus fruits. **Flavanones** are found in citrus fruits, primarily in the membrane structure and peel. **Isoflavones** are characteristically found in legumes including soy and are stable to cooking and processing, which is reflected in high levels found in soy products such as tofu, tempeh, and soy flours (Figures 2.8 and 2.9).

Polyphenols are susceptible to oxidation during processing and storage and to leaching during washing and blanching due to their water-soluble nature (Rickman, Barrett, et al., 2007). In general, most phenolic compounds are well preserved in fresh and frozen storage in most fruit and vegetable products studied (Bouzari et al., 2015a; Rickman, Barrett, et al., 2007). Minor losses have been observed in vegetables including broccoli, peas, corn and, cherries during frozen storage, likely due to oxidation (Bouzari et al., 2015a). Phenolic compounds found in fruit products tend to be well preserved during refrigerated storage and in some products, such as frozen raspberries, have been reported to increase during freezing, which could be related to higher amounts being available to the analytical assay after blanching (Rickman, Barrett, et al., 2007). A separate study observed that frozen blueberries had higher phenolic levels than fresh ones potentially due to enzymatic degradation in the fresh samples that would have been minimized during frozen storage (Bouzari et al., 2015a).

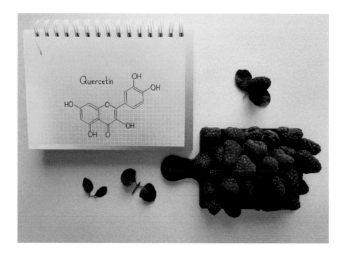

FIGURE 2.8   Molecular structure of quercetin and common food sources.

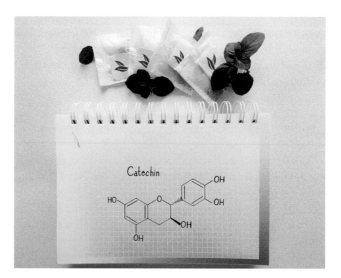

FIGURE 2.9   Molecular structure of catechin and common food sources.

The effect of canning on the content of phenolic compounds in fruits and vegetables is not completely understood. Most phenolic compounds are water soluble, which makes them susceptible to losses into the surrounding cooking liquid. For instance, substantial losses of total phenolic compounds have been reported in canned cherries, peaches, and beets compared to their fresh versions; however, most of these losses were explained by leaching out into the brine or syrup surrounding the product (Rickman, Barrett, et al., 2007). However, losses seem to be dependent on the specific commodity. For example, beets experienced little change in phenolic levels after canning, whereas decreases of about 30% were observed in green beans (Jirantanan & Liu, 2004). Furthermore, there may be differential losses depending on the type of phenolic compound of interest, which needs to be researched in more detail to yield consistent results (Rickman, Barrett, et al., 2007). Other studies have reported increased concentrations of total phenolics in fruit and vegetable, specifically in corn products, due to release of bound phenolics from plant wall materials (Dewanto, Wu, & Liu, 2002).

Dietary Fiber: The term dietary fiber encompasses a heterogeneous group of plant-based carbohydrates that offer resistance to enzymatic hydrolysis in mammalian digestive systems. Dietary fiber includes plant cell wall material including cellulose, hemicellulose, lignin, pectins, and other polysaccharides. Cellulose is characterized for being a group of glucose polymers found in many cell walls consisting of beta 1–4 linkages, which human amylases cannot hydrolyze. Several definitions of dietary fiber exist in the literature. According to the Food and Nutrition Board of the US Institute of Medicine, **dietary fiber** consists of nondigestible carbohydrates and lignin that are intact in plants; **functional fiber** consists of isolated, nondigestible carbohydrates that have beneficial physiological effects in humans; and **total fiber** is the sum of both (Institute of Medicine, 2001). The distinction is important because their ability to survive in various food processing and cooking steps varies by type and the commodity of which they are part.

In general, frozen fruits and vegetables have lower fiber levels than fresh products; this may be related to losses and/or degradation during the blanching process (Bouzari et al., 2015a). Storage of either frozen or canned products does not seem to affect the fiber content in various fruits and vegetables (Rickman, Bruhn, et al., 2007). A separate study measured acid-digestible fiber in six different fruits and vegetables observing that either fresh or frozen storage did not have significant effects on fiber levels (Bouzari et al., 2015a). There were some product-specific changes that were noteworthy. For instance, broccoli showed an increase in fiber content during fresh storage (possibly due to thickening of cell walls during storage), whereas carrots showed a decrease in fiber content, possibly due to degradation of cell wall components including cellulose, hemicellulose, pectin, and lignin (Bouzari et al., 2015a). Soluble fiber was not affected by freezing of corn, peas, and green and yellow beans (Rickman, Bruhn, et al., 2007). Other products such as blueberries and peas experienced some fiber losses during the blanching step, but those levels remained relatively stable during frozen storage (Bouzari et al., 2015a).

Canned vegetables contain lower fiber content than their fresh counterparts; however, these loses occur during operations such as peeling and trimming prior to canning (Martín-Belloso & Llanos-Barriobero, 2001; Rickman, Bruhn, et al., 2007). For instance, crude fiber losses in the range of 20%–27% were observed in mushrooms, tomatoes, and asparagus (Martín-Belloso & Llanos-Barriobero, 2001; Rickman, Bruhn, et al., 2007). Other products, such as lentils, corn, peas, and green and yellow beans, which do not undergo a preparation step prior to canning, did not experience fiber losses during the canning process (Martín-Belloso & Llanos-Barriobero, 2001; Rickman, Bruhn, et al., 2007) (Figure 2.10).

Dehydration increases the shelf life of fruits and vegetables by removing water via evaporation making it unavailable for enzymatic reactions or microbial growth (Sumonsiri & Barringer, 2014). Dehydration can be accomplished by sun drying, tunnel or cabinet drying, and freeze drying. Sun drying is a slow process whereby fruits and

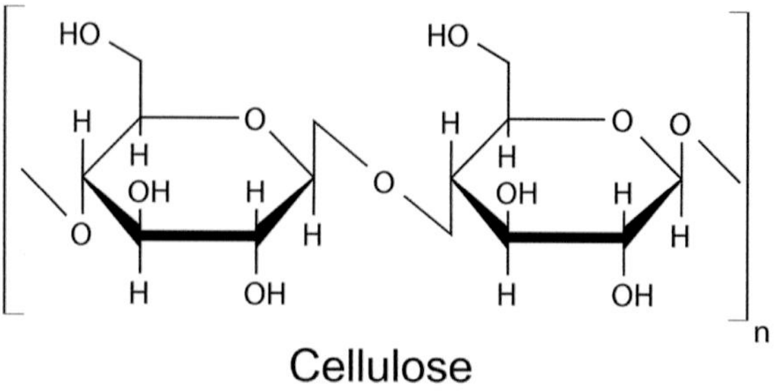

FIGURE 2.10 Molecular structure of cellulose.

vegetables are left to dry in product beds in open fields. This process is slow and exposes the product to contamination and results in losses of product attributes (color and flavor) and nutrients. Industrial drying exposes products to a stream of hot air (between 40°C and 60°C) until the product is dried to the desired moisture content. The process can be conducted continuously in conveyor belts and tunnels or in batches by drying the product in drawers inside drying cabinets where the interaction between the product and hot air occurs. Freeze drying is a complex process that removes water by sublimation. Thus, the product must be frozen first and then exposed to a low temperature, low pressure environment to enable the transition from ice to water vapor (Sumonsiri & Barringer, 2014). This process helps preserve color and flavor attributes as well as nutrients by preventing exposure to high temperatures (Bhatta, Stevanovic Janezic, & Ratti, 2020).

Of note, there is limited evidence comparing nutrient retention using these three methods (Bhatta et al., 2020; Siriwattananon & Maneerate, 2016). One study compared the effect of sun drying to cabinet drying of green leafy vegetables and observed that products dried using cabinet drying retained a higher proportion of beta-carotene and vitamin C than those dehydrated using sun drying (Lakshmi & Vamala, 2000). The levels of these vitamins were lower than those found in the fresh products. The study also observed higher retention of fiber and no differences in the levels of protein, iron, copper, and magnesium between drying methods and good overall retention of these nutrients compared to the fresh product (Lakshmi & Vamala, 2000). Another study examining nutrient changes during cherry tomato dehydration (using cabinet drying) reported that beta-carotene, vitamin C, and lycopene were substantially lower in dehydrated samples compared to their fresh counterparts. Furthermore, the rate of degradation increased with increasing dehydration temperatures (Muratore, Rizzo, Licciardello, & Maccarone, 2008). A few studies have observed better retention of phenolic compounds and vitamin C in berries (blueberries, cherries, cranberries and strawberries) (Nemzer, Vargas, Xia, Sintara, & Feng, 2018) and tomatoes (Bhatta et al., 2020) in freeze drying compared to conventional air drying. However, the retention may vary for specific compounds and treatments. One study observed similar lycopene levels between samples dehydrated using oven drying and freeze drying (Ke et al., 2020), whereas another study observed that conventional drying preserved a higher proportion of lycopene compared to freeze drying while both processes produced substantial losses (albeit similar in magnitude) in total polyphenols (Zunli Ke et al., 2021). With regard to dietary fiber, sun drying has been reported to result in better retention of dietary fiber than cabinet drying or freeze drying of cabbage, pumpkin, and guava but not of tomatoes (Siriwattananon & Maneerate, 2016).

Novel technologies including microwave drying (dehydration by heating the product via electromagnetic radiations), vacuum drying (dehydration under partial vacuum, which allows to use lower temperatures), and other emerging technologies (infrared drying) may contribute to better micronutrient retention (Hasan et al., 2019). However, evidence is still sparse, and these technologies are not widely used in food processing due to elevated capital costs.

FRUIT AND VEGETABLE COOKING METHODS

Vegetables are cooked to produce desirable flavors and textures and improve their digestibility by breaking down cellulose and gelatinize starches. Most fruits can be consumed without cooking; however, they are sometimes cooked to improve their flavor and texture (i.e., poached pears). Fruits and vegetables should be cooked for the shortest possible amount of time that allows the development of flavors and textures while minimizing nutrient and color losses. Fruits and vegetables can be cooked using a variety of methods as outlined in this section.

Boiling and steaming are wet-cooking methods used extensively in vegetable cooking. Boiled vegetables can be served immediately after cooking, or they can be further processed into purees or undergo other cooking steps (sautéing, roasting) to develop additional flavors. Boiling is commonly used to cook starchy vegetables but can be used to prepare a wide range of vegetables such as carrots, green beans, asparagus, cabbage, beets, broccoli, and cauliflower. Vegetables can be cooked whole or in evenly shaped pieces (text box 2).

It is important to chill the product immediately after boiling by rinsing with cold water (or submerged in ice water if not to be consumed immediately). This step stops heat transfer and prevents vegetables from being overcooked by their retained heat. At this point, vegetables can be seasoned and served or kept cold and reheated to be served at a later time. Boiling is an appropriate cooking method for cooking green vegetables. Steaming is appropriate for vegetables such as broccoli that break easily in boiling.

TEXT BOX 2

General cooking steps to cook vegetables by boiling:

1. Wash, trim, peel, and cut vegetables into even-sized pieces
2. Prepare the steaming liquid and bring it to a boil
3. Place vegetables in the intended basket or perforated pan, and place it over the boiling liquid
4. Cook until desired doneness is achieved
5. Drain vegetables quickly
6. Cool vegetables with cold water, season, and serve

Steaming is an efficient method to cook vegetables with minimal loss of nutrients. Steaming takes advantage of the heat transferred from steam to the product as it condenses into a liquid. Steaming is usually conducted in a basket, perforated pan or rack suspended over a boiling liquid in a pot, pan, or wok (text box 3). With this type of set-up, the product is only in contact with the steam produced by the boiling liquid and thus produces vegetables with a clean flavor. Alternatively, vegetables may be cooked in a covered pot or pan with a small amount of liquid, which allows some contact between the product and the cooking liquid. Thus, any flavors added to the cooking liquid, such as herbs and spices, are transferred to the steamed vegetables.

TEXT BOX 3

General cooking steps to cook vegetables by steaming:

1. Wash, trim, peel, and cut vegetables into even-sized pieces
2. Add water (2–3 times the volume of vegetables) and bring to a boil. A little bit of salt (1 tablespoon per gallon) may be added to season the cooking liquid; add other seasonings to taste
3. Once water has begun boiling, add vegetables and return water to a boil
4. Reduce heat to simmer and cook to desired doneness. Green beans, asparagus, broccoli, and cauliflower cut in small pieces usually require 2–4 minutes to cook
5. Drain vegetables quickly
6. Cool vegetables with cold water, season, and serve

When using a wet-cooking method, it is important to consider the type of vegetable to decide whether to cook covered or uncovered. White vegetables such as onions, cauliflower, and potatoes contain pigments called flavones, and these pigments retain their color in acidic conditions and may turn yellow in alkaline water. Thus, preserving natural acids or adding acid to white vegetables is helpful. White vegetables may be cooked with the lid on to keep some of the natural acids in the cooking water. Alternatively, a very small amount of acid, such as vinegar or lemon juice, may be added. Cook for a short period of time, and cool quickly to prevent white pigments from turning gray.

Green vegetables owe their color to the natural pigment chlorophyll, which is an essential molecule in photosynthesis. The structure of chlorophyll is a porphyrin ring containing four pyrrole rings and a magnesium ion attached to the center of these four rings. This structure is similar to that of hemoglobin, where an iron ion is placed at the center of the pyrrole rings. The removal of the magnesium ion in the central position causes irreversible changes in color. Some of the factors that can cause color changes include heat from various cooking processes, the presence of acids, and some minerals such as zinc and copper. Exposure to these conditions, particularly cooking at higher temperatures or for longer times in combination to the presence of acids, causes color loss turning green vegetables to an olive-green color and in extreme cases resulting in brown color (Karadeniz, Burdurlu, & Koca, 2007).

Furthermore, the addition of acids, such as lemon juice, vinegar, or wine to the cooking liquid can produce firmer vegetables.

This is because some cellulose components, particularly hemicellulose, are not soluble in acidic environments and thus will take much longer to break down. Conversely, cooking vegetables in an alkaline liquid decreases their micronutrient content, creates a soft, mushy texture, and imparts bitter flavors. In general, adding acids or baking soda or using hard water as the cooking liquid should be avoided.

Green vegetables should be cooked as briefly as possible and in the absence of acids. During the initial stages of cooking, air pockets are removed from plant cells creating a bright green color. As cooking continues, the natural organic acids present in vegetables are released. When these acids interact with the chlorophyll molecule, they displace the magnesium ion and introduce a hydrogen ion producing dark green pigments called pheophytins (Nihal Turkmen, Poyrazoglu, Sari, & Sedat Velioglu, 2006). These color changes become more evident with longer cooking times. One way to minimize this color change is to cook green vegetables uncovered, especially in the first few minutes of cooking, to allow the short-chain organic acids to escape (Figure 2.11).

Conversely, the addition of alkalis such as baking soda produces a bright green color, but this practice is detrimental to vitamin stability and texture preservation as mentioned previously and thus, should be discouraged. On the other hand, carotenoids are stable in a wide range of pH levels. Thus, cooking vegetables such

Plant chlorophylls

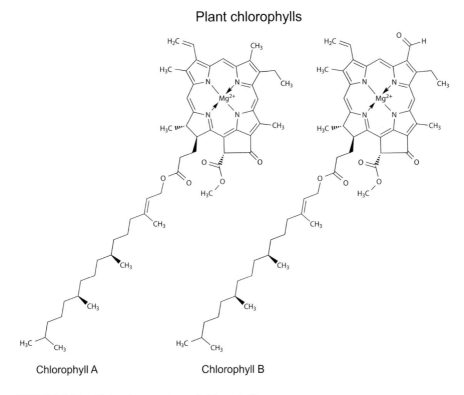

Chlorophyll A   Chlorophyll B

FIGURE 2.11   Molecular structure of chlorophyll.

as carrots, squash, or sweet potatoes in environments with acid or alkali has little impact on their stability. Nonetheless, cook all vegetables for short periods of time and in a small volume of water to prevent color and nutrient losses. Cooking carotenoid-rich vegetables covered or uncovered does not substantially affect their color or flavor.

Anthocyanins are extremely sensitive to the presence of acids or alkalis in the cooking environment. Cooking red cabbage with a small amount of acid turns the finished product bright red. This last principle also applies to white vegetables, such as cauliflower, which retains its flavor and texture in the presence of a small amount of acid. Alternatively, red, blue, and white fruits and vegetables may be cooked covered to retain organic acids and produce bright colors and firm textures.

Sautéing, stir-frying, panfrying, and deep-frying: Frying is a common cooking technique used in both industrial settings and home kitchens that relies on the use of oil as a cooking medium. The main advantage of frying, from a processing perspective, is that it allows cooking at high temperatures, which makes it a quick cooking method. The temperatures reached during frying (160°C–190°C) are notably higher than what can be reached using water as a cooking medium (poaching, simmering, or boiling), which are limited by its boiling temperature. Furthermore, heat transfers more readily in oil than in air, making frying a more efficient cooking method than baking or roasting at the same oven temperature. Exposure of foods to the high temperatures used in frying results in dehydration and allows some of the oil to be absorbed into the food. Frying results in important changes to the micronutrient content of foods depending on the food product, the temperature of the oil, and the time that the food is left in contact with the oil. Frying is particularly damaging for heat-sensitive micronutrients such as vitamin C in foods such as carrots, broccoli, and eggplant when comparing frying to wet-cooking methods such as boiling and steaming.

Sautéing is a quick cooking method that uses a small amount of fat in which the product is tossed over high heat with quick movements of the sautéing pan. Stir-frying is similar to sautéing in that it is a quick cooking technique over high heat. The main difference is that the cooking pan is left stationary, and the product is stirred using spatulas. When sautéing or stir-frying vegetables, it is important to complete all preparation steps before cooking because these methods take little time to fully cook the products. Both methods are appropriate for a wide range of vegetables. Root vegetables, Brussels sprouts, and cauliflower may be precooked using a blanching or baking step and then sautéed to finish cooking and develop flavor. Please refer to text box 4 for general instructions to sauté fruits and vegetables.

Panfrying typically uses a larger amount of fat that partially covers the product and usually requires longer time at a lower heat than sautéing, and the product is not tossed (text box 5). Conversely, during **deep-frying,** vegetables are submerged in hot oil (160°C–175°C or 325°F–350°F), which is used to develop textures and flavors that cannot be achieved using other methods (text box 6). Some vegetables are breaded or dipped in a batter or coating before frying, and some others like root vegetables can be fried without a coating.

TEXT BOX 4

General cooking steps for sautéing vegetables:

1. Wash, trim, peel, and cut vegetables
2. Place the pan over high heat, and add a small amount of oil to cover the bottom of the pan
3. Once the oil is hot, add vegetables being careful not to overload the pan. Overloading will prevent the product from cooking at high temperature and will promote the release of a larger amount of moisture, which will simmer the product rather than allowing the product to cook in hot oil. If necessary, cook in batches
4. Flip the pan, and toss the vegetables to ensure even cooking, and remove when they reach the desired level of doneness. Do not toss more than necessary to make sure the pan remains in contact with the heat source
5. Season to taste

TEXT BOX 5

General cooking steps for panfrying vegetables:

1. Place a pan over medium to high heat and add oil
2. Once the oil is hot, place the product in the pan and cook to desired doneness on one side
3. Turn the product to continue cooking
4. Remove from the pan when cooking is complete

TEXT BOX 6

General cooking steps for deep-frying vegetables:

1. Preheat oil to (160°C–175°C or 325°F–350°F)
2. Prepare vegetables. This includes cutting them into even pieces to ensure uniform cooking and applying breading or batter if needed
3. Cook in small batches to avoid overloading the fryer and letting the oil temperature drop
4. Fry until desired doneness. Hold the cooked product over the fryer to allow excess fat to drain
5. Remove and serve immediately

Roasting and baking: The terms roasting and baking are used interchangeably in vegetable cooking. Baking involves cooking vegetables in dry heat with the objective of developing texture and flavor characteristics such as those produced by nonenzymatic browning and caramelization, which cannot be produced with wet-cooking methods. Baking is typically used to cook root vegetables, which contain enough moisture to be fully cooked. Vegetables can be baked whole or cut into uniform pieces (text box 7). Baking can also be used to finish cooking vegetable dishes that were initially cooked using a separate method such as simmering or steaming. Examples of these dishes include vegetable casseroles.

TEXT BOX 7

General for roasting or baking vegetables:

1. Wash, trim, peel, and cut vegetables
2. Season vegetables, and brush with oil (if desired)
3. Preheat oven, place vegetables in a baking dish, and cook until done

---

Broiling and grilling: Both boiling and grilling use high heat to develop unique caramelized flavor notes while preserving most nutrients. Grilling allows for quick cooking of thin vegetable pieces to produce desirable flavors (text box 8).

TEXT BOX 8

General steps for grilling vegetables:

1. Preheat the grill, and remove burnt particles
2. Cut vegetables into even-sized pieces, and brush them with oil
3. Grill vegetables until desired texture and color have developed
4. Serve immediately

Broiling is a cooking method that uses radiant heat to finish cooking vegetables at very high temperatures, and it is suitable for soft or small vegetables (i.e., cherry tomatoes) that cannot be handled properly in the grill. The preparation steps are similar to those used in grilling, and the products should be served immediately after cooking. Broiling is also used to finish cooking casseroles or grating dishes that would not develop the same color using other cooking methods.

Combination cooking methods: Braising vegetables combines the addition of vegetables to a braising pan that has oil in it. Depending on the recipe, the vegetable maybe cooked in the oil before adding liquid. The product is then partially covered in a cooking liquid (water or vegetable stock) followed by covered cooking at moderate temperature. Examples of dishes that use braising include braised cabbage and Ratatouille.

EFFECTS OF COOKING METHODS ON RETENTION LEVELS OF VARIOUS NUTRIENTS

Nutrient changes during cooking depend on the food product and the specific nutrient in question. The same principle holds true when comparing nutrient retention levels across several industrial processing steps. The next section includes a short comparison of nutrient retention profiles among several cooking methods.

Carotenoids: The choice of cooking methods influences not only the resulting sensory properties of flavor and texture but also the micronutrient profile of the cooked dish. Interestingly, **wet-cooking methods**, particularly **boiling** and **steaming**, are reported to leave the carotenoid content of fruits, vegetables and starchy roots either unchanged or even increased compared to the levels in the raw vegetable form (Palermo, Pellegrini, & Fogliano, 2014; Taleon, Sumbu, Muzhingi, & Bidiaka, 2019). This increase is likely related to the denaturation of protein-carotenoid complexes, which leave more carotenes available for consumption (Palermo et al., 2014). Wet-cooking methods are also responsible for increases in the *cis* form of carotenoids in contrast to the naturally occurring *trans* form (Imsic, Winkler, Tomkins, & Jones, 2010). The health effects of this change are inconclusive.

On the other hand, dry cooking methods such as **baking and frying** are responsible for substantial decreases in total carotenoid concentrations (Palermo et al., 2014). The primary factors driving carotene loss during frying are frying time and vegetable cut size (Imsic et al., 2010). Longer frying times result in higher carotenoid losses, and smaller cut sizes expose more surface area to high-temperature oil during frying and allow more heat to be transferred into the food pieces. It is also likely that longer frying times could promote the formation of free radicals and accelerate carotenoid degradation (Mayeaux, Xu, King, & Prinyawiwatkul, 2006). Frying has been shown to decrease the concentrations of individual carotenoids including beta-carotene, beta-cryptoxanthin, and lycopene (Miglio, Chiavaro, Visconti, Fogliano, & Pellegrini, 2008). Carotenoid losses are evident at the relatively lower temperatures used in pan frying (145°C–165°C); even exposures as short as 1–2 minutes to oil in this temperature range result in >60% lycopene loss with little variation due to frying time or temperature (Mayeaux et al., 2006). The same study observed that lycopene losses during baking ranged between 40% and 60% with longer baking time (45 minutes vs. 15 minutes), and higher oven temperatures (218°C/425°F vs. 177°C/350°F) are associated with more pronounced losses (Mayeaux et al., 2006).

An open question remains as to whether these cooking methods have any effects on the bioavailability of beta-carotene, despite the changes in absolute levels. One study examined the content of beta-carotene in a group of vegetables (carrot, pumpkin, and fenugreek) and amaranth after boiling, stir-frying, and pressure-cooking (Veda, Platel, & Srinivasan, 2010). The authors defined "bioaccessibility" as the proportion of intact beta-carotene remaining after a simulated digestion process *in vitro* (Veda et al., 2010). Despite the observed losses in absolute content of beta-carotene in the cooked samples compared to the fresh product, they did observe an increased bioaccessibility of beta-carotene after cooking, which made the total bioaccessible beta-carotene comparable between the fresh and cooked products (Veda et al., 2010). These results would need to be replicated *in vivo* and confirmed in other studies. However, they pose an interesting hypothesis regarding the role of cooking on nutrient availability independent of their absolute levels.

B vitamins: Thiamin losses of 13%–46% have been reported during fresh storage, whereas riboflavin is relatively stable (Bouzari et al., 2015b; Rickman, Barrett, et al., 2007). Storage at refrigeration temperatures helps improve their retention, but this is highly dependent on the food product (Bouzari et al., 2015b; Rickman, Barrett, et al., 2007).

Vitamin C: Fruits and vegetables have their highest vitamin C content immediately after harvest, and after this point, its levels begin to degrade. For instance, losses in the range of 27%–100% are common in vegetables stored for up to 7 days at 20°C; these losses are mitigated in refrigerated storage (4°C) but are still substantial (0%–75%) (Rickman, Barrett, et al., 2007). Other studies suggest that vitamin C levels are better preserved in whole fruits such as blueberries or strawberries, while substantial losses are observed in vegetables such as green beans and corn (Bouzari et al., 2015b). Cooking fresh vegetables rich in vitamin C such as broccoli, green beans, and fresh spinach using boiling, steaming, or pressure-cooking resulted in losses >46%; conversely, folate levels were not impacted by these cooking methods (Rumm-Kreuter & Demmel, 1990).

Polyphenols: In general, polyphenol degradation has been observed using wet and dry cooking methods including boiling, steaming, microwaving, baking, and frying (Palermo et al., 2014). However, there is considerable variability by product type and phenolic compound (Rickman, Barrett, et al., 2007). A study comparing the effect of boiling, steaming, and microwaving found that most of the variability in the levels of phenolic compounds and their antioxidant activity was related to the type of commodity, while there were only small differences among cooking methods (N. Turkmen, Sari, & Velioglu, 2005). For instance, increases in phenolic levels were observed in peppers, green beans, broccoli, and spinach, whereas all three cooking methods led to losses in squash, peas, and leeks (N. Turkmen et al., 2005). It is unclear whether this variability was due to the specific types of phenolic compounds or the structure of each type of food.

Other phytochemicals: water-soluble nutrients including **glucosinolates**, which give Brussels sprouts their characteristic bitter taste, are degraded in wet-cooking methods, possibly due to their leaching out into the cooking liquid (Palermo et al., 2014). A study comparing the effect of boiling, steaming, and microwaving on flavonoid retention in broccoli pieces observed substantial flavonoid losses with boiling, modest losses with steaming, and modest gains with microwaving (Wu, Zhao, Haytowitz, Chen, & Pehrsson, 2019). Few studies have studied the survival of these nutrients in dry cooking methods; thus, the evidence is limited and inconclusive.

Dietary Fiber: Limited evidence shows that small fiber losses (<10%) are expected in cooked vegetables compared to their fresh counterparts, but more research is needed to include a wide range of commodities and cooking methods (Rickman, Bruhn, et al., 2007).

General considerations: Fresh fruits and vegetables provide nutritional benefits including micronutrients such as dietary fiber, vitamins, minerals, and phenolic compounds and ideally should be the first choice. In general, frozen fruits and vegetables may represent viable alternatives when fresh fruits and vegetables are not available. Frozen fruits and vegetables represent nutritionally viable alternatives to fresh produce subjected to typical postharvest holding times. Total phenolics, fiber, and minerals were for the most part well conserved in frozen samples as compared to fresh. Canned fruits and vegetables are the next option to consider. In addition to the degradation of some nutrients due to the thermal process and precanning processing steps, it is important to consider the amount of sodium added in the brining liquid of canned vegetables and the amount of sugar added to the syrup that surrounds canned fruits. Overall, the scientific evidence shows that frozen and canned fruits and vegetables should not be excluded from recommendations. These processed forms offer added convenience to the consumer and offer diversity to the diet with a small compromise in nutritional quality compared to fresh produce.

Cooking methods to enable preparation and cooking of vegetables should consider the desired flavor and texture of the finished product while optimizing the retention of micronutrients and phytochemicals. Whereas some nutrient losses are inevitable, following some basic preparation principles, such as those which follow, can help achieve all these goals.

1. Use wet-cooking methods such as boiling, simmering, or steaming as they tend to minimize nutrient losses
2. Cook vegetables in small batches; this results in shorter cooking times and results in evenly cooked vegetables
3. Cut vegetables into uniform pieces to allow for even cooking. Smaller pieces help reduce cooking time but produce a greater surface area, which promotes nutrient loss
4. Do not overcook vegetables
5. In general, do not use acids or alkalis to vegetables. Some exceptions may apply to red, blue, and white vegetables, which may be cooked with small amounts of acid to help retain color
6. Cook vegetables as close as possible to consumption time. When cooking ahead of time, stop cooking before desired doneness is achieved and chill to stop cooking. Then reheat at the time of consumption.
7. For mixed vegetable dishes, cook each vegetable separately, and combine at the time of consumption

PROCESSING OF CEREALS AND GRAINS

Cereals and grains undergo several processing steps before reaching our supermarket shelves and kitchen tables. Cereals include a wide range of commodities including wheat, corn, rice, oats, rye, barley, sorghum, and many more used throughout the world. From a botanical perspective, cereals are a form of cultivated grass, which produces an edible seed. Cereals can be processed into breads, flat breads and tortillas, ready-to-eat cereals, pasta, starch, and oils. This section will discuss the primary steps involved in industrial cereal processing and the consequences of these processes on the nutritional content of various cereal products. This section will include the impact of cooking methods on the nutritional attributes of several cereals and grains used in commercial or home kitchens.

The structure of grain kernels is remarkably similar for most grains and it is composed of three edible parts: the germ, the endosperm, and the bran. The kernel is usually covered and protected by the husk, which is an inedible fibrous layer that is removed during cleaning and processing. Whole grains contain the endosperm, bran, and germ; removal of the bran and germ from the kernel during milling produces a refined grain. The endosperm makes up about 83% of the kernel; it contains most of the carbohydrate and protein and contains some B vitamins. The bran is the outer layer of the kernel, and it makes up about 14.5% of the weight of the kernel. The bran contains most of the fiber, B vitamins, minerals, and polyphenols. The germ makes up about 2.5% of the weight of the kernel. It contains about 10% fat, which is prone to oxidation and may decrease the shelf life of products that keep the germ portion.

Whole grains contain all three components of the kernel. According to the Global Whole Grain Ingredient Definition agreed upon during the 6th International Whole Grain Summit (Vienna, 13–15 November 2017), the following definition was proposed: "Whole grains shall consist of the intact, ground, cracked, flaked or otherwise processed kernel after the removal of inedible parts such as the hull and husk. All anatomical components, including the endosperm, germ, and bran, must be present in the same relative proportions as in the intact kernel" (Cereals & Grains Association, 2017). Whole grains are sources of macronutrients and several micronutrients including protein, fat, and carbohydrates, which includes dietary fiber. Whole grains are sources of several micronutrients including B vitamins, vitamin E, magnesium, iron, zinc, copper, and manganese as well as sources of many phenolic compounds (Rebello, Greenway, & Finley, 2014). A detailed list of various cereals and grains and basic cooking methods is included in Chapter 6, Cooking for Diabetes Prevention (Figure 2.12).

ANATOMY OF A GRAIN

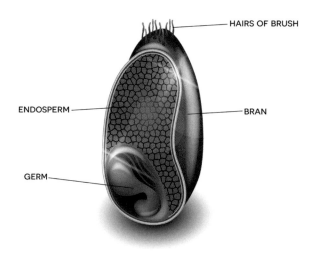

FIGURE 2.12   Main components of a grain kernel.

Cereal processing: The main processing steps for cereals and grains include postharvest storage and handling, milling, and separation of the components of the kernel, which are common for many grains and other specialized steps such as nixtamalization for corn.

Postharvest storage and handling of cereal grains: Proper postharvest storage and handling of cereal crops are essential to preserve the integrity, quality, and safety of the grains during long-term storage. Proper cereal grain storage is essential to prevent spoilage and to preserve their nutritional content, particularly vitamins and polyphenols.

Short-term grain storage: Temporary storage of grains at the farm level has the main aim of keeping the product in bulk for short-term storage before drying it and transferring it to long-term storage in silos. The main control point is to keep the product at below 18% moisture to prevent the growth of molds that may produce toxins such as ochratoxin A. If the moisture content exceeds 18%, the grain may need to be dried or kept at cool temperatures. Long-term storage requires a drying step to bring the moisture content to less than 14.5% to prevent damage and spoilage of the cereal grains.

Drying prior to long-term storage: There are two primary methods to dry grain: high-temperature drying used primarily for feed grain and near-ambient drying. Both have the objective of decreasing the moisture content of the harvested grain to below 14.5%. For reference, freshly harvested wheat contains 18%–20% moisture. High-temperature drying is conducted at about 40°C in special equipment that allows warm air to come in contact with a bed of grain to effectively remove moisture. Drying of grain kernels must be conducted gradually; prolonged heating or excessive temperature can form stress cracks in grain kernels. In turn, these cracks may affect the milling process and are possible entry points for mold, insects, and other pests. Near-ambient drying is a slower process, which may take several days; it involves using air 5°C warmer than the grain. Near-ambient drying carries a higher risk of product spoilage than high-temperature drying, but it has the advantage of preventing the grain from becoming over-heated. This is important to avoid exceeding the germination temperature of the grain, which is essential to produce malted barley and other germinated grains.

Long-term storage of grains: Once dried, cereal grains may be stored for several months in concrete silos. It is essential to carefully control the moisture and temperature of the grains with proper ventilation. Additionally, leaks should be avoided to prevent external moisture to enter the silo and increase the moisture content of the grains. Mold growth and insects are the main risks to which grains are exposed during long-term storage. Thus, proper handling procedures are required to avoid crop losses or damage of product integrity. Suitable conditions for mold growth are present when the moisture content of the cereal is above 14.5% in a relatively wide range of storage temperatures. A few examples of molds and their associated crop and health-related effects include *Aspergillus* species, which require cereal moisture content ranging from 15% to 20% and may damage germination and cause slow heating of the product, and *Penicillium* species, which may produce mycotoxins under the appropriate moisture and temperature.

Other organisms of concern during grain storage are mites, which can cause damage to the grain by eating the germ and hollowing out seeds. Their growth can be easily prevented by controlling the cereal moisture content to less than 14.5% and/or cooling the grains to less than 5°C. Several types of insects including grain beetles, spider beetles, and grain weevils may cause commercial damage by breaking and/ or hollowing out the grain. Proper hygiene and adequate storage temperatures may prevent insect growth.

The aforementioned strategies to improve cereal grain storage can substantially improve postharvest losses of cereal grains. In developing countries, these losses may account for a substantial proportion of the total harvest of commodities such as rice (5%–25%), corn (40%–50%), and wheat (3%–25%) (Kumar & Kalita, 2017). Addressing these fundamental storage issues can not only increase economic productivity but also improve food security, help alleviate hunger, aid in sustainable agricultural production, and improve the livelihoods of the farmers who depend on these products (Kumar & Kalita, 2017). Moreover, improvement in storage conditions may also decrease exposure to mycotoxins from *Aspergillus flavus* and *A. parasiticus*, which are associated with the incidence of liver cancer in adults and may affect growth in children (Kumar & Kalita, 2017) (Figure 2.13).

Milling is conducted to achieve size reduction of several cereal kernels to produce flour. The conventional milling process includes a cleaning step to remove dirt and rocks. The kernels continue through two more cleaning steps, one to remove impurities using an air aspirator and another one to remove traces of other grains using separators. A further step removes traces of metals using a magnetic separator. Subsequent steps include washing to separate any additional foreign materials followed by a conditioning step to adjust the moisture content of the grain and to achieve separation of several components of the kernel. The next stage of the process is the first break producing coarse grain particles and separates the bran (containing the fiber) from the germ and the endosperm (containing most of the starch). The rest of the process consists of successive grinding states to produce the desired particle size (A. Singh et al., 2015).

Once the desired particle size has been obtained, the protein content of the flour is carefully adjusted by mixing flour streams from wheat varieties with varying levels

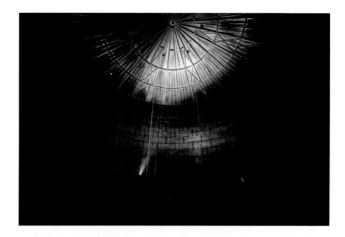

FIGURE 2.13   Inside view of a grain silo.

of protein content. Flours with less protein content such as cake or pastry flours are produced from soft wheat varieties containing 7%–9% protein. These flours are used in pastry products, cakes, and muffins. On the other hand, flours with higher protein content are produced from hard wheat varieties. For instance, bread flour contains 10%–14% and is used in applications where gluten development is important. All-purpose flour is a blend of flour made from hard and soft wheat creating a product with about 10% protein designed for use in a wide variety of products. The process of balancing the protein content is quite delicate and complex because the raw materials have a wide range of protein content depending on the variety, season, growing region, and year-to-year variation due to weather patterns.

CHANGES IN NUTRIENT CONTENT WITH CEREAL GRAIN PROCESSING AND HANDLING

Storage: Cereal storage temperature is important to preserve its micronutrient and phenolic content in addition to helping preserve grain integrity. The effect of temperature on carotenoid content has been evaluated in a few studies. In general, carotenoid content increases in cereal stored at 4°C, possibly due to breakdown of the cellulose structures that bind to carotenoids, which allows more carotenoids to be available for analysis (Mellado-Ortega, Atienza, & Hornero-Méndez, 2015; Trono, 2019). In contrast, no changes in carotenoid content were observed with storage at 20°C, and carotenoid losses were observed with storage at 37°C (Mellado-Ortega et al., 2015; Trono, 2019). Vitamin B losses during storage are also common. For instance, folate reduction of 20% to 30% has been observed in wheat flour depending on storage time and conditions (Liang, Wang, Shariful, Ye, & Zhang, 2020). The concentration of total phenolic compounds decreases during cereal storage with similar degradation observed for various classes of phenolic compounds (Ragaee, Seetharaman, & Abdel-Aal el, 2014). Temperature seems to play a role in stability during storage. For instance, bigger phenolic compound losses were observed in rice, i.e., the loss is greater in products stored at 37°C compared to cereal stored at 4°C (Ragaee et al., 2014).

Milling: In milling of refined flours, the bran and germ are separated from the endosperm. For instance, the pericarp, and aleurone layers are all removed from the rest of the flour fraction. During milling, the germ and bran layer are removed from the grain. As a result, the dietary fiber, protein, and the vitamins, minerals, and phenolic compounds concentrated in those layers are lost, resulting in refined grains with decreased nutritional content compared to the original intact kernel (A. Singh et al., 2015). Substantial losses of B vitamins occur during milling, and up to 70% folate is lost during this processing step due to the removal of the bran (Liang et al., 2020).

Micronutrient losses during milling are direct result of the loss of the cereal bran layer. In the production of durum flour, up to 8% of carotenoids are lost during milling (Trono, 2019). Most of the phenolic compounds in wheat kernels are in the cereal bran, and loss of this layer results in substantial decreases in phenolic compound content (Calinoiu & Vodnar, 2018). Pearling, which is primarily carried out to remove the hull, also results in decreases in phenolic compound concentrations due to the fact that part of the bran layer is lost to in this process in both wheat and barley kernels (Calinoiu & Vodnar, 2018). Cereal grains such as oats and rye, which are often consumed in their whole-grain forms, observed minimal phenolic compound losses during milling.

Baking: Several steps in baking are associated with nutrient changes. For instance, kneading and dough formation are associated with 15%–50% decreases in carotenoid content; bread baking leads to an additional 30%–40% loss (Trono, 2019). Bread baking resulted in losses of vitamins, particularly 3%–19% of folate (Liang et al., 2020). Of note, folate levels increase during the dough fermentation process prior to baking; this is believed to be due to increases in one of the forms of folate (5-methyltetrahydrofolate) during yeast fermentation (Liang et al., 2020). Increases in folate levels and other B vitamins have been observed in fermented products as a result of lactic acid bacteria (Holasova, Fielderova, Roubal, & Pechacova, 2005; LeBlanc et al., 2011). Interestingly, the content of several phenolic compounds, particularly phenolic acids, increases during baking. However, it is unclear whether this is related to release from other starch and fiber components or due to the thermal process (Calinoiu & Vodnar, 2018). Increases in both baking temperature and temperature time are linked to increases in phenolic compound levels (Calinoiu & Vodnar, 2018).

Roasting: Grain roasting is carried out to change the flavor profile of various grains. However, roasting of barley and buckwheat is linked to marked reductions in phenolic compounds (Calinoiu & Vodnar, 2018).

Extrusion: Food extrusion is a process whereby mixed ingredients are conveyed by rotating screws inside a barrel and then forced through an opening in a perforated plate, called a die used to control its shape. A set of blades then cuts the pieces at a specific length to produce the desired three-dimensional shape (Harper, 1978). Extrusion is used to make several types of products including pasta, ready-to-eat cereal, snacks, and pet food, among others. Dry ingredients (flour, cornmeal, wheat) are fed through a hopper, and water is added to keep the moisture and consistency of the mix constant and at a level to produce the desired texture.

There are two primary types of extrusion; the first one is called forming extrusion, which is mainly used to shape the product with minimal cooking. Pasta manufacture is a prime example of a product manufactured with forming of extrusion. The second type of extrusion is called cooking extrusion. In this process, the rotating screws shear the product against the barrel walls, and the resulting friction cooks the product. This type of extrusion is used in cereal and snack products and results in substantial changes to its nutritional content (Figure 2.14).

The effects of extrusion on the concentration of phenolic compounds are unclear. Extrusion may free some of these compounds from fiber and starchy material, whereas the high temperature may contribute to degradation of total antioxidant capacity (Calinoiu & Vodnar, 2018). Most studies observed decreases in phenolic content in grains including corn, corn products, rye, oats, barley, and sorghum during extrusion (Calinoiu & Vodnar, 2018).

Pasta and noodles: Various forms of pasta products are subsequently cooked in water for final consumption that may lead to losses of water-soluble vitamins that may leach out. For instance, cooking noodles in water resulted in folate losses of up to 22% (Liang et al., 2020). Cooking wheat noodles resulted in slightly lower losses (16%) possibly due to reduced leaching of vitamins (Liang et al., 2020). It is

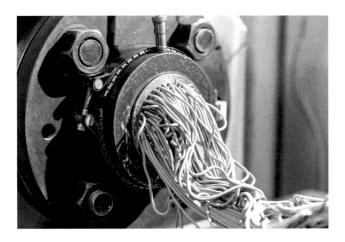

FIGURE 2.14   Extrusion of pasta.

important to note that durum wheat for pasta is bred for high carotenoid content driven in part by consumer preferences (Trono, 2019).

Canning: There are a few grain products that undergo canning, including corn, sorghum, and barley. It has been observed that total phenolic content and in particular ferulic acid, increased in canned corn, potentially explained due to the release of these compounds from cell wall materials during cooking (Dewanto et al., 2002).

Corn processing: Corn is one of the most widely consumed grains in the world. Corn can be processed and prepared using a wide range of methods, resulting in products with unique properties and final nutritional content. Corn has the highest content of carotenoids among cereal grains of which zeaxanthin is the main carotenoid. Other carotenoids include lutein, beta-carotene and beta-cryptoxanthin (Ortiz, Rocheford, & Ferruzzi, 2016). Most carotenoids in corn are contained in the endosperm (92%–100%) (Ortiz et al., 2016). In contrast, in most other grains, carotenoids are concentrated in the bran in addition to the endosperm (Trono, 2019). Other vitamins include thiamin, riboflavin, niacin, and vitamin E. Most of the minerals including calcium, iron, magnesium potassium, and zinc are found in the endosperm (Suri & Tanumihardjo, 2016).

Corn storage: Corn is usually dried after harvest to maintain its moisture content below 14%–15% to prevent spoilage and infestation during storage. Most drying treatments result in carotenoid losses in the range of 15%–45% regardless of drying temperature, which can range from room temperature to 90°C (Trono, 2019). Laboratory experiments have shown that freeze drying improves the retention of total carotenoids, but it is a very expensive process to use routinely in most commercial settings (Suri & Tanumihardjo, 2016). Corn can be stored for periods ranging from 6 to 18 months. Like other cereals, temperature and moisture conditions must be carefully controlled to avoid product spoilage and infestation. Corn storage has been associated with carotenoid losses in the range of 30% to 40% regardless of storage temperature and time (Suri & Tanumihardjo, 2016; Trono, 2019). However, several studies have shown that higher retention (20%–40%) was observed with storage at 4°C and 20°C compared to higher storage temperatures for up to 53 months (Ortiz et al., 2016). Similar losses (20%–40%) have been observed during 6–18-month storage of biofortified corn, specifically bred for higher content of carotenoids (Bechoff & Dhuique-Mayer, 2017).

Corn milling is the most common processing step before undergoing further transformation. **Dry milling** produces a range of products depending on the desired particle size including corn grits, cornmeal, and corn flour in increasing degrees of fineness (Suri & Tanumihardjo, 2016). Dry milling removes part of the bran and the germ leaving only the starchy endosperm; however, traditional stone grinding keeps some of the germ (Suri & Tanumihardjo, 2016). The removal of the germ and bran during dry milling results in decreased fiber content in the corn flour product, and it decreases the levels of several micronutrients. In general, carotenoid content is not affected by milling because the majority are located in the endosperm (Suri & Tanumihardjo, 2016). However, the concentrations of most B vitamins are 40%–76% lower in degermed corn. Most of vitamins C and E and minerals such as copper, magnesium, manganese, and zinc are substantially lower in milled degermed corn (Suri & Tanumihardjo, 2016). Dry milling results in substantial losses of phenolic compounds because the bran is one of the primary layer that contains them although the germ also contains a smaller fraction of phenolic acids and flavonoids (Calinoiu & Vodnar, 2018).

Wet milling is used to separate corn into various component streams such as starch, protein, oil, and fiber (Suri & Tanumihardjo, 2016). In wet milling, corn kernels are hydrated in water for 24–40 hours to soften them and improve the ease and efficiency of the milling step (N. Singh & Eckhoff, 1996). Additives such as lactic acid and sulfur dioxide are used to break down the protein matrix and separate starch granules more efficiently (N. Singh & Eckhoff, 1996). In the first grind, oil is separated from the kernels, followed by a second grind that separates the germ and finished by a final grind to extract the starch materials. The starch extracted by wet milling is used to manufacture industrial ingredients including corn syrup, glucose, and various native and modified starches for use in food product applications. The soaking step of wet milling decreases carotenoid levels by 7.0%–9.5% in corn kernels and produces substantial decreases in the levels of most micronutrients (Suri & Tanumihardjo, 2016).

Nixtamalization is a traditional process developed in Mexico and Central America. To prepare corn following this process, corn first is soaked overnight and then cooked in an alkaline solution made with lime (calcium hydroxide) and then washed and hulled. The resulting product, the nixtamal, is the starting ingredient to make tamales, corn tortillas, and tortilla chips. Several chemical changes take place during the nixtamalization process because of the increased pH produced by the calcium hydroxide. Several pigments in corn including carotenoids and anthocyanins produce more intense colors in the alkaline pH environment. The alkaline environment degrades the plant cell wall material, allowing the outer layer, or pericarp, to be removed (Figure 2.15).

The nixtamalization process changes the concentrations of several nutrients found in corn. For instance, masa made with nixtamalized corn retained about 64% of its original carotenoid content compared to the original raw material (Trono, 2019). The alkaline environment during nixtamalization results in substantial polyphenol losses (54%–66% of total polyphenols and almost all of anthocyanins) (Suri &

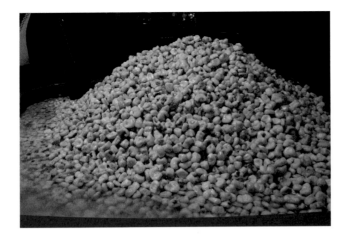

FIGURE 2.15   Corn produced from nixtamal.

Tanumihardjo, 2016). Nixtamalization tends to decrease the overall concentration of most vitamins. For instance, levels of thiamin, riboflavin, and niacin decrease by 30%–50%. However, nixtamalization increases the bioavailability of niacin by releasing it from cell wall materials (Suri & Tanumihardjo, 2016). Nixtamalization results in small decreases in concentrations of iron, magnesium, phosphorus, and copper, but it substantially increases its calcium content because of the calcium contributions of limewater (calcium hydroxide) (Suri & Tanumihardjo, 2016).

Cooking Methods

Whole-grain corn is consumed in various forms including boiled, roasted on the cob, frozen, and canned as popcorn. Cooking whole-grain corn using wet-cooking methods retained most of its carotenoid content (>70%), and in some cases, increases were observed due to the release of bound carotenoids from fibrous materials (Suri & Tanumihardjo, 2016; Trono, 2019). For instance, steam cooking and boiling corn on the cob results in significant increases in levels of total carotenoids, lutein, zeaxanthin, beta-cryptoxanthin, and beta-carotene (Trono, 2019). Other dishes including corn porridge dishes retained 63%–97% of beta-carotene, beta-cryptoxanthin, and 90%–120% total carotenoids (Suri & Tanumihardjo, 2016). Similar retention levels (75%) have been observed in biofortified corn varieties bred specifically for their carotenoid content (Bechoff & Dhuique-Mayer, 2017). Micronutrient retention during cooking varies widely depending on the method used. Baked corn products (muffins, cornbread) lose 25%–35% of total carotenoids (Trono, 2019). Deep-fat frying also results in substantial carotenoid losses (22%–50%) (Suri & Tanumihardjo, 2016; Trono, 2019). Other dry cooking methods including roasting (with extrusion and flaking preprocessing steps) led to decreases of 40%–60% in carotenoid content (Trono, 2019).

Industrial processing methods: Refined products produced via extrusion (corn puffs) or deep-frying (corn chips) result in carotenoid losses of 40%–60% in the former and almost 100% in the latter (Suri & Tanumihardjo, 2016; Trono, 2019). Laminated and toasted cornflakes result in similar carotenoid losses (~80%) (Trono, 2019). Polyphenol content is also greatly decreased in products that undergo extrusion and/or frying (75% to 80% losses) (Suri & Tanumihardjo, 2016). Extrusion is associated with decreases of thiamin (16%), niacin (25%) and tocopherols (63% to 94%) (Suri & Tanumihardjo, 2016). Extrusion and deep-frying have a noticeable effect in the concentration of most minerals with decreases of close to 50% in levels of copper, iron, manganese, and selenium and minimal losses for zinc and magnesium (Suri & Tanumihardjo, 2016).

RICE PROCESSING

Harvesting and storage: Rice harvesting involves four primary steps including reaping (cutting the rice straws), threshing to separate the grain (also called paddy) from the rest of the crop, cleaning to remove immature grains, and hauling to transport it for postharvest (Atungulu & Pan, 2014). From that point, the main postharvest operations are similar to those of other grains including cleaning, drying, storage, and milling. As with other grains, proper drying is important to minimize contamination and postharvest losses. Rice drying may be performed in open-air fields or by heated air systems.

The husk comprises about 20% of the weight of rice. Once it is removed, the resulting brown rice is comprised of about 10% bran, 90% endosperm, and 1% germ (Atungulu & Pan, 2014). In single-step milling processes, the husk is removed to produce brown rice, or both the bran and husk are removed to make white rice. In processes where the removal of the husk is conducted first, an additional cleaning step is performed to remove foreign material like stones. From that point forward, the bran is removed from brown rice by polishing whereby mild abrasion removed a specified amount of bran to produce a desired level of whiteness (A. Singh et al., 2015).

Arsenic in rice: In addition to the nutrient changes that result from various postharvesting and processing options, an issue is relevance for rice cultivation and processing. Arsenic has been used in pesticides for many decades, which can persist in the soil and underground water reservoirs for many decades in arsenic endemic areas. Arsenic has been associated with the incidence of cardiovascular disease, diabetes, and bladder, lung, and skin cancers (Huang et al., 2015). The primary sources of arsenic in endemic areas include the soil, the irrigation water, and the cooking water (Kumarathilaka, Seneweera, Ok, Meharg, & Bundschuh, 2019). Arsenic is of particular concern for rice cultivation because this crop is grown in many places using flooded paddies. This system helps solubilize the arsenic in the soil, which contributes to its uptake by the rice plant. Moreover, the water used to flood the paddies may contribute additional arsenic. Furthermore, well water for home use may also contain elevated arsenic levels, which contributes additional arsenic during the cooking process.

Few options are available to decrease arsenic content of harvested rice. At the postharvest stage, rice polishing can decrease inorganic arsenic levels by 51%–70% compared to brown rice (Kumarathilaka et al., 2019). The primary disadvantage of this method is the removal of the bran which leads to nutrient losses. At the kitchen level, washing up to three times with deionized or tap water decreased arsenic levels by 16%–19% in brown rice and by 17%–29% in white rice (Kumarathilaka et al., 2019). The effectiveness of this process is driven by the arsenic content of the water source. For instance, sequential washing of rice with well water with traces of arsenic added 30% arsenic for every wash cycle (Kumarathilaka et al., 2019). A disadvantage of this method is the loss of water-soluble vitamins and minerals due to leaching out to the washing water.

Parboiled rice is made by cooking rice (usually by boiling) while is its still in its husk. This process entails overnight soaking at room temperature, boiling or steaming to partially cook the rice, and drying to achieve the desired moisture content for storage. It is estimated that the parboiling process leads to losses of protein and of 7%–15% thiamine, 12%–15% riboflavin, and 10%–13% niacin (Atungulu & Pan, 2014). More recent technologies have optimized the temperature of the cooking step to achieve starch gelatinization while minimizing vitamin losses.

Sprouted rice is produced by germinating brown rice in water at 30°C–40°C for about 20 hours. It has been reported that this process increases the availability of several nutrients, primarily B vitamins, vitamin E, potassium, zinc, and magnesium and of several phenolic compounds including ferulic acid (Atungulu & Pan, 2014).

OAT PROCESSING

The main structural components of the oat kernel are similar to other grains: a protective hull that surrounds the groat, which is comprised of the barn, germ, and endosperm. The endosperm contains most of the starch, whereas the bran contains most of the dietary fiber, vitamins, and minerals (Grundy, Fardet, Tosh, Rich, & Wilde, 2018). In addition to cellulose, oats and barley contain a special type of fibers called beta-glucans, which are glucose polysaccharides arranged in a repeating pattern of three glucose units linked by a beta (1–4) linkages followed by a beta (1–3) linkage (Henrion, Francey, Le, & Lamothe, 2019). Cereal beta-glucans comprise about 4.5% of the mass of barley, and oats also occur in whole wheat and rye (Henrion et al., 2019).

Beta-glucans generate viscosity during their transit through the intestinal tract, which slows down the rate of gastric emptying. It is believed that the increased viscosity slows down the absorption of simple carbohydrates, which results in a slower rise of blood glucose and insulin levels after a meal (Regand, Chowdhury, Tosh, Wolever, & Wood, 2011; Regand, Tosh, Wolever, & Wood, 2009). Both the concentration and the molecular weight of the beta-glucan chains are a primary determinant of the viscosity level produced in the intestinal tract (Regand et al., 2011). In turn, higher viscosity decreased blood glucose response as evidenced by reduced peak glucose levels after a meal (Regand et al., 2009).

Oats are available in several forms such as steel-cut oats, rolled oats, quick-cook oats, and instant oatmeal. Steel-cut oats are produced by cutting the oat groats into 2–4 smaller pieces with steel blades. Steel-cut oats are usually coarse and produce a chewy texture. Because they are not precooked, they require soaking and cooking for 20–30 minutes. Rolled oats are made by steam cooking the whole kernels and subsequently passing them through a pair of rollers, which reduces their size. Because this process partially cooks them and decreases their thickness, they only need to be cooked at home for 7–10 minutes. Quick-cook oats are made in a similar fashion but with a thinner gap between the rollers so that the resulting product is smaller in size and only needs a few minutes to cook with home methods (stovetop or microwave). Instant oatmeal is a smaller particle size version of rolled oats that are cooked at higher temperature than rolled oats so that the starch gelatinizes almost completely, and they require little additional home cooking. Other products are muesli, which is produced form oat flakes and granola, which is made by toasting the oat flakes.

Cooking and industrial processing of oats influence the molecular weight of beta-glucans and thus, their physicochemical characteristic including its viscosity. These changes may alter their sensory properties and physiological effects in several food products. The addition of beta-glucan extracts to food products may improve their glycemic response, and it is determined by their concentration, the preserved molecular weight of the beta-glucan chains, and the resulting viscosity (Regand et al., 2009).

Consumption of beta-glucans has been associated with improvements in blood lipid levels in processes where the molecular weight of beta-glucan polymers is preserved. Addition of high and medium molecular weight beta-glucans to ready-to-eat cereals has shown decreases of LDL cholesterol levels compared to the same products made with an equivalent amount wheat bran (Wolever et al., 2010). Similar studies conducted in vivo and in vitro have produced similar results (Grundy et al., 2018). The mechanisms linking beta-glucan consumption to blood lipid levels are complex. It has been proposed that viscosity plays a role by decreasing the absorption of dietary cholesterol and bile acids, which slows down their return to the liver, which in turn may lead to conversion of hepatic cholesterol to bile acids, thereby decreasing blood cholesterol levels (Grundy et al., 2018).

Cooking Methods

Beta-glucan added to pasta largely preserved its molecular weight and produced high viscosity, which resulted in favorable glycemic response as evidenced by low postprandial peak blood glucose levels (Regand et al., 2009). On the other hand, the addition of beta-glucans to bakery products such as breads and muffins resulted in substantial decreases in its molecular weight and resulting viscosity, which produced less favorable glycemic responses (Regand et al., 2009). The beta-glucan molecular weight reduction seems to be a direct effect of mixing and fermentation, resulting from enzymatic hydrolysis, rather than on the baking process itself (Aman, Rimsen, & Andersson, 2004). For instance, the molecular weight of beta-glucan strands decreased with increased fermentation time; however, cooking preparations including of oat products including porridges, pancakes, and nonfermented baked products did not alter the molecular weight of beta-glucan chains nor their resulting viscosity (Aman et al., 2004).

Industrial Processing Methods

Industrial processing such as the production of rolled oats or the extraction of oat bran does not seem to alter the molecular weight of beta-glucans (Aman et al., 2004). The molecular weight of beta-glucans in granola products made from industrially processed oats was well preserved and resulted in higher viscosity and favorable glycemic responses (Regand et al., 2009). A review of oat products and their resulting glycemic index (GI; text box 9) showed that there were substantial differences in the glycemic response to these products (Tosh & Chu, 2015). Steel-cut and rolled oats produced medium glycemic responses (GI: 50–60) whereas quick oats and instant oatmeal had a GI or 70–90, which indicates a less favorable glycemic response than the less processed products (Tosh & Chu, 2015). Muesli and granola exhibited medium glycemic responses (Tosh & Chu, 2015). The differences were likely

---

TEXT BOX 9

The **GI** is a measure to characterize carbohydrate quality. The GI is a relative measure of the incremental blood glucose response (measured as the area under the glucose curve) per gram of carbohydrate compared to the same amount of carbohydrate from glucose (Jenkins, 1981).

---

explained by the particle size and degree of starch gelatinization. For instance, quick oats and instant oatmeal had a higher percentage of gelatinized starch as a result of the additional processing (Tosh & Chu, 2015).

The incorporation of beta-glucans into bakery products that undergo freeze-thaw cycles may attenuate their postprandial glycemic response. For instance, the glycemic response of muffins made with beta-glucan extracts showed similar responses after 2 freeze-thaw cycles; however, the benefit was lost after 4 cycles (Lan-Pidhainy, Brummer, Tosh, Wolever, & Wood, 2007). This difference was explained by decreased viscosity produced by beta-glucans, rather than by changes in its molecular weight, which may in turn increase starch digestibility and increase the postprandial glycemic response (Lan-Pidhainy et al., 2007; Regand et al., 2011).

Extrusion cooking influence the molecular weight of beta-glucan chains. A study of various extrusion conditions of oat bran extrudates showed that increasing temperature and shear stress led to increasing cell wall disruption and decreased beta-glucan molecular weight distributions even when the total levels of beta-glucan and dietary fiber were not affected (Tosh et al., 2010).

FERMENTATION

Fermentation is a biochemical process in which glucose or other carbohydrates are broken down in the absence of oxygen. In the context of food production, it encompasses changes in flavor and texture brought about microbial activity, which under anaerobic conditions transforms available carbohydrates to produce lactic and other organic acids, alcohol and carbon dioxide. Fermentation can be applied to a wide range of food substrates such as fruits, vegetables, legumes, grains, dairy products and meat products to enhance flavor, texture and extend their shelf life. Additionally, fermentation enriches the nutritional value of many foods and improves their palatability. For instance, levels of B vitamins and phenolic compounds increase in fermented whole-grain products as compared to their raw materials (Adebo & Gabriela Medina-Meza, 2020). Changes in phenolic compounds have been observed in the fermentation of fruits and vegetables due to the breakdown of plant cell walls as a result of microbial enzymatic activity, which helps release these compounds (Adebo & Gabriela Medina-Meza, 2020; Hidalgo & Zamora, 2017).

In the context of fruits and vegetables, fermentation is often conducted by microbial communities that naturally occur in fruits and vegetables. Pickling is a special case of fermentation in which the product is submerged in brine, which creates optimal growth conditions for specific lactic acid bacteria and suppresses the growth of competing microorganisms, and it is employed in the production of fermented olives, sauerkraut, and kimchi. Fermentation is also used for cereal, grains, and legumes as the substrate material. For instance, soy sauce and miso are products of fermentation of soybeans. Other products include natto, tofuyo (Japan), douchi, sufu, doubanjiang (China), cheonggukjang, doenjang, kanjang, meju (Korea), tempeh (Indonesia), thua nao (Thailand), kinema, hawaijar, and tungrymbai (India) (Sanjukta & Rai, 2016). In the production of soy sauce, complex carbohydrates and proteins are broken down by the action of *Aspergillus oryzae* mold (koji). Several species of *Bacillus*, lactic acid bacteria, and yeasts further breakdown these compounds into components that provide flavor (peptides, lactic acid, and simple sugars). Fermentation of soybeans increases levels of peptides with antioxidant, antimicrobial, and potentially antihypertensive properties (Sanjukta & Rai, 2016) (Figure 2.16).

The production of organic acids may help release antioxidant molecules from plant cell walls and hydrolyze large polyphenol molecules, which increases their antioxidant activity (Hur, Lee, Kim, Choi, & Kim, 2014). Several other compounds are increased in various foods including the release of bioactive peptides in cereals, peanuts, rapeseed, and lentils; increased phenolic levels in olives, soybeans, cranberry and apple pomace, blueberry, and wheat; increased isoflavone levels in various fermented soybean products; increased anthocyanin levels in fermented mulberry and increased level of various vitamins in soybeans (Hur et al., 2014).

Cereal grains are sources of many classes of phenolic compounds including phenolic acids, flavonoids, and tannins (Adebo & Gabriela Medina-Meza, 2020). Several studies have documented increases in total phenolic compounds in the fermentation of barley, corn, millet, quinoa, rye, and wheat, which are attributed to the release of these compounds from plant cell walls and complex carbohydrates as they are broken

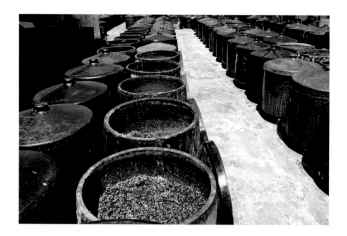

FIGURE 2.16   Soybean fermentation vessels.

down by fermentation from endogenous microorganisms or by using starter cultures (Adebo & Gabriela Medina-Meza, 2020).

However, the fermentation of sorghum was reported to result in higher levels of catechin, gallic acid, and quercetin while levels of total phenolic compounds as well as total flavonoid and tannin content decreased (Adebo & Gabriela Medina-Meza, 2020). This decrease was attributed to the degradation of phenolic compounds after fermentation with *Lactobacillus* strains (Adebo & Gabriela Medina-Meza, 2020). Various strains of lactic acid bacteria have been shown to metabolize phenolic compounds, which may explain the changes in levels of specific molecules (Adebo & Gabriela Medina-Meza, 2020). Fermentation of cereals and legumes may increase the bioavailability of minerals including copper, manganese, and chromium due to the breakdown of plant cell wall materials (Kumari & Platel, 2020).

Sensory properties of fermented foods can be influenced by various variables including fermentation temperature, time, humidity, and the choice of microorganisms. Thus, these conditions have the potential to increase levels of antioxidant and bioactive compounds in addition to improving flavor and texture and extending the shelf life of fermented foods.

REFERENCES

Adebo, O. A., & Gabriela Medina-Meza, I. (2020). Impact of fermentation on the phenolic compounds and antioxidant activity of whole cereal grains: A mini review. *Molecules, 25*(4). doi:10.3390/molecules25040927.

Alvi, S., Khan, K. M., Sheikh, M. A., & Shahid, M. (2003). Effect of peeling and cooking on nutrients in vegetables. *Pakistan Journal of Nutrition, 2*(3), 189–191.

Aman, P., Rimsen, L., & Andersson, P. (2004). Molecular weight distribution of beta-glucan in oat-based foods. *Cereal Chemistry, 81*(3), 356–360.

Atungulu, G. G., & Pan, Z. (2014). Rice industrial processing worldwide and impact on macro- and micronutrient content, stability, and retention. *Annals of the New York Academy of Sciences, 1324*, 15–28. doi:10.1111/nyas.12492.

Barth, M. M., & Zhuang, H. (1996). Packaging design affects antioxidant vitamin retention and quality of broccoli florets during postharvest storage. *Postharvest Biology and Technology, 9*, 141–150.

Bechoff, A., & Dhuique-Mayer, C. (2017). Factors influencing micronutrient bioavailability in biofortified crops. *Annals of the New York Academy of Sciences, 1390*(1), 74–87. doi:10.1111/nyas.13301.

Bhatta, S., Stevanovic Janezic, T., & Ratti, C. (2020). Freeze-drying of plant-based foods. *Foods, 9*(1). doi:10.3390/foods9010087.

Blumberg, J. B., & Milbury, P. E. (2006). Dietary Flavonoids. In B. A. Bowman & R. M. Russell (Eds.), *Present Knowledge in Nutrition* (Vol. 1, pp. 361–370). Washington, D.C.: ILSI Press.

Bouzari, A., Holstege, D., & Barrett, D. M. (2015a). Mineral, fiber, and total phenolic retention in eight fruits and vegetables: A comparison of refrigerated and frozen storage. *Journal of Agriculture and Food Chemistry, 63*(3), 951–956. doi:10.1021/jf504890k.

Bouzari, A., Holstege, D., & Barrett, D. M. (2015b). Vitamin retention in eight fruits and vegetables: A comparison of refrigerated and frozen storage. *Journal of Agriculture and Food Chemistry, 63*(3), 957–962. doi:10.1021/jf5058793.

Calinoiu, L. F., & Vodnar, D. C. (2018). Whole grains and phenolic acids: A review on bioactivity, functionality, health benefits and bioavailability. *Nutrients, 10*(11). doi:10.3390/nu10111615.

Cefola, M., Carbone, V., Minasi, P., & Pace, B. (2016). Phenolic profiles and postharvest quality changes of fresh-cut radicchio (Cichorium intybus L.): Nutrient value in fresh vs. stored leaves. *Journal of Food Composition and Analysis*, 51, 76–84. doi:10.1016/j.jfca.2016.06.004.

Cereals & Grains Association. (2017). Proposed definition of whole grain as food ingredient. http://online.cerealsgrains.org/initiatives/definitions/Pages/HarmonizedWGFood IngredientDefinition.aspx.

Code of Federal Regulations, 21CFR1.227 C.F.R. (2019).

Dewanto, V., Wu, X., & Liu, R. H. (2002). Processed sweet corn has higher antioxidant activity. *Journal of Agriculture and Food Chemistry, 50*, 4959–4964.

Ekinci, N., Aydin, F., & Şeker, M. (2016). Effects of modified atmosphere conditions on beta carotene and anthocyanin contents of arbutus unedu fruits. *Proceedings of the VII International Scientific Agriculture Symposium*, "Agrosym 2016", 6–9 October 2016, Jahorina, Bosnia and Herzegovina, 1415–1421.

Erturk, E., & Picha, D. H. (2002). Modified atmosphere packaging of fresh-cut sweetpotatoes (Ipomoea Batatas L.). *Acta Horticulturae*, 583, 223–230. doi:10.17660/ActaHortic.2002.583.25.

Granado-Lorencio, F., Olmedilla-Alonso, B., Herrero-Barbudo, C., Sánchez-Moreno, C., de Ancos, B., Martínez, J. A., et al. (2008). Modified-atmosphere packaging (MAP) does not affect the bioavailability of tocopherols and carotenoids from broccoli in humans: A cross-over study. *Food Chemistry*, 106(3), 1070–1076. doi:10.1016/j.foodchem.2007.07.038.

Grundy, M. M., Fardet, A., Tosh, S. M., Rich, G. T., & Wilde, P. J. (2018). Processing of oat: The impact on oat's cholesterol lowering effect. *Food & Function, 9*(3), 1328–1343. doi:10.1039/c7fo02006f.

Harper, J. M. (1978). Food extrusion. *Critical Reviews in Food Science and Nutrition, 11*(2), 155–215.

Hasan, M. U., Malik, A. U., Ali, S., Imtiaz, A., Munir, A., Amjad, W., & Anwar, R. (2019). Modern drying techniques in fruits and vegetables to overcome postharvest losses: A review. *Journal of Food Processing and Preservation, 43*(12). doi:10.1111/jfpp.14280.

Henrion, M., Francey, C., Le, K. A., & Lamothe, L. (2019). Cereal B-Glucans: The impact of processing and how it affects physiological responses. *Nutrients, 11*(8). doi:10.3390/nu11081729.

Hidalgo, F. J., & Zamora, R. (2017). Food processing antioxidants. *Advances in Food and Nutrition Research*, 81, 31–64. doi:10.1016/bs.afnr.2016.10.002.

Holasova, M., Fielderova, V., Roubal, P., & Pechacova, M. (2005). Possibility of increasing natural folate content in fermented milk products by fermentation and fruit component addition. *Czech Journal of Food Science, 23*(5), 196–201.

Huang, Y., Wang, M., Mao, X., Qian, Y., Chen, T., & Zhang, Y. (2015). Concentrations of inorganic arsenic in milled rice from china and associated dietary exposure assessment. *Journal of Agriculture and Food Chemistry, 63*(50), 10838–10845. doi:10.1021/acs.jafc.5b04164.

Hur, S. J., Lee, S. Y., Kim, Y. C., Choi, I., & Kim, G. B. (2014). Effect of fermentation on the antioxidant activity in plant-based foods. *Food Chemistry, 160*, 346–356. doi:10.1016/j.foodchem.2014.03.112.

Imsic, M., Winkler, S., Tomkins, B., & Jones, R. (2010). Effect of storage and cooking on beta-carotene isomers in carrots (Daucus carota L. cv. 'Stefano'). *Journal of Agriculture and Food Chemistry, 58*(8), 5109–5113. doi:10.1021/jf904279j.

Institute of Medicine. (2001). *Institute of Medicine (US) Panel on the Definition of Dietary Fiber and the Standing Committee on the Scientific Evaluation of Dietary Reference Intakes. Dietary Reference Intakes Proposed Definition of Dietary Fiber*. Washington, DC: National Academies Press. Available from: https://www.ncbi.nlm.nih.gov/books/NBK223587/ doi: 10.17226/10161

Jenkins, D. (1981). Glycemic index of foods: A physiological basis for carbohydrate exchange. *American Journal of Clinical Nutrition, 34*(3), 363–366.

Jirantanan, T., & Liu, R. H. (2004). Antioxidant activity of processed table beets (Beta vulgaris var, conditiva) and green beans (Phaseolus vulgaris L.). *Journal of Agriculture and Food Chemistry, 52*, 2659–2670.

Karadeniz, F., Burdurlu, H. S., & Koca, N. (2007). Effect of pH on chlorophyll degradation and colour loss in blanched green peas. *Food Chemistry, 100*(2), 609–615.

Ke, Z., Chai, D., Miao, Y., Luo, K., Tan, S., & Li, W. (2020). Lycopene, polyphenols and antioxidant activities of three characteristic tomato cultivars subjected to two drying methods. *Food Chemistry, 338*, 128062. doi:10.1016/j.foodchem.2020.128062; PMID: 32950009.

Kumar, D., & Kalita, P. (2017). Reducing postharvest losses during storage of grain crops to strengthen food security in developing countries. *Foods, 6*(1). doi:10.3390/foods6010008.

Kumarathilaka, P., Seneweera, S., Ok, Y. S., Meharg, A., & Bundschuh, J. (2019). Arsenic in cooked rice foods: Assessing health risks and mitigation options. *Environment International, 127*, 584–591. doi:10.1016/j.envint.2019.04.004.

Kumari, M., & Platel, K. (2020). Impact of soaking, germination, fermentation, and thermal processing on the bioaccessibility of trace minerals from food grains. *Journal of Food Processing and Preservation, 44*(10). doi:10.1111/jfpp.14752.

Lakshmi, B., & Vamala, V. (2000). Nutritive value of dehydrated green leafy vegetable powders. *Journal of Food Science and Technology, 37*(5), 465–471.

Lan-Pidhainy, X., Brummer, Y., Tosh, S. M., Wolever, T. M., & Wood, P. (2007). Reducing beta-glucan solubility in oat bran muffins by freeze-thaw treatments attenuates its hypoglycemic effect. *Cereal Chemistry, 85*(5), 512–517.

LeBlanc, J. G., Laino, J. E., del Valle, M. J., Vannini, V., van Sinderen, D., Taranto, M. P., et al. (2011). B-group vitamin production by lactic acid bacteria--current knowledge and potential applications. *Journal of Applied Microbiology, 111*(6), 1297–1309. doi:10.1111/j.1365-2672.2011.05157.x.

Li, L., Pegg, R. B., Eitenmiller, R. R., Chun, J.-Y., & Kerrihard, A. L. (2017). Selected nutrient analyses of fresh, fresh-stored, and frozen fruits and vegetables. *Journal of Food Composition and Analysis, 59*, 8–17. doi:10.1016/j.jfca.2017.02.002.

Liang, Q., Wang, K., Shariful, I., Ye, X., & Zhang, C. (2020). Folate content and retention in wheat grains and wheat-based foods: Effects of storage, processing, and cooking methods. *Food Chemistry, 333*, 127459. doi:10.1016/j.foodchem.2020.127459.

Manach, C., Scalbert, A., Morand, C., Rémésy, C., & Jiménez, L. (2004). Polyphenols: Food sources and bioavailability. *American Journal of Clinical Nutrition, 79*, 727–747.

Martín-Belloso, O., & Llanos-Barriobero, E. (2001). Proximate composition, minerals and vitamins in selected canned vegetables. *European Food Research and Technology, 212*, 182–187.

Mayeaux, M., Xu, Z., King, J. M., & Prinyawiwatkul, W. (2006). Effects of cooking conditions on the lycopene content in tomatoes. *Journal of Food Science, 71*(8), C461–C464. doi:10.1111/j.1750-3841.2006.00163.x.

Mellado-Ortega, E., Atienza, S. G., & Hornero-Méndez, D. (2015). Carotenoid evolution during postharvest storage of durum wheat (Triticum turgidum conv. durum) and tritordeum (×Tritordeum Ascherson et Graebner) grains. *Journal of Cereal Science, 62*, 134–142. doi:10.1016/j.jcs.2015.01.006.

Miglio, C., Chiavaro, C., Visconti, A., Fogliano, V., & Pellegrini, N. (2008). Effects of different cooking methods on nutritional and physiochemical characteristics of selected vegetables. *Journal of Agriculture and Food Chemistry, 56*, 139–147.

Mujumdar, A. S. (2019). Chemical and physical pretreatments of fruits and vegetables: Effects on drying characteristics and quality attributes – a comprehensive review. *Critical Reviews in Food Science and Nutrition, 50*, 1408–1432.

Muratore, G., Rizzo, V., Licciardello, F., & Maccarone, E. (2008). Partial dehydration of cherry tomato at different temperature, and nutritional quality of the products. *Food Chemistry, 111*(4), 887–891. doi:10.1016/j.foodchem.2008.05.001.

Nemzer, B., Vargas, L., Xia, X., Sintara, M., & Feng, H. (2018). Phytochemical and physical properties of blueberries, tart cherries, strawberries, and cranberries as affected by different drying methods. *Food Chemistry, 262*, 242–250.

Ngobese, N. Z., Workneh, T. S., & Siwela, M. (2017). Effect of low-temperature long-time and high-temperature short-time blanching and frying treatments on the French fry quality of six Irish potato cultivars. *Journal of Food Science and Technology, 54*(2), 507–517. doi:10.1007/s13197-017-2495-x.

Ogawaa, Y., & Suzuki, Y. (2016). Effect of CO_2 gas concentration on quality of packaged fresh-cut bell pepper during cold storage. *Paper Presented at the CIGR-AgEng Conference*, Aarhus, Denmark.

Ortiz, D., Rocheford, T., & Ferruzzi, M. G. (2016). Influence of Temperature and Humidity on the Stability of Carotenoids in Biofortified Maize (Zea mays L.) Genotypes during Controlled Postharvest Storage. *Journal of Agriculture and Food Chemistry, 64*(13), 2727–2736.

Palermo, M., Pellegrini, N., & Fogliano, V. (2014). The effect of cooking on the phytochemical content of vegetables. *Journal of the Science of Food and Agriculture, 94*(6), 1057–1070. doi:10.1002/jsfa.6478.

Park, S. H., Lamsal, B. P., & Balasubramaniam, V. M. (2014). Principles of Food Processing. In S. Clark, S. Jung, & B. Lamsal (Eds.), *Food Processing: Principles and Applications* (pp. 1–15). New York: John Wiley & Sons, Incorporated.

Ragaee, S., Seetharaman, K., & Abdel-Aal el, S. M. (2014). The impact of milling and thermal processing on phenolic compounds in cereal grains. *Critical Reviews in Food Science and Nutrition, 54*(7), 837–849. doi:10.1080/10408398.2011.610906.

Rebello, C. J., Greenway, F. L., & Finley, J. W. (2014). Whole grains and pulses: A comparison of the nutritional and health benefits. *Journal of Agriculture and Food Chemistry, 62*(29), 7029–7049. doi:10.1021/jf500932z.

Regand, A., Chowdhury, Z., Tosh, S. M., Wolever, T. M. S., & Wood, P. (2011). The molecular weight, solubility and viscosity of oat beta-glucan affect human glycemic response by modifying starch digestibility. *Food Chemistry, 129*(2), 297–304. doi:10.1016/j.foodchem.2011.04.053.

Regand, A., Tosh, S. M., Wolever, T. M., & Wood, P. J. (2009). Physicochemical properties of beta-glucan in differently processed oat foods influence glycemic response. *Journal of Agriculture and Food Chemistry, 57*(19), 8831–8838. doi:10.1021/jf901271v.

Rickman, J. C., Barrett, D. M., & Bruhn, C. M. (2007). Nutritional comparison of fresh, frozen and canned fruits and vegetables. Part 1. Vitamins C and B and phenolic compounds. *Journal of the Science of Food and Agriculture, 87*(6), 930–944. doi:10.1002/jsfa.2825.

Rickman, J. C., Bruhn, C. M., & Barrett, D. M. (2007). Nutritional comparison of fresh, frozen, and canned fruits and vegetables II. Vitamin A and carotenoids, vitamin E, minerals and fiber. *Journal of the Science of Food and Agriculture, 87*(7), 1185–1196. doi:10.1002/jsfa.2824.

Rumm-Kreuter, D., & Demmel, I. (1990). Comparison of vitamin losses in vegetables due to various cooking methods. *Journal of Nutritional Science and Vitaminology, 36*, S7–S15.

Sanjukta, S., & Rai, A. K. (2016). Production of bioactive peptides during soybean fermentation and their potential health benefits. *Trends in Food Science & Technology, 50,* 1–10. doi:10.1016/j.tifs.2016.01.010.

Singh, A., Karmakar, S., Jacob, B. S., Bhattacharya, P., Kumar, S. P., & Banerjee, R. (2015). Enzymatic polishing of cereal grains for improved nutrient retainment. *Journal of Food Science and Technology, 52*(6), 3147–3157. doi:10.1007/s13197-014-1405-8.

Singh, N., & Eckhoff, S. E. (1996). Wet milling of corn-a review of laboratory-scale and pilot plant-scale procedures. *Cereal Chemistry, 73*(6), 659–667.

Siriwattananon, L., & Maneerate, J. (2016). Effect of drying methods on dietary fiber concent in dried fruit and vegetables from non-toxic agricultural field. *International Journal of GEOMATE, 11*(28), 2896–2900.

Sumonsiri, N., & Barringer, S. A. (2014). Fruits and Vegetables –Processing Technologies and Applications. In S. Clark, S. Jung, & B. Lamsal (Eds.), *Food Processing: Principles and Applications.* New York: John Wiley & Sons, Incorporated.

Suri, D. J., & Tanumihardjo, S. A. (2016). Effects of different processing methods on the micronutrient and phytochemical contents of maize: From A to Z. *Comprehensive Reviews in Food Science and Food Safety, 15*(5), 912–926. doi:10.1111/1541-4337.12216.

Taleon, V., Sumbu, D., Muzhingi, T., & Bidiaka, S. (2019). Carotenoids retention in biofortified yellow cassava processed with traditional African methods. *Journal of the Science of Food and Agriculture, 99*(3), 1434–1441. doi:10.1002/jsfa.9347.

Tareke, E., Rydberg, P., Karlsoon, P., Eriksson, S., & Tornqvist, M. (2002). Analysis of acrylamide, a carcinogen formed in heated foodstuffs. *Journal of Agriculture and Food Chemistry, 50,* 4998–5006.

Tosh, S. M., Brummer, Y., Miller, S. S., Regand, A., Defelice, C., Duss, R., et al. (2010). Processing affects the physicochemical properties of beta-glucan in oat bran cereal. *Journal of Agriculture and Food Chemistry, 58*(13), 7723–7730. doi:10.1021/jf904553u.

Tosh, S. M., & Chu, Y. (2015). Systematic review of the effect of processing of whole-grain oat cereals on glycaemic response. *British Journal of Nutrition, 114*(8), 1256–1262. doi:10.1017/S0007114515002895.

Traber, M. G. (2006). Vitamin E. In B. A. Bowman & R. M. Russell (Eds.), *Present Knowledge in Nutrition* (Vol. 1, pp. 211–219). Washington, D.C.: ILSI Press.

Trono, D. (2019). Carotenoids in cereal food crops: Composition and retention throughout grain storage and food processing. *Plants, 8*(12). doi:10.3390/plants8120551.

Turkmen, N., Poyrazoglu, E. S., Sari, F., & Sedat Velioglu, Y. (2006). Effects of cooking methods on chlorophylls, pheophytins and colour of selected green vegetables. *International Journal of Food Science and Technology, 41*(3), 281–288. doi:10.1111/j.1365-2621.2005.01061.x.

Turkmen, N., Sari, F., & Velioglu, Y. (2005). The effect of cooking methods on total phenolics and antioxidant activity of selected green vegetables. *Food Chemistry, 93*(4), 713–718. doi:10.1016/j.foodchem.2004.12.038.

US Food and Drug Administration. (2020). Code of Federal Regulations Title 21. April 1, 2020. Available at: https://www.accessdata.fda.gov/scripts/cdrh/cfdocs/cfcfr/cfrsearch.cfm

Vaclavik, V. A., & Christian, E. W. (2014). Food Packaging. In *Essentials of Food Science,* 4th edition (pp. 367–390). New York: Springer.

Vallejo, F., Tomas-Barberan, F., & Garcia-Vigurea, C. (2003). Health-promoting compounds in broccoli as influenced by refrigerated transport and retail sale period. *Journal of Agriculture and Food Chemistry, 51,* 3029–3034.

Veda, S., Platel, K., & Srinivasan, K. (2010). Enhanced bioaccessibility of β-carotene from yellow-orange vegetables and green leafy vegetables by domestic heat processing. *International Journal of Food Science & Technology, 45*(10), 2201–2207. doi:10.1111/j.1365-2621.2010.02385.x.

Villanueva, M. J., Tenorio, M. D., Sagardoy, M., Redondo, A., & Saco, M. D. (2005). Physical, chemical, histological and microbiological changes in fresh green asparagus (Asparagus officinalis, L.) stored in modified atmosphere packaging. *Food Chemistry, 91*(4), 609–619. doi:10.1016/j.foodchem.2004.06.030.

Wolever, T. M., Tosh, S. M., Gibbs, A. L., Brand-Miller, J., Duncan, A. M., Hart, V., et al. (2010). Physicochemical properties of oat beta-glucan influence its ability to reduce serum LDL cholesterol in humans: A randomized clinical trial. *American Journal of Clinical Nutrition, 92*(4), 723–732. doi:10.3945/ajcn.2010.29174.

Wu, X., Zhao, Y., Haytowitz, D. B., Chen, P., & Pehrsson, P. R. (2019). Effects of domestic cooking on flavonoids in broccoli and calculation of retention factors. *Heliyon, 5*(3), e01310. doi:10.1016/j.heliyon.2019.e01310.

Zunli, Ke, Chai, D., Yiwen, M., Kui, L., Si, T., & Wenfeng, L. (2021). Lycopene, polyphenols and antioxidant activities of three characteristic tomato cultivars subjected to two drying methods. *Food Chemistry, 338*, 128062. doi:10.1016/j.foodchem.2020.128062.

3 An Overview of Molecular Nutrition

Vincent W. Li, Catherine Ward, and Delaney K. Schurr
The Angiogenesis Foundation

CONTENTS

INTRODUCTION: HEALTH DEFENSE SYSTEMS

Molecular nutrition encompasses the processes by which the body breaks down foods into their separate components and absorbs the components and the effects these components exert on the body. Building on the fields of molecular biology and cellular biology, molecular nutrition allows for the investigation of fundamental questions about health related to our diet by offering mechanistic explanations.

WHY MOLECULAR NUTRITION

The USDA Dietary Guidelines for Americans are a set of dietary recommendations released by the United States Department of Agriculture (USDA) together with the US Department of Health and Human Services (HHS) every 5 years. The guideline outlines healthy components of food to include in the diet and unhealthy components that should be avoided. The most recent version of the dietary guidelines is known as MyPlate, which is a visual representation of how the diet should be balanced, depicted in Figure 3.1 as a place setting divided into five food groups. It replaced the food pyramid schematic in 2011.

MyPlate is a useful guide for information on the basic building blocks of the diet, but to go beyond this and understand the differences within each category of food requires a deeper understanding of nutrition. A basic understanding of molecular nutrition and how the constituents of foods contribute to health can be broken down

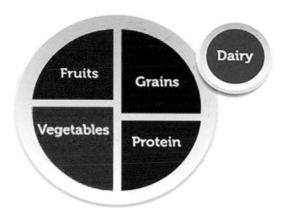

FIGURE 3.1 The most recent version of the USDA's "MyPlate", featured in the Dietary Guidelines for Americans, to provide a practical and simple template of the components of a generally balanced meal.

into sections, each with unique effects on the body. Grasping this knowledge can help inform decisions made about food every day. Understanding what foods are made of, how they get into the body, and what they do once they're inside provide key understandings necessary to make the best dietary choices given a specific personalized health situation. Thus, molecular nutrition informs decisions on how to choose and combine a variety of health-promoting foods to make up the diet.

The best way to learn about molecular nutrition is to integrate fundamental concepts with the latest research applying these concepts to human health, through the effects of food on various self-defense systems of the body. Five of the major health defense systems are **angiogenesis**; the **immune system**; **DNA protection**, **expression**, and **repair**; the gut **microbiome**; and stem cell **regeneration**. (Li, 2019)

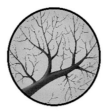

Angiogenesis is the process by which the body grows new blood vessels. There are 60,000 miles of blood vessels winding through the body that bring oxygen and nutrients to tissues and organs. Angiogenesis is essential for processes like wound healing, but grows abnormally in the context of diseases such as cancer. Tumors hijack the angiogenesis process and grow new blood vessels to feed themselves, expand, and spread via metastases. Because of this, the angiogenesis system must be kept in balance. Food can play a role in this.

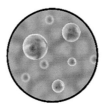

Regeneration is the process by which the body grows vital new cells. Stem cells are special cells that are able to divide and turn into different types of tissue, depending on what the body needs. The body is constantly maintaining, repairing, and regenerating itself using its stem cells. Like angiogenesis, regeneration must be kept in balance, especially because otherwise cells would grow without control, like tumors. Certain foods can boost the regenerative capacity of normal stem cells, while other foods can suppress or even destroy cell growing out of control such as cancer cells.

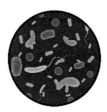

Our **microbiome** is made up of 37 trillion bacteria, which means that there are more microorganisms than human cells in the body. When the term "microbiome" is used, it usually refers to the gut microbiome, but there are bacteria in many other body parts, such as the skin microbiome and oral (mouth) microbiome. The bacteria in the gut microbiome use the food that makes it through to the large intestine for its own food, so diet is particularly important for maintaining healthy gut microbiome. Keeping a healthy microbiome also means feeding the healthy bacteria with dietary fibers, which keeps harmful bacteria at bay.

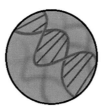

DNA is the genetic material that determines every aspect of the body. Each strand of DNA is made of nucleotides linked together. The nucleotides are then translated into proteins needed for the body's structure and function. While DNA itself cannot be changed – i.e., the same DNA at birth is kept throughout the entire lifespan – but how DNA is used, or expressed, can be changed. Lifestyle factors like diet, exercise, sleep, and stress can all affect how DNA is used and translated into the proteins it codes. In general, healthy behaviors equate to a greater number of healthy proteins created and the suppression of unhealthy proteins.

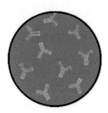

The **immune system** is perhaps the most well-known defender against disease. This defense system is made up of immune cells such as white blood cells, natural killer cells, T cells, and others that work together to protect the body from foreign invaders. During illness, boosting the immune system can help the body recover faster. Sometimes, the immune system can get out of control. For example, in the case of autoimmune disease, the immune system turns against and attacks the body. In the case of chronic inflammation, the immune system constantly fires at a low level, which over time can lead to negative health effects. In these cases, calming the immune system is often beneficial to health. A healthy diet can help achieve both of these goals.

Together, these health defense systems interact in ways to defend the body from conditions stemming from inflammation, as well as long-term diseases like cardiovascular disease and cancer. Food plays an integral role through its effect on these systems on many levels, from overall content of the diet and dietary patterns down to the specific actions of beneficial phytochemicals.

MACRONUTRIENTS

Macronutrients include food components that most people are familiar with, such as carbohydrates, fats, and protein. Macronutrients can be described as large molecules in food, needed in relatively large quantities, that contribute energy to the diet. For example, carbohydrates and protein each contribute 4 calories per gram. Fat is more energy-dense and contributes 9 calories per gram.

Carbohydrates are, in most diets, the most abundant macronutrient, and typically make up 45%–65% of total daily intake.[1] There are several different types of carbohydrates:

- **Fiber**: Fiber is made up of long strings of glucose molecules. The glucose linkages in fiber consist of beta-1,4 linkages, which the body cannot easily break down. This makes fiber indigestible. The extreme linearity of these strings also allows for close packing, adhered by hydrogen bonds, and therefore high mechanical strength. Plants contain fiber in the form of cellulose, which provides a structure for the plant. Other forms of fiber found in plants

[1] Manore MM. Exercise and the Institute of Medicine recommendations for nutrition. *Curr Sports Med Rep.* 2005 Aug;4(4):193–8.

and plant food include hemicellulose, lignin, pectin, and beta-glucans. Because it is not absorbed or digested, fiber adds bulk to a meal and slows the progress of food through the digestive tract. These qualities contribute to its many health benefits, including the two dietary indications proposed by the U.S. Food and Drug Administration (FDA) for fiber: protection of many types of cancers as well as lowering of cardiovascular disease risk.

An example of a cardiovascular health benefit of fiber is that high fiber intake helps lower cholesterol (Manore, 2005). It does this by binding to cholesterol and bile acids in the small intestine. Not only is the cholesterol not absorbed from the food, but the body also has to make more bile acids to replace the ones carried off by the fiber and excreted. Because bile acids are made using cholesterol, the body therefore eliminates more cholesterol from the blood.

Health Defense Connection: **Microbiome**

Fiber has recently received increased attention for the crucial role it plays in maintaining gut health, including laxative effects. In addition, because fiber isn't absorbed and can resist gastric acids and digestive enzymes, fiber can make its way through the digestive tract into the large intestine, where the majority of gut bacteria reside. Certain fibers are sometimes called "prebiotics" because bacteria are able to break down the fiber as a food source to generate energy through fermentation and release beneficial chemicals (metabolites) that go on to have a myriad of healthy effects throughout the body. Certain fibers such as inulin and oligofructose (both found in onion, garlic, Jerusalem artichoke, and asparagus) are well-known prebiotics. The most common beneficial bacteria that are stimulated are Bifidobacterium (Holscher, 2017). Among the healthy chemicals generated are short-chain fatty acids. The importance of the microbiome has been continuously supported by recent research; a healthy gut can influence the immune system, brain, and even how well people respond to certain treatments for cancer (Geuking et al., 2014; Wang & Wang, 2016; Routy et al., 2018)

- **Starches**: Starches are made up of long strings of glucose molecules connected primarily by bonds called alpha-1,4 linkages. These bonds are broken down by enzymes during digestion, releasing glucose into the blood. Starches are an important source of energy, accounting for more than 50% of total carbohydrate intake, and foods containing starch often provide B vitamins, iron, calcium, and folate (https://www.nutrition.org.uk/healthy-living/basics/carbs.html). Starchy foods are also typically high in fiber, which aids with digestion and benefits the microbiome as described below. Starchy foods include peas, corn, potatoes, rice, and beans. Although potatoes are often thought of as starchy, other foods contain more starch (potato 15%, wheat 55%, corn 65%, rice 75%).

- **Sugars**: Simple sugars consist of the unbound simple sugar molecules (monosaccharides) glucose, fructose, and galactose. These monosaccharides can also bind together to form combinations (e.g., disaccharides) such as lactose or milk sugar, maltose or malt sugar, and sucrose or table sugar.

FACTOID 3.1 MACRONUTRIENTS – CARBOHYDRATE SECTION:

Why milk is sweeter when heated

- When milk is heated, the longer chain lactose sugar breaks down into simple sugars, galactose and glucose, which taste sweeter.

Although the World Health Organization recommends limiting free sugars to less than 10% of daily intake (WHO, 2015), most Americans get too much sugar from processed sources. Excessive sugar intake contributes to the rising rates of obesity. Rising intake of processed foods high in sugar has certainly advanced the issue of obesity. But it is under-recognized that many health-promoting foods also contain natural sugars. For example, fruit is sweet and fairly high in sugar. Nevertheless, it also contains natural fibers, vitamins, minerals, and phytochemicals and is recommended as part of a healthy diet.

Health Defense Connection: **Regeneration**

Foods that are low in fiber and high in sugar are sometimes called "hyperglycemic," because they cause a rapid rise in blood glucose after being eaten. As a result, frequent spikes in blood glucose can slow down the body's production of stem cells, which can hinder the body's ability to repair itself (Kang et al., 2017). According to the American Diabetes Association, hyperglycemic foods are typically highly processed foods; examples include soda, candy, refined grains like white bread and rice, and sugary cereals (ADA, 2022).

Rapid spikes in blood glucose can be avoided by making sure food contains enough fiber. Fiber will slow the absorption of glucose into the blood, which results in a more gradual increase in blood sugar.

So, when it comes to simple sugars, ensure that they are paired with a fiber and even better, with a fiber that contains health-promoting molecules like vitamins, minerals, and polyphenols.

Digestion, absorption, and metabolism of sugars and starches:

The absorption and digestion of carbohydrates varies by the type of carbohydrate. For both sugars and starches, the absorption and digestion processes are dependent upon a series of enzymes located throughout the digestive tract. The long chains of sugars or starches are broken down into shorter chains of carbohydrates. Starting in the mouth, starch polysaccharides are made into shorter chains of dextrin by the salivary enzyme, amylase. Dextrin then is broken down into maltose by pancreatic amylase. Sugars, such as sucrose and lactose, are broken down at the pancreatic stage also by amylase. The resultant sugars from amylase are monosaccharides – glucose, galactose, fructose – are then absorbed in the small intestine. Once through the small intestine enterocytes, the monosaccharides enter the blood stream and through the portal vein circulate to the liver.

Within the liver, the primary metabolism of sugar or starch carbohydrates occurs to meet the body's energy needs. When the absorbed glucose amount exceeds the body's needs, the liver will make glycogen through the process of glycogenosis to store the glucose for later use. The production of glycogen also occurs in skeletal muscle. In the liver, glycogen is changed into glucose when energy is needed in a process called gluconeogenesis. In the muscle, glycogen is utilized in its branched polysaccharide form when energy is needed.

Maintaining a level of available glucose for the cell's energy need occurs under the control of an anabolic versus catabolic hormone system involving insulin, epinephrine, growth hormone, and cortisol. Lastly, glucagon is a pancreatic hormone that can increase glycogen release when low levels of circulating glucose occur.

Fats, otherwise known as lipids, are typically the second-most common macronutrient in the diet and make up 20%–30% of daily calories in a Western-style diet (Manore, 2005). There are many different types of fats, with a wide variety of health effects between them. Likewise, common cooking and salad oils differ greatly in their fat content, as shown in Figure 3.2.

Triglycerides are the most common type of fat consumed in the diet. They have one central glycerol molecule with three fatty acid chains extending from it. The length of these chains and the types of bonds they contain are what determine the type of fat and the effect it will have on the body.

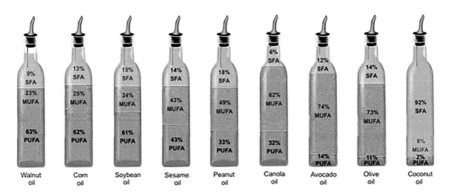

FIGURE 3.2 Fatty acid content varies in different cooking oils. In the oils depicted from left to right, there is a relative increase in MUFA content and decrease in PUFA content, while SFA-content is significantly higher in coconut oil. Both PUFAs and MUFAs are considered to have cardioprotective effects. *SFA (in blue) = Saturated Fatty Acid; MUFA (in yellow) = Monounsaturated Fatty Acid; PUFA (in green) = Polyunsaturated Fatty Acid.*

Fat is the main source of energy for the body. In fact, when dietary carbohydrate, protein, and fat are digested and processed by the body, if the body doesn't need the energy right away, it will be stored in the form of fat to provide fuel for the body at a later time. Therefore, eating *any* macronutrient in excess will result in increased fat storage. In addition to storage, fat actually has important functions in health as well. For example, cholesterol is an important gatekeeper in cell membranes to allow certain molecules to pass into cells while keeping others out. Dietary fat is also necessary for the absorption of fat-soluble vitamins (vitamins A, D, E, and K) and plays a role in several other processes such as blood clotting, muscle movement, and inflammation. Nevertheless, the health benefit or detrimental effects of fat are based on their chemical structure. Figure 3.3 shows the structural difference between unsaturated, saturated, and trans fat.

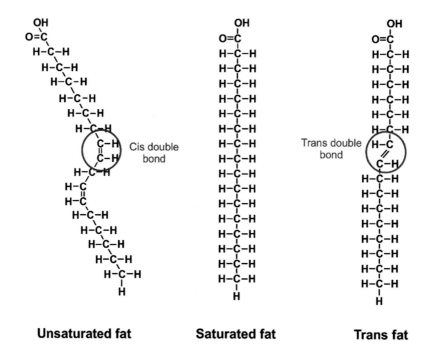

Unsaturated fat   **Saturated fat**   **Trans fat**

FIGURE 3.3 Structural Components of Fatty Acid Types. Fats contain a long hydrocarbon chain which is deemed either "saturated" or "unsaturated". Saturated fatty acids (middle structure) contain only single bonds between the neighboring carbons, creating rigid chains, and explains why foods high in saturated fats (such as butter and bacon fat) are more solid at room-temperature. Unsaturated fats (far left structure) contain cis-double bonds (hydrogen on same side of the carbon double bond), leading to kinks in the chain and an overall flexible structure, resulting in liquid form at room temperature. Trans fats (far right structure) are unsaturated fats that are artificially-processed to manipulate the cis-double bond into a trans-configuration (hydrogens on different sides of the carbon double bond) to achieve a desirable solid texture and prolong shelf life. Trans fats are common in highly-processed foods.

- **Unsaturated fats**: Unsaturated fats can either be monounsaturated (MUFA) or polyunsaturated (PUFA). "Unsaturated" means that some carbon molecules contain less than the maximum amount of hydrogen, which allows for one or a few double bonds between carbon atoms in the fatty acid chain, i.e., the chain is not *saturated* with hydrogen. This double bond in the fatty acid chains allows the chains to spin and thus be fluid and flexible, which then keeps them liquid at room temperature.

  There is one double bond in MUFAs, whereas PUFAs have two or more double bonds. Although there are slight differences in the structure of unsaturated fats, both MUFA and PUFA have been shown to reduce low-density lipoprotein (LDL) cholesterol when saturated fat is swapped out for these healthy fats in the diet (Mozaffarian and Clarke, 2009). Improving cholesterol in this way reduces the risk of cardiovascular diseases, type 2 diabetes, and high blood pressure. A common and well recognized MUFA is oleic acid, which is found in olive oil (60%–80% oleic acid). Other foods high in MUFA are peanut oil, avocados, peanut butter, nuts, and seeds. Foods high in PUFA are fatty fish like salmon, mackerel, and tuna, walnuts, sunflower seeds, and flaxseed.

Omega-3 fatty acids: Perhaps the most well-known form of PUFAs is omega-3 fatty acids. Omega-3 fatty acids are PUFAs that have their first double bond on the third carbon of the fatty acid chain. Because the body cannot create these fatty acids on its own, omega-3s must be consumed in the diet. High omega-3 intake has been associated with a number of health benefits, such as heart health, lower inflammation, DNA protection, and improving the health of stem cells. Omega-3s are also antiangiogenic (Kang & Liu, 2013).

Omega-3 fatty acids have long been associated with a lower risk of pancreatic, colon, breast, and prostate cancer in many populations (Gong et al., 2010; Szymanski et al., 2008). Laboratory studies have showed that omega-3 fatty acids, particularly eicosapentanoic acid (EPA) and docosahexaenoic acid (DHA), inhibit the blood vessels that feed cancers, by inhibiting many angiogenesis growth factors (Szumczaki et al., 2008).

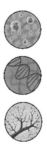

Health Defense Connection: ***DNA + Regeneration + Angiogenesis***
Omega-3s have antioxidant effects, which protect DNA from oxidation by free radicals. A study done using human cells found that when cells were treated

with EPA and DHA omega-3s, the cells were protected from oxidative damage when challenged with a molecule that damages DNA (Sakai et al., 2017).
Omega-3 fatty acids may even boost the ability of stem cells to migrate, or, in
other words, travel to their target tissues. A research group from Montreal
found that when mice were fed a diet high in fish oil (a source of omega-3),
the numbers of stem cells increased, and those stem cells were better at
moving through the body (Turgeon et al., 2013).

Food sources of omega-3 fatty acids include cold water oily fish, like salmon,
mackerel, herring, anchovies, and sardines, nuts (particularly walnuts), seeds (such
as chia or flax), soybeans, and avocados.

FACTOID 3.2 FATS SECTION:

Is coconut oil healthy?

Coconut oil has seen popularity as a healthy oil due to its phytochemicals and the similarity of coconut's lauric acid to medium chain triglycerides
(MCTs)[2] – which in some studies appear to improve "good" HDL cholesterol
and peripheral insulin resistance and reduce adiposity. However, many coconut
oil products are refined and have limited MCTs, and its saturated fat content
(coconut oil is ≥90% saturated fat) may outweigh any beneficial effects.

- **Saturated fats**: Saturation of a fat refers to the hydrogens surrounding a carbon. A fat is considered "saturated" if there are no double
  bonds between the carbons of the fatty acid chain, and hydrogens fill
  all the bonds. This structure makes the fatty acid very rigid, as the
  extra hydrogen molecules take up space and prevent the chain from
  being flexible. Because of this rigid structure, saturated fats can be
  easily identified as being solid at room temperature (e.g., butter is
  50% saturated fat).

  Saturated fats increase the risk of heart disease by raising the so-
  called "bad" LDL cholesterol levels in the blood while also decreasing LDL turnover. Figure 3.4 illustrates the fate of saturated fats in
  the body after consumption. When fats are absorbed into the bloodstream from the small intestine, they are turned into triglycerides and
  travel to the liver.

  In the liver, the triglycerides are broken down and packaged into
  very-low-density lipoprotein (VLDL), which is then further processed in the blood to form LDL cholesterol. LDL is removed from
  the bloodstream by binding to the LDL receptor on cells. Saturated
  fat has been shown to downregulate, or decrease, the amount of LDL

---

[2] Dayrit FM. Lauric acid is a medium-chain fatty acid, coconut oil is a medium-chain triglyceride. *Phil J Sci* 2014;143(2):157–66.

receptor (Fernandez & West, 2005). This in turn decreases LDL turn-over, so LDL concentrations in the blood remain high.

When LDL levels are chronically elevated, they are more likely to infiltrate artery linings where they can be turned into foam cells by oxidation, and eventually form atherosclerotic plaques (http://www.fao.org/docrep/v4700e/V4700E08.htm). A study done at Harvard using a large group of volunteers found that replacing 5% of calories from saturated fat with an equal amount of unsaturated fat can reduce the risk of coronary heart disease by 43% (Hu et al., 1999).

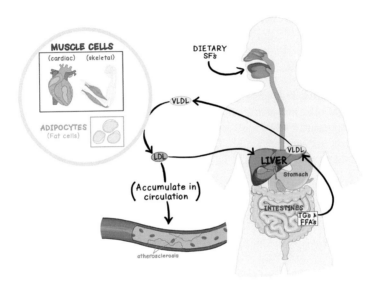

FIGURE 3.4 Basic Overview of the Metabolism of Dietary Saturated Fats (SF). Saturated fats are broken down in the stomach and intestines and absorbed into the bloodstream as tri-glycerides (TG) or free fatty acids (FFA). In the liver, fats can be packaged into transport molecules called lipoproteins. Most commonly, they will be packaged into Very-Low Density Lipoproteins (VLDL), which are made in the liver and sent out through the circulation to muscle tissue or adipose tissue (where it deposits its contents for energy or storage, respec-tively). Once this task is complete, the emptied VLDL is known as an Low Density Lipoprotein (LDL). This remnant LDL contains mostly cholesterol, so it is imperative for the healthy body to remove it from the circulation to avoid accumulation of cholesterol in the blood stream. For that reason, the liver has receptors that recognize and take in the LDL particles and remove 70–80% of the LDL from the blood. However, the number of these receptors that our liver is able to express is highly dependent on our diet, body composition, and genetics.

Health Defense Connection: **Regeneration**

According to animal models, diets high in saturated fats can be damaging to stem cells (Mana et al., 2017). A study done in Taiwan found that mice fed diets high in saturated fat had lower circulating stem cells in their blood than mice on a regular chow diet. The lower stem cells resulted in poor blood flow and capillary growth necessary for wound healing (Chen, 2012b).

Saturated fats can be found in animal products, such as meat, poultry, and dairy, and in coconut and palm oil.

FACTOID 3.3 OMEGA-3 FATTY ACID SECTION:

Choosing fish

Fish and shellfish vary in their healthy omega-3 PUFA level, and also in their level of toxic mercury concentrated from water pollution. It's best to balance healthy fats and lowest mercury which can be found in fish such as anchovies, herring, sardines, salmon, mackerel, oysters, and clam

- **Trans fats**: Trans fats are created when unsaturated fats, such as vegetable oils, are artificially hydrogenated to form a solid. Although they occur in very small amounts in nature, their presence in modern foods was primarily a product of industrial manufacturing. The artificial production of trans fats became a widely used technique in the 1950s to extend the shelf-life of foods (CSPI). Trans fats are created from the hydrogenation of unsaturated fat. In the process of artificial hydrogenation, the natural *cis* structure of the unsaturated fats' bonds is changed into a *trans* structure. This small change in structure makes the fat solid at room temperature and more stable against challenges like heat and oxidation. They are resistant to the natural oxidation process that breaks down other fats, so products could last for longer periods of time before spoiling.

  Trans fats have a very negative effect on health; intake of trans fats is associated with increased risk of death, risk of coronary heart disease, and risk death from coronary heart disease (de Souza et al., 2015). A large population study called the Nurses' Health Study found that for every 2% increase in calories from trans fats consumed, the risk for coronary heart disease doubled (Hu et al., 1997). A more recent study that included participants from the Nurses' Health Study and Health Professional's Follow-up Study found that for every 2% increase in trans fat intake, risk of overall mortality increased by 16% when compared with calories from carbohydrate (Wang et al., 2016). Due to the overwhelming evidence of their detrimental effects, trans fats were ruled unsafe to eat by the U.S. FDA in 2015, and artificial trans fats were banned from the U.S. food supply as of June, 2018. (https://www.fda.gov/Food/IngredientsPackagingLabeling/FoodAdditivesIngredients/ucm449162.htm).

Digestion, absorption and metabolism of fat

As with sugars and starches, the digestion of fat starts in the mouth. Lingual lipase is released upon chewing. Although human studies have yet to support that this lipase release can turn on satiety signals early in a meal, animal studies do show this as a potential satiety signal.

Once in the stomach, gastric lipase, amongst other digestive enzymes, is released. However, gastric lipase is responsible for only the initial and minimal breakdown of ingested fats. The large majority of fat digestion does not occur in the stomach, but later on in the small intestine. Once released from the food matrix, fat is now bound to bile salts to undergo its main form of digestion in the small intestine. Pancreatic lipase works to break down triglyceride fats into monoglycerides and fatty acids. The efficient activity of the lipase is dependent on the presence of bile salts on fat droplets. Multiple bile salts with the complexed triglyceride components spontaneously form micelles. Micelles then enter enterocytes where the bile is broken down and chylomicrons are packaged and extruded from the basolateral enterocyte wall to enter the lymphatics. This is the mechanism for absorption of triglycerides which represent 90% of dietary fat. Dietary cholesterol undergoes a similar process except it requires a transport protein in order to enter the enterocyte. Lastly, MCTs, such as coconut oil, when extruded from the enterocyte go directly into the blood stream, by passing the lymphatic system. Therefore, MCTs are suspected of having a favorable metabolic profile.

Protein is the third macronutrient and typically makes up 10%–35% of our diets (Manore, 2005). The average person needs 7 g of protein for every 20 pounds of body weight. Most people know of protein as the "building blocks of the body," but the functions of protein go far beyond their role in forming structural components: functional proteins, enzymes, catalyze reactions responsible for metabolism, DNA replication, and transportation of molecules between cells.

Not only are proteins used as the body's building blocks, but they do so also because they are made of building blocks. At their most basic level, proteins are combinations of chains of 22 naturally occurring amino acids. These combinations may be long chains, branched, sheets, or helixes. If not in any of the aforementioned forms, amino acids also serve multiple functions. Certain single amino acids (aspartic acid, glutamic acid, gamma-aminobutyric acid, glycine, taurine) can function as neurotransmitters. Two amino acid combinations, called dipeptides, may function as cell-to-cell communicators. Because of these different functions for amino acids, clinically there are several uses of amino acids: for example, L-tryptophan for sleep. This clinical use also provides a basis for the role of certain amino acids naturally found at higher combinations in certain foods. For example, arginine is an amino acid with vasodilation capabilities. The Mayo Clinic recommends an arginine-rich diet for patients suffering from poor blood perfusion, such as peripheral artery disease (Mayo Clinic, 2021). Arginine-rich foods include walnuts, brazil nuts, and almonds and may thus be beneficial to this patient population.

Our body can make certain amino acids on its own, but there are nine so-called "essential" amino acids that the body cannot make and thus must come from food (https://www.nap.edu/read/10490/chapter/12#591). Protein can come from a variety of sources such as animal products, seafood, soy, nuts, grains, and legumes. Both soy as well as animal sources of protein contain all nine of the essential amino acids and are called "complete proteins." Other vegetarian proteins like nuts, grains, and legumes do not contain all of the essential amino acids and must complement each other to fulfill the body's protein needs. This can easily be achieved by including a variety of foods in the diet. For this reason, vegetarians with limited soy intake are often advised to complement their diet with these "complete-protein" combinations. This is generally an effective approach because many plant-based foods vary in their amino acid compositions; Thus, combining two foods in your meal with varying amino acid compositions makes for a more complete intake of the essential amino acids are body needs.

Although important in terms of describing what may be nutritionally necessary for most, the categorization of essential and nonessential amino acids may not provide information about individual level needs for certain amino acids. For example, the production of both glycine and serine, although nonessential amino acids, is dependent on vitamins B6, B3, and folic acid. Therefore, deficiencies in these B vitamins will lead to reduction in ability of the body to produce these nonessential amino acids.

During digestion, protein is broken down into its constituent amino acids from hydrochloric acid and enzymes within the stomach. Thus, the first step in protein digestion is dependent on the presence of stomach acid. It is important to note that stomach acid may be reduced by use of antacid medications, chronic stress, and with age (particularly after the age of 60) (Holt et al., 1989). After digestion, peptide chains are then absorbed across the membrane of the small intestine. The first part of the small intestine produces the enzyme trypsin, which converts the peptide chains into shorter peptide chains (dipeptides and tripeptides). The role of trypsin is a necessary step in protein digestion as without trypsin amino acid chains remain too large for absorption. Trypsin release is dependent upon function of the gallbladder's release of cholecystokinin. Thus, protein digestion is inherently linked to digestion of fat within the diet, as well as gallbladder function. Amino peptidases in the small intestine then convert dipeptides into single amino acids. There is a preference for absorption of dipeptides first, then single amino acids, and then tripeptides across the small intestine wall into the blood stream. Once in the blood, amino acids are available to be absorbed by other tissues (https://www.ncbi. nlm.nih.gov/books/NBK22600/). The first stop after absorption is to the liver through the portal vein circulation. The liver's role is key in protein metabolism. The liver is the regulator of how proteins are made and broken down daily.

Overall, three-fourths of absorbed amino acids are used to form proteins needed for body function – enzymes, hormones, antibodies, and muscle. Everyday endogenous amino acids are made through the breakdown (catabolism) or synthesis (anabolism) of protein throughout the body. Exogenous amino acids that are digested then are utilized based on this need. This balance of amino acids between endogenous amino acids and exogenous (dietary) amino acids is important as excess protein is converted into fat for future energy use or stored in the liver as glycogen. Conversely, when not enough protein is part of the diet or if digestion is not adequate, a deficiency of protein occurs, which can lead to weight loss or systemic problems such as loss of needed hormone production.

Health Defense Connection: **Inflammation**

When choosing between different sources of protein, it's best to keep a healthy balance between animal and plant proteins. Having a diet too high in animal protein and low in plant-based foods can be pro-inflammatory and increases your risk for disorders such as inflammatory bowel disease (Jantchou et al., 2010). Plant-based proteins can be found abundantly in legumes (e.g., lentils, beans, peas, soybeans, and soy products), nuts, seeds, and whole grains (including quinoa and oats).

MICRONUTRIENTS

There are approximately 30 essential vitamins and minerals, or micronutrients, that the body cannot produce on its own. Micronutrients are needed in much smaller amounts to fulfill the body's needs compared to macronutrients. Micronutrients do not provide energy (calories); rather, they participate in important bodily functions such as cell division, maintenance of tissue function, and metabolism.

Vitamins: Vitamins are categorized into water-soluble and fat-soluble vitamins. As the names imply, water-soluble vitamins dissolve into water, and fat-soluble vitamins dissolve into fat. These differences can have a large impact on how well the body absorbs them. Water-soluble vitamins are easily absorbed through the intestinal membrane, whereas fat-soluble vitamins need to cross the membrane inside fat globules. Because of this, the absorption of fat-soluble vitamins can be greatly increased by taking them with a meal containing a source dietary fat.

- Water-soluble vitamins include the B vitamins (**thiamine, riboflavin, niacin, vitamin B6, folate, vitamin B12, biotin, and pantothenic acid**) and **vitamin C**. See Table 3.1 for their functions and food sources:

Absorption of water-soluble vitamins occurs within the intestine. In the small intestine, the water-soluble vitamins enter into enterocytes on the lumen side and then are released into the bloodstream on the basal side of enterocytes. There are some water-soluble vitamins that are unlike others. For instance, niacin can be produced from the metabolism of the amino acid tryptophan. And all water-soluble vitamins except for vitamin C can be made from bacterial sources within the large intestine.

Health Defense Connection: **Immune**

Vitamin C plays an important role in the body as a coenzyme and an antioxidant and even in immune function. Vitamin C calms the immune system by increasing the levels of regulatory T cells (Tregs) that calm the immune system to prevent inflammatory responses from getting out of hand. Consuming foods high in vitamin C may be beneficial for people with autoimmune disorders, such as lupus (Minami et al., 2003).

TABLE 3.1

Functions and food sources of major water-soluble vitamins. The water-soluble vitamins include thiamine (vitamin B1), riboflavin (vitamin B2), niacin (vitamin B3), pyridoxine (vitamin B6), folate (vitamin B9), cobalamin (vitamin B12), and ascorbic acid (vitamin C).

Vitamin	Important Functions	Food Sources
Thiamine	Necessary for the oxidation of carbohydrates and for the metabolism of pyruvate.	Grains, wheat germ, pork, liver.
Riboflavin	Energy release from protein and necessary for red blood cell production.	Milk, cheese, eggs, liver, kidney, legumes, mushrooms, almonds.
Niacin	Essential in all cells for energy production and metabolism of carbohydrates, fat, and protein.	Protein, peanuts, cereals, chicken, rice, yeast, milk.
Folate	Cofactor in DNA synthesis, forms red blood cells in bone marrow, and prevents neural tube defects in fetal development.	Fortified cereal, liver, kidney, green leafy vegetables, lentils, beans.
Vitamin B6	Coenzyme in amino acid metabolism, glucose metabolism, and lipid metabolism.	Meat, wheat, yeast, fortified cereals, bananas, chickpeas.
Vitamin B12	Coenzyme in protein synthesis and forms red blood cells	Liver, meat, milk, eggs, fish, cheese.
Vitamin C	Acts as an antioxidant, and is necessary for wound healing, collagen formation, and increases iron absorption.	Citrus fruits, potatoes, papaya, dark green and yellow vegetables.

Fat-soluble vitamins include **vitamin A, vitamin D, vitamin E, and vitamin K**. See Table 3.2 for their functions and food sources:

Fat-soluble vitamins are absorbed similar to fat molecules. Fat-soluble vitamins are complexed with fats within micelles and are transported through the lymphatic system after absorption in the small intestine. In addition, some fat-soluble vitamins such as vitamin K may be made by bacteria within the large intestine.

*Health Defense Connection: **Angiogenesis***

Vitamin K1, or phytomenadione, is the most common form of vitamin K in the diet and is found mainly in green leafy vegetables. It's most commonly known for its role in blood clotting. There is another less recognized form of vitamin K known as vitamin K2 (menaquinone) that is particularly notable for its antiangiogenic properties. In 2009, a research group in Japan found that vitamin K2 was capable of suppressing blood vessel growth and through this mechanism also suppressing colon cancer cells (Kayashima et al., 2009). Another study demonstrated this antiangiogenic effect in prostate cancer cells (Samykutty et al., 2013). Vitamin K2 is found in specific

TABLE 3.2

Functions and food sources of major fat-soluble vitamins. The fat-soluble vitamins include vitamin A (retinoic acid/retinol), vitamin D (calciferol), tocopherols/tocotrienols (vitamin E), and phylloquinone/menaquinone (vitamin K1/2).

Vitamin	Important Functions	Food Sources
Vitamin A	Important for growth, development, immune health, skin health, and vision.	Yellow and orange fruits, dark green leafy vegetables, fish, carrots, fortified milk, sweet potato.
Vitamin D	Necessary for bone health; increases absorption of calcium, magnesium, and phosphate.	Fatty fish, irradiated mushrooms, fortified milk, egg yolk.
Vitamin E	Acts as an antioxidant and protects red blood cells against hemolysis.	Vegetable oils, whole grains, nuts, and seeds.
Vitamin K	Necessary for blood clotting and calcium metabolism.	Dark green leafy vegetables, broccoli.

age-ripened hard cheeses like Gouda, Edam, and Müenster cheese but not in other cheeses such as feta, mozzarella, Pecorino, or Parmesan (Vermeer et al., 2018).

FACTOID 3.4 MICRONUTRIENTS SECTION:

Foods that are high in interesting micronutrients

- Fermented foods, chicken, and cheese all contain vitamin K2
- Green leafy vegetables are a source of calcium other than milk/dairy products
- Surprising food sources of vitamin D are fatty fish, eel, maitake mushrooms, and fortified yogurt

Minerals: Like vitamins, minerals are natural nonnutritive substances that are necessary for the body to function. The essential minerals are calcium, phosphorus, potassium, sulfur, sodium, chloride, magnesium, iron, zinc, copper, manganese, iodine, and selenium, molybdenum, chromium, and fluoride.

In order to become bioavailable, minerals have to enter the small intestine, much like vitamins and macronutrients. There are two mechanisms that minerals may use for absorption, directly through the enterocyte or moving through the spaces in between enterocytes (paracellular). Either mechanism leads to minerals entering into the blood stream for circulation throughout the body. Factors that may increase absorption of some minerals such as magnesium are linked to dietary factors, including meal components. For example, the presence of some types of fiber (fructo-oligosaccharides) in a meal may increase magnesium absorption (Schuchardt & Hahn, 2017) (Table 3.3).

TABLE 3.3

Functions and food sources of major dietary minerals. The dietary minerals include calcium (Ca), phosphorus (P), potassium (K), sulfur (S), sodium (Na), chloride (Cl), magnesium (Mg), iron (Fe), zinc (Zn), copper (Cu), manganese (Mn), iodine (I), selenium (Se), molybdenum (Mo), chromium (Cr), and fluoride (F).

Mineral	Important Functions[a, b]	Food Sources
Calcium	Important for growth and maintenance of bones and teeth, nervous system function, muscle contraction and relaxation, hormone secretion, and blood clotting.	Green leafy vegetables, tofu, yogurt, milk, cheese, canned seafood with bones, fortified cereals, and juices.
Phosphorous	Involved in most of the chemical reactions in the body and is also important for bone development and hormone activation.	Legumes, beans, dairy products, whole grains, nuts and seeds, seafood, poultry, meats.
Potassium	Regulates blood pressure and fluid balance, along with sodium. It's also important in nervous system function, carbohydrate metabolism, protein formation, muscle contraction, and heart function.	Bananas, fruit and vegetable juices, milk, potatoes and sweet potatoes, spinach, tomatoes, white beans, yogurt.
Sulfur	Necessary for protein synthesis.	Meats, poultry, fish, eggs, milk, legumes, nuts.
Sodium	Regulates blood pressure and fluid balance, along with potassium. It's also important for maintaining the body's acid-base balance, muscle contraction, and nervous system function.	Cheese, processed meat, processed and/or packaged foods, restaurant foods, soups, breads and baked goods, table salt.
Chloride	Enables the conversion of food to energy and digestion and is important for acid-base balance, fluid balance, and nervous system function.	Celery, lettuce, olives, rye, table salt, tomatoes.
Magnesium	Magnesium has a broad range of roles in blood pressure regulation, bone formation, energy production, hormone secretion and immune function, muscle contraction, nervous system function and protein formation.	Avocados, bananas, beans, green leafy vegetables, dairy products, potatoes, wheat bran, and whole grains.
Iron	Important for energy production, red blood cell formation, growth and development, reproduction, wound healing, and immune function.	Beans and peas, dark green vegetables, meats, poultry, seafood, whole grains, enriched and fortified cereals, and breads.
Zinc	Has roles in immune function, growth and development, reproduction, protein formation, nervous system function, wound healing, and taste and smell	Beans and peas, seafood, beef, dairy, poultry, nuts, whole grains.
Copper	Copper is an antioxidant, and has important roles in bone and collagen formation, energy production, iron metabolism, and nervous system function.	Chocolate and cocoa, shellfish, lentils, nuts and seeds, whole grains.
Manganese	Necessary for carbohydrate, protein and cholesterol metabolism, cartilage and bone formation, and wound healing.	Beans, nuts, pineapple, spinach, sweet potato, whole grains.

(Continued)

TABLE 3.3 (*Continued*)
Functions and food sources of major dietary minerals. The dietary minerals include calcium (Ca), phosphorus (P), potassium (K), sulfur (S), sodium (Na), chloride (Cl), magnesium (Mg), iron (Fe), zinc (Zn), copper (Cu), manganese (Mn), iodine (I), selenium (Se), molybdenum (Mo), chromium (Cr), and fluoride (F).

Mineral	Important Functions[a, b]	Food Sources
Iodine	Needed for thyroid hormone production, growth and development, metabolism, reproduction.	Iodized salt, breads and cereals, dairy products, potatoes, seafood, turkey.
Selenium	Acts as an antioxidant, and plays a role in immune function, reproduction, and thyroid function.	Brazil nuts, eggs, meats, poultry, seafood, whole grains, enriched pasta and rice.
Molybdenum	Important for enzyme production.	Beans and peas, nuts, whole grains.
Chromium	Important for muscle function, and plays a role in carbohydrate and fat metabolism. It even can increase the effect of insulin.	Whole grains, broccoli, shellfish, brazil nuts.
Fluoride	Role in bone formation, tooth and enamel resistance.	Fluoridated water, shellfish, canned fish with bones, whole grains, legumes, tea.

[a] https://www.accessdata.fda.gov/scripts/InteractiveNutritionFactsLabel/factsheets/Vitamin_and_Mineral_Chart.pdf.

[b] https://www.uofmhealth.org/health-library/ta3912.

PHYTOCHEMICALS

Phytochemicals (or phytonutrients) are substances found in foods (generally in fruits, vegetables, grain, beans, and other plants) that have beneficial health effects beyond conventional nutrition. They are different from vitamins and minerals in that they are not necessary for the body to function. Thus, there are no recommended daily amounts for phytochemicals. Figure 3.5 shows different types of phytochemicals and their classification. Although phytochemicals are most well known for their antioxidant capabilities, a wide range of scientific benefits are being discovered as further research is conducted into this exciting new field of molecular nutrition. For example, studies have shown that a number of phytonutrients suppress tumor angiogenesis (Li, 2012b). Some phytonutrients can also interact with DNA to protect DNA from harm. Others increase the activity of DNA repair mechanisms to fix errors occurring in DNA replication. And others upregulate genes that can suppress cancer development. Furthermore, studies have investigated the effects of phytonutrients on the microbiome and found that they can increase beneficial bacteria and overall health of the gut.

In relation to food and dietary intake and health, carotenoids, phenolics, and organosulfur compounds likely represent the most widely investigated phytochemicals. Among the phenolic phytochemicals, flavonoids are divided into several groups

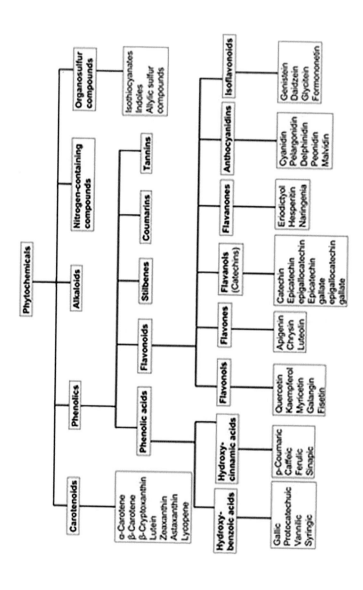

FIGURE 3.5 Classification of dietary phytochemicals. (From Liu RH. Potential synergy of phytochemicals in cancer prevention: mechanisms of action. *J Nutr* 2004;134(12):3479S–3485S.)

(Figure 3.5), among which flavonols, flavones, and flavanols are the most common in foods that are related to health. In fact, flavonols are the most ubiquitous flavonoids in foods. Quercetin is one of the major flavonoids found in foods. Flavonol biosynthesis is stimulated by light within the plant. Thus, fruit often contains more flavonols in the outer (skin) or aerial tissues (leaves). For example, cherry tomatoes have higher flavonol content than standard tomatoes because they have different proportion of skin to whole fruit. Flavones are less common than flavonols in fruit and vegetables. Most flavones in foods are luteolin and apigenin. Like flavonols, the skin of fruits and vegetables contain the largest amounts of flavones (Figure 3.6).

Phytochemicals that are the most common in the human diet are not necessarily the most active within the body, because of lower intrinsic activity or because they are poorly absorbed from the intestine, highly metabolized, or rapidly eliminated (Manach et al., 2004). Most polyphenols are too hydrophilic (attracted to water) to penetrate the small intestinal wall by passive diffusion. To date, transporters for polyphenols have not yet been identified in humans. However, there are exceptions. Flavonoid phytochemicals in the form of aglycones or glucosides are easily absorbed

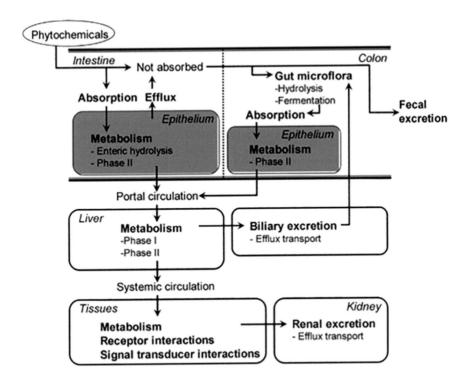

FIGURE 3.6 Source of variation in phytochemical metabolism and disposition in the body. From Lampe JW, Chang JL. Interindividual differences in phytochemical metabolism and disposition. Semin Cancer Biol. 2007;17(5):347–353.

in the small intestine. For example, the glucoside flavonol quercetin reaches maximum absorption 0.5–0.7 hours after ingestion. However, rutin, a glycoside flavonol has 15% of the absorption of quercetin.

During the course of absorption, phytochemicals such as polyphenols are conjugated in the small intestine and later in the liver. This process mainly includes methylation, sulfation, and glucuronidation. This is a metabolic detoxication process common to many xenobiotics that restricts their potential toxic effects and facilitates their biliary and urinary elimination by increasing their hydrophilicity. Quercetin, catechin, caffeic acid, and luteolin are some of the polyphenols known to undergo this metabolism process. Dietary fiber is generally associated with phytonutrients in plant foods. Fiber may stimulate intestinal fermentation, which could influence the production of particular microbial metabolites. Hydroxy-cinnamic acids, which are naturally esterified in foods and thus cannot be absorbed in the small intestine, depend upon colonic microflora to break the ester bonds to allow for absorption in the large intestine. And the flavonoid, rutin, is complexed with the polysaccharide rhamnose. This linkage prevents absorption from occurring until colonic microflora can break the rhamnose molecule.

Cooking may lead to changes in the bioavailability of phytochemicals. For example, onions, especially red onions, are a rich in quercetin; while boiling them may result in a 30% loss in quercetin, it is transfered to the boiled water (Ioku, 2001), giving scientific rationale to the health benefits of onion soups and stocks that utilize the boiled water.

In general, the more intense the color of the uncooked food, the more phytochemicals it will have. This is because phytochemicals are often pigments that give the food its color. Some well-known sources of phytochemicals are berries, tomatoes, green tea, grapes, red wine, and green tea. Some potentially surprising sources of phytochemicals are coffee, dark chocolate, and beer. But it is important to note that with cooking or heating, the bioavailability of some phytochemicals, notably lycopene, is increased.

FACTOID 3.5 PHYTONUTRIENTS SECTION:

Ways to cook foods to make phytonutrients more available

- Lycopene exists in two forms in tomatoes: cis and trans. Cis-lycopene is harder to absorb, while trans-lycopene is easier to absorb. Lycopene in raw tomatoes is almost always in the cis form, but cooking the tomato can change it to the trans form. Lycopene is also fat-soluble, so cooking it in olive oil can increase its absorption even more (Unlu et al., 2007).

Some examples of phytochemicals in relation to the major health defense systems follow below.

Health Defense Connection:

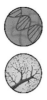

- **Lycopene**: Lycopene is a natural pigment carotenoid found in tomatoes, watermelon, and papayas (Graff et al., 2016). Lycopene plays a role in DNA protection (Jang et al., 2012) as well as inhibits angiogenesis by suppressing growth factor signaling (Chen, 2012a). In the Health Professionals Follow-up Study, men who consumed the lycopene as tomato sauce twice weekly had a 23% reduced risk for developing prostate cancer compared to those who consumed only once weekly (Chen et al., 2001).

- **EGCG**: EGCG, or epigallocatechin-3-gallate, is a polyphenol found in green tea. EGCG inhibits angiogenesis in laboratory and animal studies. Mice consuming the equivalent of 2–3 cups of tea/day show suppression of blood vessels and reduction of tumor cell invasion by 50% (Cao & Cao, 1999). Inhibition of angiogenesis in fat may also explain the antiobesity effects of green tea in human intervention studies (Huang et al., 2014). EGCG also has been shown to have anti-inflammatory properties (Dona et al., 2003) and neuroprotective effects in Alzheimer's and Parkinson's disease (Weinreb et al., 2004).

- **Anthocyanins**: Anthocyanins can appear as red, purple, or blue pigments in foods depending on the pH. They are at the highest levels in purple potatoes, berries, and grapes and also are present in red wine. More than just adding color, they have been shown to be bioactive cancer-fighting molecules on multiple levels. Anthocyanins suppress antiangiogenesis (Bagchi et al., 2004) and have been shown to kill colon cancer stem cells (Charepalli et al., 2015).

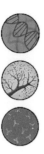

- **Caffeic acid**: Caffeic acid is a hydroxy-cinnamic phenolic acid found in coffee, red wine, chamomile tea, and apples. It is the most abundant of phenolic acids in the diet. Laboratory studies show that caffeic acid inhibits DNA methylation and activates the tumor suppressor gene RARB2, which is protective against cancer (Lee & Zhu, 2006). Caffeic acid also inhibits angiogenesis in a model of eye retinopathy (Kim et al., 2009). Furthermore, caffeic acid, in combination with another phytochemical ellagic acid, reduced inflammatory mediators and attenuated arthritis in an animal model, with comparable efficacy to the drug celecoxib (Fikry et al., 2019).

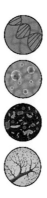

- **Chlorogenic acid**: In addition to suppressive effects on DNA expression, chlorogenic acid affects almost all of the health defense systems. For example, it enhances normal stem cell function (Li, 2012a) while crippling cancer cells (Yamagata et al., 2018), promotes the growth of a beneficial bacterium in the gut (Zhang et al., 2017), and also has antiangiogenic properties (Lin et al., 2017). Chlorogenic acid is found in coffee, black tea, blueberries, peaches, fresh and dried plums, eggplants, bamboo shoots, and many other plant foods.

SUMMARY

Molecular nutrition is an emerging, important area in nutrition science. With advances in laboratory research at the molecular and cellular level and the ability to assess nutrient-driven changes in gene expression and regulation, signal transduction, and protein modifications, there is now a growing understanding about the body's response to food consumption. Macronutrients, micronutrients, and phytochemicals all play key roles in sustenance, maintenance of health, and prevention of disease. Food is able to impact the major health defense system component of angiogenesis, the immune system, DNA protection, expression, and repair, the gut microbiome, and stem cell regeneration. Molecular nutrition can help inform decisions on how best to choose and consume a variety of health-promoting foods that make up the diet.

REFERENCES

American Diabetes Association. http://www.diabetes.org/food-and-fitness/food/what-can-i-eat/understanding-carbohydrates/glycemic-index-and-diabetes.html.

Bagchi D, Sen CK, Bagchi M, et al. Anti-angiogenic, antioxidant, and anti-carcinogenic properties of a novel anthocyanin-rich berry extract formula. *Biochemistry (Mosc)*. 2004 Jan;69(1):75–80, 1 p preceding 75.

Cao Y, Cao R. Angiogenesis inhibited by drinking tea. *Nature* 1999;398(6726):381.

Charepalli V, Reddivari L, Radhakrishnan S, et al. Anthocyanin-containing purple-fleshed potatoes suppress colon tumorigenesis via elimination of colon cancer stem cells. *J Nutr Biochem* 2015 Dec;26(12):1641–9.

Chen L, Stacewicz-Sapuntzakis M, Duncan C, et al. Oxidative DNA damage in prostate cancer patients consuming tomato sauce-based entrees as a whole-food intervention. *J Natl Cancer Inst* 2001;93(24):1872–9.

Chen ML, Lin YH, Yang CM, et al. Lycopene inhibits angiogenesis both in vitro and in vivo by inhibiting MMP-2/u PA system through VEGFR2-mediated PI3K-Akt and ERK/p38 signaling pathways. *Mol Nutr Food Res* 2012a;56(6):889–99.

Chen YL, Chang CL, Sun CK, et al. Impact of obesity control on circulating level of endothelial progenitor cells and angiogenesis in response to ischemic stimulation. *J Transl Med* 2012b July 11;10:86.

CSPI. "About Trans Fat and Partially Hydrogenated Oils". https://cspinet.org/sites/default/files/attachment/trans_q_a.pdf.

Dayrit FM. Lauric acid is a medium-chain fatty acid, coconut oil is a medium-chain triglyceride. *Phil J Sci* 2014;143(2):157–66.

de Souza RJ, Mente A, Maroleanu A, et al. Intake of saturated and trans unsaturated fatty acids and risk of all cause mortality, cardiovascular disease, and type 2 diabetes: systematic review and meta-analysis of observational studies. *BMJ* 2015 Aug 11;351:h3978.

Dona M, Dell'Aica I, Calabrese F, et al. Neutrophil restraint by green tea: inhibition of inflammation, associated angiogenesis, and pulmonary fibrosis. *J Immunol* 2003;170:4335–41.

Fernandez ML, West KL. Mechanisms by which dietary fatty acids modulate plasma lipids. *J Nutr* 2005 Sep;135(9):2075–8.

Fikry EM, Gad AM, Eid AH, et al. Caffeic acid and ellagic acid ameliorate adjuvant-induced arthritis in rats via targeting inflammatory signals, chitinase-3-like protein-1 and angiogenesis. *Biomed Pharmacother* 2019;111:878–86.

Geuking MB, Köller Y, Rupp S, et al. The interplay between the gut microbiota and the immune system. *Gut Microbes* 2014 May-Jun;5(3):411–8.

Gong Z, Holly EA, Wang, J, et al. Intake of fatty acids and antioxidants and pancreatic cancer in a large population-based case control study in the San Francisco Bay area. *Int J Cancer* 2010;127(8):1893–904.

Graff RE, Pettersson A, Lis RT, Ahearn TU, Markt SC. Wilson KM, Rider JR, Fiorentino M, Finn S, Kenfield SA, Loda M, Giovannucci EL, Rosner B, Mucci LA. Dietary lycopene intake and risk of prostate cancer defined by ERG protein expression. *Am J Clin Nutr* 2016 Mar;103(3):851–60.

Holscher, HD. Dietary fiber and prebiotics and GI microbiota. *Gut Microbes* 2017;8(2):172–84

Holt PR, Rosenberg IH, Russell RM. Causes and consequences of hypochlorhydria in the elderly. *Dig Dis Sci* 1989 Jun;34(6):933–7.

http://www.fao.org/docrep/v4700e/V4700E08.htm.

https://www.accessdata.fda.gov/scripts/InteractiveNutritionFactsLabel/factsheets/Vitamin_ and_Mineral_Chart.pdf.

https://www.fda.gov/Food/IngredientsPackagingLabeling/FoodAdditivesIngredients/ ucm449162.htm.

https://www.nap.edu/read/10490/chapter/12#591.

https://www.ncbi.nlm.nih.gov/books/NBK22600/.

https://www.nutrition.org.uk/healthyliving/basics/carbs.html.

https://www.uofmhealth.org/health-library/ta3912.

Hu FB, Stampfer MJ, Manson JE, et al. Dietary fat intake and the risk of coronary heart disease in women. *N Engl J Med* 1997 Nov 20;337(21):1491–9.

Hu FB, Stampfer MJ, Manson JE, et al. Dietary saturated fats and their food sources in relation to the risk of coronary heart disease in women. *Am J Clin Nutr* 1999 Dec;70(6):1001–8.

Huang J, Wang Y, Xie Y, et al. The anti-obesity effects of green tea in human intervention and basic molecular studies. *Eur J Clin Nutr* 2014;68:1975–1087.

Ioku K, Aoyama Y, Tokuno A, Terao J, Nakatani N, Takei Y. Various cooking methods and the flavanoid content in onion. *J Nutr Sci Vitaminol (Tokyo)* 2001 Feb;47(1):78–83.

Jang SH, Lim JW, Morio T, Kim H. Lycopene inhibits Helicobacter pylori-induced ATM/ATR-dependent DNA damage response in gastric epithelial AGS cells. *Free Radic Biol Med* 2012 Feb 1;52(3):607–15.

Jantchou P, Morois S, Clavel-Chapelon F, et al. Animal protein intake and risk of inflammatory bowel disease: the E3N prospective study. *Am J Gastroenterol* 2010 Oct;105(10):2195–201.

Kang H, Ma X, Liu J, et al. High glucose-induced endothelial progenitor cell dysfunction. *Diab Vasc Dis Res* 2017 Sep;14(5):381–394.

Kang JX, Liu A. The role of the tissue omega-6/omega-3 fatty acid ratio in regulating tumor angiogenesis. *Cancer Metastasis Rev* 2013 Jun;32(1–2):201–10.

Kayashima T, Mori M, Yoshida H, et al. 1,4-Naphthoquinone is a potent inhibitor of human cancer cell growth and angiogenesis. *Cancer Lett* 2009 Jun 8;278(1):34–40.

Kim JH, Yu YS, Kim KW. Anti-angiogenic effect of caffeic acid on retinal neovascularization. *Vascul Pharmacol* 2009;51(4):262–7.

Lampe JW, Chang JL. Interindividual differences in phytochemical metabolism and disposition. *Semin Cancer Biol.* 2007;17(5):347–53. doi:10.1016/j.semcancer.2007.05.003.

Lee WJ, Zhu BT. Inhibition of DNA methylation by caffeic acid and chlorogenic acid, two common catechol-containing coffee polyphenols. *Carcinogenesis* 2006 Feb;27(2):269–77.

Li S, Bian H, Liu Z, Wang Y, et al. Chlorogenic acid protects MSCs against oxidative stress by altering FOXO family genes and activating intrinsic pathway. *Eur J Pharmacol* 2012a Jan 15;674(2–3):65–72.

Li WW, Li VW, Hutnik M, et al. Tumor angiogenesis as a target for dietary cancer prevention. *J Oncol* 2012b: article ID 879623, 23 pages.

Li WW. *Eat to Defeat Disease: The New Science of How Your Body Can Heal Itself.* New York: Grand Central Publishing. 2019.

Lin S, Hu J, Zhou X, et al. Inhibition of vascular endothelial growth factor-induced angiogenesis by chlorogenic acid via targeting the vascular endothelial growth factor receptor 2-mediated signaling pathway. *J Funct Foods.* 2017 May;32:285–295

Mana MD, Kuo EY, Yilmaz ÖH. Dietary regulation of adult stem cells. *Curr Stem Cell Rep* 2017 Mar;3(1):1–8.

Manach C, Scalbert A, Morand C, Rémésy C, Jiménez L. Polyphenols: food sources and bioavailability. *Am J Clin Nutr* May 2004;79(5):727–47. doi:10.1093/ajcn/79.5.727.

Manore MM. Exercise and the Institute of Medicine recommendations for nutrition. *Curr Sports Med Rep* 2005 Aug;4(4):193–8.

Mayo Clinic. L-Arginine. Last updated Feb. 2021. Retrieved from https://www.mayoclinic. org/drugs-supplements-L-arginine/art-20364681.

Minami Y, Sasaki T, Arai Y, et al. Diet and systemic lupus erythematosus: a 4 year prospective study of Japanese patients. *J Rheumatol* 2003 Apr;30(4):747–54.

Mozaffarian D, Clarke R. Quantitative effects on cardiovascular risk factors and coronary heart disease risk of replacing partially hydrogenated vegetable oils with other fats and oils. *Eur J Clin Nutr* 2009 May;63(Suppl 2):S22–33.

Routy B, Le Chatelier E, Derosa L, et al. Gut microbiome influences efficacy of PD-1-based immunotherapy against epithelial tumors. *Science* 2018 Jan 5;359(6371):91–7.

Sakai C, Ishida, M, Ohba, H, et al. Fish oil omega-3 polyunsaturated fatty acids attenuate oxidative stress-induced DNA damage in vascular endothelial cells. *PLoS One* 2017;12(11):e0187934. doi:10.1371/journal.pone.0187934.

Samykutty A, Shetty AV, Dakshinamoorthy G, et al. Vitamin k2, a naturally occurring menaquinone, exerts therapeutic effects on both hormone-dependent and hormone-independent prostate cancer cells. *Evid Based Complement Alternat Med* 2013;2013:287358.

Schuchardt JP, Hahn A. 2017. Intestinal absorption and factors influencing bioavailability of magnesium: an update. *Curr Nutr Food Sci* 13(4):260–78.

Szumczak M, Murray M, Petrovic N. Modulation of angiogenesis by omega-3-polyunsaturated fatty acids in mediated by cyclooxygenases. *Blood* 2008;111(7):3514–21.

Szymanski KM, Wheeler DC, Mucci LA. Fish consumption and prostate cancer risk: a review and meta-analysis. *Am J Clin Nutr* 2010;92(5):1223–33.

Turgeon J, Dussault S, Maingrette F, et al. Fish oil-enriched diet protects against ischemia by improving angiogenesis, endothelial progenitor cell function and postnatal neovascularization. *Atherosclerosis* 2013 Aug;229(2):295–303.

Unlu NZ, Bohn T, Francis DM, Nagaraja HN, Clinton SK, Schwartz SJ. Lycopene from heat-induced cis-isomer-rich tomato sauce is more bioavailable than from all-trans-rich tomato sauce in human subjects. *Br J Nutr* 2007 July;98(1):150–6.

Vermeer C, Raes J, Hoofd CV, et al. Menaquinone content of cheese. *Nutrients* 2018;10(4):446.

Wang DD, Li Y, Chiuve SE, et al. Association of specific dietary fats with total and cause-specific mortality. *JAMA Intern Med* 2016;176(8):1134–45. doi:10.1001/jamainternmed.2016.2417.

Wang HX, Wang YP. Gut Microbiota-brain Axis. *Chin Med J (Engl)* 2016 Oct 5;129(19):2373–80.

Weinreb O, Mandel S, Amit T, et al. Neurological mechanisms of green tea polyphenols in Alzheimer's and Parkinson's diseases. *J Nutr Biochem* 2004;15:506–516.

WHO. 2015. Guideline: sugar intake for adults and children (PDF). Geneva: World Health Organization: 4. Archived (PDF) from the original on July 4, 2018.

Yamagata K, Izawa Y, Onodera D, et al. Chlorogenic acid regulates apoptosis and stem cell marker-related gene expression in A549 human lung cancer cells. *Mol Cell Biochem* 2018 Apr;441(1–2):9–19.

Zhang Z, Wu X, Cao S, et al. Chlorogenic acid ameliorates experimental colitis by promoting growth of akkermansia in mice. *Nutrients* 2017 Jun 29;9(7). pii: E677. doi:10.3390/nu9070677.

4 Cooking for Diabetes Prevention

Andres Victor Ardisson Korat
Harvard T.H. Chan School of Public Health

Grace Rivers
Nutrition Works, Inc.

CONTENTS

DOI: 10.1201/b22377-4

INTRODUCTION

Diabetes is a chronic metabolic condition that occurs when the body cannot produce enough insulin or utilize the insulin it produces effectively (International Diabetes Federation, 2019). The main feature of diabetes is hyperglycemia (elevated blood glucose levels) that results from deficient insulin secretion or action (The Expert Committee on the Diagnosis and Classification of Diabetes Mellitus, 1997). When left untreated, chronic elevated blood glucose levels can lead to several other conditions including damage to the heart, blood vessels, kidneys, eyes, and nerves (The Expert Committee on the Diagnosis and Classification of Diabetes Mellitus, 1997).

The main categories of diabetes are type 1 diabetes (T1D), type 2 diabetes (T2D), and gestational diabetes (American Diabetes Association, 2019). T1D is characterized by the body's inability to produce insulin or sufficient insulin. T1D can develop at any point in life, but it arises more commonly during childhood or adolescence. T1D results from a cellular-mediated autoimmune destruction of the beta cells of the pancreas, which leads to diminished beta-cell function and decreased insulin secretion (The Expert Committee on the Diagnosis and Classification of Diabetes Mellitus, 1997). Many people with T1D require daily insulin injections to manage blood glucose levels. T2D, which is the main focus of this chapter, is more common in adults, and it is defined by the body's inability to use the insulin that it produces. T2D is defined by the American Diabetes Association (ADA) as fasting glucose concentration ≥ 126 mg/dL (7.0 mmol/L) or nonfasting glucose levels ≥ 200 mg/dL (11.1 mmol/L) (American Diabetes Association, 2019; The Expert Committee on the Diagnosis and Classification of Diabetes Mellitus, 1997) (Figure 4.1).

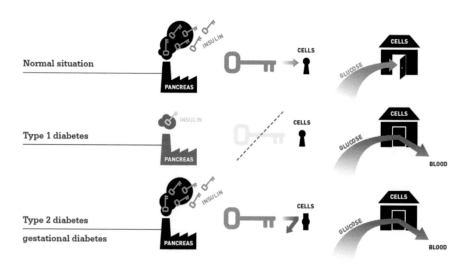

FIGURE 4.1   The role of insulin in diabetes. (International Diabetes Federation (IDF). *Diabetes Atlas*, 6th edition.)

The criteria for diagnosis of T2D by the ADA include the following (American Diabetes Association, 2019):

1. Fasting glucose concentration ≥126 mg/dL (7.0 mmol/L) or
2. 2-hour plasma glucose concentration ≥200 mg/dL during an oral glucose tolerance test (OGTT), which measures the glucose concentration in plasma after the consumption of 75-g anhydrous glucose dissolved in water or
3. HbA1c ≥6.5% (48 mmol/mol) or
4. Presenting with symptoms of diabetes (polyuria, polydipsia, and unexplained weight loss) plus a plasma glucose concentration of ≥200 mg/dL (11.1 mmol/L) without regard for the timing since the last meal.

Elevated blood glucose levels are the result of the body's inability to utilize the insulin produced by the pancreas. This condition is called insulin resistance, and it is one of the hallmark features of T2D (American Diabetes Association, 2019). As the disease progresses, insulin deficiency becomes manifest as the pancreas is increasingly unable to produce extra insulin to compensate for insulin resistance and keep blood sugar at normal levels (International Diabetes Federation, 2019). The term "prediabetes" is used to describe a condition of increased insulin resistance or impaired glucose metabolism that results in elevated glucose levels that do not yet rise to the fasting glucose threshold used to define T2D (American Diabetes Association, 2019; International Diabetes Federation, 2019). The ADA recommends not considering prediabetes as its own clinical entity but a state of increased risk for diabetes and cardiovascular disease (CVD) (American Diabetes Association, 2019).

ADA defines prediabetes as fasting plasma glucose levels between 5.6 and 6.9 mmol/L (100–125 mg/dL) or 2-hour plasma glucose during an OGTT of 140 mg/dL (7.8 mmol/L) to 199 mg/dL (11.0 mmol/L) or HbA1c levels between 5.7% and 6.4% (whereas T2D patients have ≥6.5%) (American Diabetes Association, 2019). Individuals with prediabetes are at increased risk of developing T2D and its complications in the future compared to the general population. T2D can be managed with lifestyle interventions including dietary changes, physical activity, weight management, and medications (Knowler et al., 2002). However, as the disease progresses, medication and in some cases, insulin injections are required to manage blood glucose levels (Centers for Disease Control and Prevention, 2020). Finally, gestational diabetes is characterized by elevated blood glucose levels during pregnancy, which may resolve after pregnancy but places women at risk of developing T2D later in life (The Expert Committee on the Diagnosis and Classification of Diabetes Mellitus, 1997) (Figure 4.2).

PATHOPHYSIOLOGY

T2D is a disease of complex etiology involving the interaction of several genetic and environmental risk factors. The glucose metabolism abnormalities that accompany a T2D diagnosis include (1) insulin resistance in muscle, fat, and liver, which are the peripheral tissues of insulin action, (2) defective insulin secretion by the pancreas in response to glucose stimulus from peripheral cells and (3) increased glucose

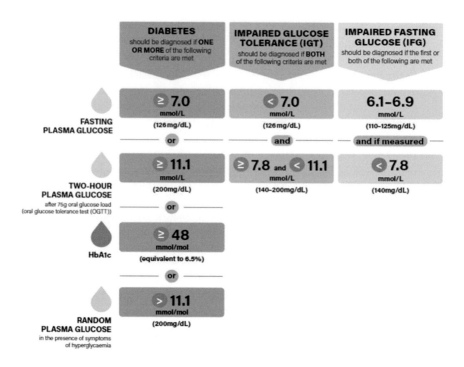

FIGURE 4.2   Diagnostic criteria for T2D. (International Diabetes Federation (IDF). *Diabetes Atlas*, 6th edition.)

production by the liver, which leads to hyperglycemia in the fasting state (Kahn, Ferris, & Brian T. O'neill, 2020).

Insulin resistance occurs when insulin-dependent cells are not able to use the insulin that the pancreas produces; thus, cells cannot use available glucose present in the bloodstream. The precise etiology of insulin resistance has not been elucidated, but it is believed to involve the interplay of several mechanisms including inflammation, oxidative stress, mutations of the insulin receptor, and mitochondrial dysfunction (Yaribeygi, Farrokhi, Butler, & Sahebkar, 2019). Once insulin reaches the target cells, it binds to the transmembrane insulin receptor. This binding initiates a cascade of cell signaling processes resulting in the translocation of glucose transporters into the cell membrane (Yaribeygi et al., 2019). Insulin-dependent cells such as adipose tissue cells, cardiomyocytes, and skeletal muscle cells produce and express glucose transporter 4 (GLUT-4). GLUT-4 resides in cytoplasmic vesicles and translocates into the cell membrane in response to insulin signaling and enables the transport of glucose into the cell, thereby decreasing plasma glucose levels after a meal (Yaribeygi et al., 2019). When the signaling mechanisms that enable insulin to express GLUT4 in cell membranes become defective, insulin resistance develops. The exact mechanisms for insulin resistance development are still unclear, but they involve heightened inflammation, reflected by increased levels of inflammatory markers, as well as increased levels of free radical production, insulin receptor mutation, and mitochondrial dysfunction (Yaribeygi et al., 2019). Excess adiposity, dietary, and lifestyle habits may contribute to the development of some of these mechanisms, which may highlight the role that environmental factors play in the etiology of insulin resistance and the eventual onset of T2D.

DEFECTIVE INSULIN SECRETION

Insulin is released by pancreatic beta cells in response to increasing plasma levels of glucose and amino acids (Yaribeygi et al., 2019). Decreased insulin secretion is believed to be a result of increased insulin resistance over time, which places increased demands on pancreatic cells, leading to beta-cell exhaustion or potential toxicity from hyperglycemia (Willett, Manson, & Liu, 2002). However, insulin resistance and defective insulin secretion often develop simultaneously in patients, which may suggest that both abnormalities may be responsible for the development of hyperglycemia (The Expert Committee on the Diagnosis and Classification of Diabetes Mellitus, 1997). From a clinical standpoint, the earliest detectable indicator of glucose metabolism dysregulation is insulin resistance, which may precede the full onset of T2D by many years. It is less clear at which point beta cells are unable to adapt to changes in insulin resistance and how this impairment contributes to the clinical onset of T2D (Kahn et al., 2020).

SYMPTOMS AND COMPLICATIONS

The most common symptoms that accompany T2D include elevated blood glucose levels (hyperglycemia), increased urination frequency (polyuria), increased thirst (polydipsia), weight loss, and blurred vision. Other more severe symptoms include hyperglycemia with ketoacidosis (a condition in which fat is metabolized into ketones), which results in blood acidification (The Expert Committee on the Diagnosis and Classification of Diabetes Mellitus, 1997).

Long-term complications of T2D include CVDs, nerve damage (neuropathy), kidney damage (nephropathy), and eye disease, which results in retinopathy and potential loss of vision and blindness (The Expert Committee on the Diagnosis and Classification of Diabetes Mellitus, 1997). The primary mechanism behind these complications is thought to be related to tissue damage resulting from glycated proteins produced by chronic hyperglycemia (The Expert Committee on the Diagnosis and Classification of Diabetes Mellitus, 1997). CVDs including acute coronary syndromes, myocardial infarction, angina (stable or unstable), arterial revascularization, ischemic attack, peripheral arterial disease, and stroke represent the primary complications of T2D and are the leading cause of death among T2D patients (American Diabetes Association, 2017). Additionally, conditions such as hypertension and dyslipidemia coexist with T2D and are independent risk factors of T2D (American Diabetes Association, 2017). General lifestyle recommendations have been issued by the ADA and American Heart Association for people with T2D, including guidelines for body weight and physical activity. The current dietary guidance is quite limited and focuses on restricting the intake of saturated fatty acids and *trans* fatty acids and emphasizing dietary fat quality by promoting the consumption of mono-unsaturated fatty acids and poly-unsaturated fatty acids (Buse et al., 2007; Evert et al., 2014).

This evidence is largely based on evidence from clinical trials (Qian, Ardisson Korat, Malik, & Hu, 2016).

Other important complications of T2D include nephropathy (affecting about 37% of patients in the U.S.) and is considered one of the main causes of renal disease (Centers for Disease Control and Prevention, 2020). T2D is the primary cause of blindness in U.S. adults with 11.7% of T2D patients reporting some vision disability including blindness in 2018 (Centers for Disease Control and Prevention, 2020). Neuropathy is a complication of T2D affecting the nervous system, which presents with a wide range of clinical manifestations including foot ulcerations (Pop-Busui et al., 2017) that can lead to other lesions and amputations (The Expert Committee on the Diagnosis and Classification of Diabetes Mellitus, 1997). Early detection is important to introduce lifestyle modifications to improve quality of life and prevent further injuries (Pop-Busui et al., 2017).

DESCRIPTIVE EPIDEMIOLOGY

Globally, 463 million adults aged 20–79 had T2D according to 2019 estimates from the International Diabetes Federation (IDF) (International Diabetes Federation, 2019). This number represents about 8.8% of the adult population and is expected to increase to 700 million by 2045. IDF further estimated that about four million deaths resulted from diabetes-related causes in 2019 among people aged 20–79 years. In the United States, estimates from the National Diabetes Statistics Report by the Centers for Disease Control (CDC) place the number of total diabetes prevalence at 30.2 million adults aged 18 or older in 2015, representing 12.2% of all U.S. adults (Centers for Disease Control and Prevention, 2020).

T2D is more common with increasing age with the prevalence of diabetes increasing sharply after age 45. 2019 data from IDF estimate that globally 135.6 million adults 65 and older (19.3%) have T2D (International Diabetes Federation, 2019). In the U.S., 25.1% of T2D cases are estimated to occur in this age group according to 2017 CDC data (Centers for Disease Control and Prevention, 2020). There are substantial disparities in diabetes prevalence among race/ethnicity groups. The prevalence is highest among American Indians/Alaska Natives (15.1% of adults 18 or older) followed by Blacks and Hispanics (12.7% and 12.1%, respectively), Asians (8.0%) and non-Hispanic whites (7.4%) from 2013 to 2015 (Centers for Disease Control and Prevention, 2020). Diabetes disproportionally affects groups with lower educational attainment (less than high school) compared to those with more than high school (Centers for Disease Control and Prevention, 2020). There are also important regional differences across the U.S. with the lowest prevalence among adults in Colorado (6.4%) to the highest in Mississippi (13.6%) (Centers for Disease Control and Prevention, 2020).

NONMODIFIABLE RISK FACTORS

Beyond the described disparities due to age and race/ethnicity, other factors including family history of T2D and genetic predisposition (both monogenic and polygenic markers) have been associated with T2D risk (Ardisson Korat, Willett, & Hu, 2014;

Kahn et al., 2020). Emerging evidence on the role of the gut microbiome has uncovered its contributions to obesity, insulin resistance, and T2D and its potential biological pathways of action, which include modulation of inflammatory and immune processes as well as having direct effects on intestinal barrier function and production and secretion of metabolites. Many of these mechanisms have been reviewed elsewhere (Kahn et al., 2020).

MODIFIABLE RISK FACTORS

ANTHROPOMETRIC FACTORS

Excess body weight is the most important modifiable risk factor of T2D and contributes to its development in conjunction with other variables such as diet, genetic predisposition, and lifestyle risk factors (Ley, Hamdy, Mohan, & Hu, 2014b). The most common measure of excess adiposity is the body mass index (BMI) expressed quantitatively as weight over height squared. BMI in the range of 18.5–24.9 kg/m^2 is considered normal weight. BMI in the range of 25–29.9 kg/m^2 is considered overweight, and BMI greater than 30 kg/m^2 falls in the obese category. Evidence from epidemiological studies has shown that individuals with obesity have a seven-fold higher risk of developing T2D compared to those with normal weight, whereas the risk for those with overweight is three times higher than those with normal weight (Abdullah, Peeters, de Courten, & Stoelwinder, 2010). Other measures of central obesity such as waist circumference or waist-to-hip ratio have been consistently shown as being associated with elevated risk of T2D (Vazquez, Duval, Jacobs, & Silventoinen, 2007). Another important factor for consideration is that excess adiposity is an important mortality risk factor among T2D patients with those in the overweight or obese range showing increasing risks of cardiovascular and overall mortality compared with those with normal weight (Zaccardi et al., 2017).

LIFESTYLE HABITS: SMOKING AND PHYSICAL ACTIVITY

There are several lifestyle factors that can help prevent the onset of T2D beyond keeping a normal body weight. Physical inactivity and habitual smoking are reported in many people diagnosed with T2D (Centers for Disease Control and Prevention, 2014). Engaging in regular physical activity is one of the most important strategies to help decrease the risk of T2D (Centers for Disease Control and Prevention, 2019). Evidence from large epidemiological studies has shown that both weight training and aerobic exercise are effective prevention strategies and are even stronger when combined (Grøntved, Pan, et al., 2014; Grøntved, Rimm, Willett, Andersen, & Hu, 2014). Conversely, sedentary behaviors such as watching television are associated with higher risk of T2D; for instance, every 2 hour/day increment of either watching television or sitting at work is associated with 14% and 7% increased risks of T2D (F. B. Hu, Li, Colditz, Willett, & Manson, 2014). Smoking is another important factor contributing to the onset of T2D, with risk increasing with the number of cigarettes smoked per day (Zhang, Curhan, Hu, Rimm, & Forman, 2011). Smoking cessation decreases risk, although elevated risk persists with time from quitting (Zhang et al., 2011) but leads to decreases in complications from T2D such as incidence of CVDs (Y. Hu et al., 2018).

DIETARY FACTORS

Many dietary risk factors are implicated in the development or prevention of T2D. This chapter will cover some of the most relevant ones as it relates to recommendations for healthy cooking.

DIETARY PATTERNS

Dietary patterns consider the total effect of dietary components rather than examining the effect of individual food items on disease incidence separately. Several dietary quality scores have been developed to characterize overall intake of nutrients or foods. For instance, the Mediterranean dietary pattern was derived from traditional culinary traditions in Crete where plant-based foods were the basis of the diet resulting in low saturated fat intake (<10% of calories) in an overall diet with 25%–35% of calories coming from fat (Willett et al., 1995). Mediterranean-style dietary patterns assign higher scores to consumption of fruits, vegetables, and whole grains and use olive oil as the main type of culinary fat. This pattern also consists of low intake of red meats and low to moderate intakes of fish, poultry, low-fat dairy, and wine with meals (de Koning et al., 2011; Schwingshackl, Missbach, König, & Hoffmann, 2015). A meta-analysis of several large observational studies including data from one randomized trial Prevencion con dieta mediterranea (PREDIMED) observed that higher adherence to Mediterranean-style diets was associated with a 25% lower risk of T2D (Schwingshackl, Missbach, et al., 2015). It is worth noting that the individuals in the PREDIMED trial were at high risk of CVD, and the trial showed that Mediterranean diets were effective at reducing the risk of T2D, especially when supplemented with extra-virgin olive oil (Salas-Salvado et al., 2014, 2011). Other dietary scores have shown benefits in terms of decreasing the risk of T2D. For instance, the Alternative Healthy Eating Index (AHEI) assigns points using a 100-point scale to the intake of whole grains, fruits, vegetables, polyunsaturated fatty acids, long-chain omega-3 fatty acids, nuts, and legumes as well as lower intakes of *trans* fat, red and processed meat, and sodium (Chiuve et al., 2012). Higher adherence to AHEI has been significantly associated with lower risk of developing T2D (Jannasch, Kroger, & Schulze, 2017). The Dietary Approaches to Stop Hypertension (DASH) was developed to manage blood pressure in individuals with hypertension. DASH is a 40-point score that assigns higher points to higher intakes of fruits, vegetables, and lean protein sources including low-fat dairy, poultry, and fish along with plant protein sources such as nuts and legumes while limiting intake of red meat, sweets, and sodium (Medina-Remón, Kirwan, Lamuela-Raventós, & Estruch, 2018). Evidence from multiple studies has shown that higher adherence to the DASH diet was associated with decreased risk of T2D and with improved glucose metabolism markers (Jannasch et al., 2017; Medina-Remón et al., 2018). Emerging evidence points to preventive benefits of plant-based diets; a meta-analysis of nine studies that compared higher adherence to plant-based dietary patterns (higher consumption of plant-based foods and lower consumption of animal-based foods) showed a 20% reduction in risk of T2D compared with those with poorer adherence (Qian, Liu, Hu, Bhupathiraju, & Sun, 2019).

The benefits of adherence to these dietary indices as potential management strategies among T2D patients have been highlighted in several studies. For instance, higher AHEI scores among patients with T2D were associated with lower risk of CVD incidence and mortality, especially in conjunction with physical activity and smoking avoidance (G. Liu, Li, et al., 2018). Higher adherence to DASH and Mediterranean diet scores has been implicated in substantial reductions in diabetes complications, including total mortality, CVD, and retinopathy (Salas-Salvadó, Becerra-Tomás, Papandreou, & Bulló, 2019). Plant-based dietary patterns including vegan diets and vegetarian and pescatarian diets are beneficial in terms of glycemic control among T2D patients (Salas-Salvadó et al., 2019). Several biological mechanisms may explain the observed benefits of these diets including improved glucose sensitivity and reduced inflammation associated with higher consumption of mono- and poly-unsaturated fats (Salas-Salvadó et al., 2019). Intake of saturated fats and heme iron from red meats has been implicated in decreases in beta-cell function and increased inflammation, which is implicated in higher insulin resistance (Salas-Salvadó et al., 2019).

In general, evidence from large observational studies points to dietary patterns that are high in cereal fiber, polyunsaturated fats, fruits, vegetables, and coffee and low in glycemic index (GI) and load, low intakes of *trans* fat, sugary beverages, and red and processed meats as beneficial in the prevention of T2D (Ley, Hamdy, Mohan, & Hu, 2014a). Evidence from short-term clinical trials of markers of glucose metabolism supports these findings (Ley et al., 2014a).

Carbohydrate Quality

Carbohydrate quality has been consistently associated with risk of T2D in multiple studies. One measure commonly used to characterize carbohydrate intake quality is the dietary GI, which is a relative measure of the incremental plasma glucose response per gram of carbohydrate (D. J. Jenkins, 1981). Another measure, glycemic load (GL), incorporates both the quantity and quality of carbohydrate (S. Liu et al., 2000). Diets with higher GI or GL have been associated with increased risk of T2D (Livesey et al., 2019). While the precise mechanism has not been elucidated, excessive insulin secretion is believed to lead to beta-cell toxicity (Salmeron et al., 1997; Willett et al., 2002).

WHOLE GRAINS

Grains are the edible seeds of grasses including wheat, rice, corn, rye, and millet, among others. Each seed consists of four parts: (1) the husk, which is an inedible fibrous layer that covers and protects the grain kernels and is removed during cleaning and processing; (2) the endosperm, a starchy mass that makes up most of the grain kernel; (3), the bran, a layer covering the endosperm containing most of the edible fiber and B vitamins; and (4) the germ, the embryo that forms a new plant if the seed sprouts and is the part of the grain that contains fat (Figure 4.3).

ANATOMY OF A GRAIN

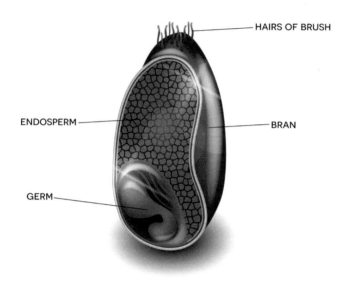

FIGURE 4.3   Main components of a grain kernel.

The transformation of grains from their harvested form into their finished form involves several processing steps (more details can be found in Chapter 2, Effects of Food Processing, Storage, and Manufacturing on Nutrients). For instance, hulling is a process in which the outer inedible hull or husk is removed from the grains. In contrast, pearling is a milling step in which the hull or husk and a portion of the bran or germ are removed. Cracking is a process in which the grains are broken open, whereas grinding is a milling process that reduces grains to powders of various degrees of coarseness.

The term whole grain refers to the intact cereal grain kernel consisting of endosperm, bran, and germ after the inedible parts (hull and husk) have been removed (Ross et al., 2017; van der Kamp, Poutanen, Seal, & Richardson, 2014). The European Union's HEALTHGRAIN consortium definition includes cereal grasses, wheat, rice, barley, corn, rye, oats, millet, sorghum, teff, triticale, canary seed, Job's tears, and fonio, and the pseudocereals amaranth, buckwheat, quinoa, and wild rice in their definition (Ross et al., 2017). Botanically, pseudocereals are nongrass plants; they produce grain-like fruits or seeds, which are similar in composition and function to those of true cereals. Whole grains are commonly processed into breads, breakfast cereals, crackers, pasta, and snacks. White rice and other refined grains have most of the bran removed and consist primarily of the endosperm (Figure 4.4).

The cereal bran includes most of the cereal micronutrients and antioxidants and virtually all of the dietary fiber; thus, its removal severely decreases the nutrient content of refined grains (Călinoiu & Vodnar, 2018). Whole grains contribute several

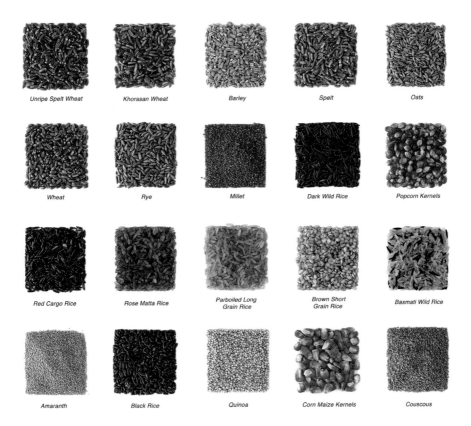

FIGURE 4.4 Cereal grains.

nutrients present in the bran including dietary fiber, vitamins, minerals, and several phenolic compounds, and the germ contains B vitamins, vitamin E, selenium, and antioxidants (Călinoiu & Vodnar, 2018; Rebello, Greenway, & Finley, 2014). For instance, whole-wheat flour contains 3–5 times more fiber, iron, magnesium, and zinc than its white flour counterpart, and higher levels of thiamine, riboflavin, niacin, and vitamin B6 (Table 4.1). In comparison, the endosperm contains most of the starch but only a small amount of B vitamins and minerals. The bran and dietary fiber help slow down the breakdown of starch into glucose and prevent sharp increases in blood glucose levels, which may contribute to its T2D preventive effects (Călinoiu & Vodnar, 2018).

EPIDEMIOLOGY

Consumption of whole grains has been linked with lower risk of T2D, even after taking the effect of body weight into account. Estimates from observational studies show that comparing higher to lower intake of whole grains or cereal fiber is associated with about 20%–30% lower risk of T2D (Della Pepa, Vetrani, Vitale, & Riccardi, 2018). Additionally, every 30 g/day serving of whole grains is associated

TABLE 4.1
Nutritional Profile of Selected Grains, Uncooked[a]

	Whole-Wheat Flour, Soft Wheat	White Wheat Flour, Unenriched	Brown Rice Flour	White Rice Flour	Hulled Barley	Pearled Barley	Whole Corn Flour	Corn Masa Flour	Quinoa, Uncooked
Carbohydrates, g	85.0	86.6	86.9	90.9	81.1	86.4	86.3	84.9	74.0
Protein, g	11.0	11.0	8.2	6.8	13.8	11.0	7.8	9.4	16.3
Fat, g	2.2	1.7	3.2	1.6	2.5	1.3	4.3	4.1	7.0
Dietary fiber, g	15.0	2.7	5.2	2.7	19.1	12.2	8.2	7.1	8.1
Thiamin, mg	0.3	0.2	0.5	1.6	0.7	0.2	0.3	0.2	0.4
Riboflavin, mg	0.2	0.1	0.1	0.0	0.3	0.1	0.1	0.1	0.4
Niacin, mg	6.1	1.4	7.2	2.9	5.1	5.1	2.1	2.8	1.8
Vitamin B6, mg	0.2	0.0	0.8	0.5	0.4	0.3	0.4	0.5	0.6
Folate, total, mg	32.0	35.2	18.2	4.5	21.0	25.6	28.1	32.1	212.2
Iron, mg	4.2	1.4	2.2	0.5	4.0	2.8	2.7	1.6	5.3
Zinc, mg	3.4	1.2	2.8	0.9	3.1	2.4	1.9	2.0	3.6
Magnesium, mg	133.6	28.4	127.2	39.7	146.9	87.9	104.4	103.1	227.2

Source: Data adapted from USDA FoodData Central: https://ndb.nal.usda.gov/fdc-app.html#/.
[a] Nutrients are expressed as percentages calculated on a dry basis (all solids without moisture).

with 13% lower risk of T2D (Schwingshackl et al., 2017). The benefits of whole grain intake extend to T2D patients, where it is associated with lower risk of mortality (He, Van Dam, Rimm, Hu, & Qi, 2010). The evidence for refined grain consumption in relation with T2D is less conclusive (Schwingshackl et al., 2017). However, there is some evidence for specific processed grains. For instance, consuming more white rice is associated with greater risk of T2D, especially in Asian populations where it is a primary source of calories (E. A. Hu, Pan, Malik, & Sun, 2012). Furthermore, replacing white rice with either brown rice or other whole grains was associated with decreased risk of T2D (Sun et al., 2010).

TYPES OF WHOLE GRAINS

- Amaranth is a yellow-brown seed with a characteristic nutty flavor. It is native to Mexico and Central America. One cup of cooked amaranth (250 g) contains 9 g protein and 5 g of fiber. Amaranth can be cooked for 20–25 minutes using 1 part of grain and 2–3 parts of water. Amaranth produces a dish with mild savory flavor that yields a creamy texture that resembles brown sugar. It may be served like rice, or it can be popped like popcorn and served as a snack.
- Barley is a whole grain in its natural state. However, most of the commercial barley is available as pearled barley which has been dehulled and polished. This process causes a portion of the outer bran to be lost, which means that pearled barley is not technically a whole grain. It is used in soups or cooked like rice using the pilaf method.
- Brown rice conserves its bran layer which gives it a light brown color. Brown rice is available as short, medium, or long grain. Because of the fiber in the bran layer, cooked brown rice has a mild nutty flavor and chewy texture. Brown rice absorbs more water than white rice and usually takes about twice as long to cook. Rice dishes are consumed around the world and are part of several national and regional cuisines.
- Buckwheat is technically the fruit of a plant with branched stems rather than a grain; however, it contains almost as much fiber as whole wheat products. The crushed grains, called buckwheat groats, can be cooked like rice. Kasha is the hulled and toasted version of buckwheat. Kasha is available whole or ground to various degrees of coarseness. Another presentation of raw buckwheat is in the form of flour, which is used to make pasta, blinis (small, savory pancakes garnished with sour cream and/or caviar), and other products. Buckwheat does not contain gluten, and thus, buckwheat flour cannot be used in lieu of whole wheat flour in traditional bakery applications.
- Corn has been used in its dried form for thousands of years and is processed into several forms including cornmeal, which is a coarse grind of dent corn that produces finished products with gritty texture. Corn products may be considered whole grains if they preserve the original bran, germ, and endosperm. Most forms of cornmeal and corn flour that retain these three constituents are whole grain products. Products such as corn starch only, containing the endosperm, are not a whole grain. Another form of corn is produced

with a traditional processing method called nixtamalization whereby corn is soaked and cooked in an alkaline solution of lime or lye. This process causes the kernels to swell and the hulls to loosen. When the hulls and germ are removed, the resulting product is called hominy or posole. Nixtamalized corn is washed and ground to form masa, which is the primary ingredient in corn tortillas, tamales, and other corn dishes. It is worth noting that the loss of part of the bran and germ during soaking means that nixtamalized corn is not a whole grain. However, nixtamalization increases the bioavailability of niacin and beta-carotene possibly due to the release of these micronutrients from complex carbohydrates in the pericarp.

- Farro (also known as emmer) is part of the grain family that includes wheat, and they are both similar in flavor. Farro has been used in countries in the Mediterranean for thousands of years where it was notably a staple of Roman armies. Farro usually requires soaking in water before cooking, and once cooked, it can be used in soups, salads, or side dishes.
- Kamut is the commercial name of the grain Kamut Khorasan, which is a relative of traditional wheat with larger berries and similar in composition and flavor. Kamut has been used for thousands of years in Central Asia and regions of modern Iran and Afghanistan. Kamut berries may be soaked overnight before cooking, which reduces the overall time needed to prepare them.
- Millet is widely used across many countries in Africa and Asia. It has a relatively bland flavor and a high protein content relative to other grains. In general, millet can be cooked, prepared, and consumed like rice. Millet can be toasted like buckwheat or processed into flour to be combined with wheat in the preparation of baked goods. Millet is generally available hulled to ease preparation.
- Oats come in several preprocessed options. Oat groats are the whole kernel with the husk removed. Steel-cut oats keep all parts of the grain and have been cut into smaller pieces to ease the cooking process. Rolled oats go through a steam-based precooking step before passing through a set of rollers than flattens them with the objective of decreasing its final cook time. Instant versions of oats are similar, except that they are completely precooked, and they only need to be rehydrated with hot water to be consumed. Cooking times for oat products vary greatly with instant requiring the shortest cooking time and groats the longest. Overnight soaking helps decrease overall cooking times.
- Spelt is related to wheat, and it has been consumed in the European continent for thousands of years. It has a sweet, nutty flavor when cooked.
- Teff is a grain consumed extensively in Ethiopia and Eritrea, and it is one of the first grains to be domesticated into a staple crop. Teff is a good source of protein and dietary fiber, and it is considered to be gluten-free. Teff is used to make the Ethiopian bread, injera.
- Triticale is a high-protein grain resulting from the hybridization of wheat and rye during the late 19th century. Triticale has a mild sweet flavor and can be cooked like rice.

- Quinoa is a high-protein seed native to the Andean region in South America covering Bolivia, Ecuador, Peru, and Chile. It comes in several colors including red, white, and black. It is worth noting that the protein in quinoa is a complete protein (it contains all nine essential amino acids) unlike most of the other grains. Quinoa contains a bitter coating of saponins, which is normally removed during processing; otherwise, the grains must be washed by placing them in a fine-meshed colander to remove it. Quinoa is considered to be a gluten-free grain.
- Wheat in its whole grain form can be consumed as whole wheatberries (with the hulls removed) or processed into flour. Wheatberries can be cooked either by simmering or by using the pilaf method as detailed below. Soaking them overnight usually helps decrease the cooking time. Other wheat products that maintain the intact bran and germ include cracked wheat in which the whole wheat kernel has been broken into a wide range of coarseness. Cooking times may be shorter for cracked wheat compared to whole berries. Bulgur is cracked whole wheat that is subsequently steam-cooked to decrease the final preparation time. Bulgur wheat can be served as a grain or in salads such as tabbouleh to which tomatoes, onions, and herbs have been added.
- Wild rice is technically a semi-aquatic grass grown in lakes and tidal rivers. Wild rice originated in the Great Lakes area between the U.S. and Canada. Wild rice has a nuttier flavor than regular rice. There are three grades of wild race available including (1) giant, which is a long grain considered to have the best quality, (2) fancy for use in most dishes, and (3) select, a short grain used primarily in soups and baked goods.

COOKING WITH WHOLE GRAINS

There are three primary methods to cook grains: the simmering method, the pilaf method, and the risotto method. These methods can be used for both whole grains and refined grains with small changes to some parameters such as the cooking time and the water-to-grain ratios.

Simmering is the most common method to cook grains. Washed whole grains are placed in a pot with water (generally one part of grain and two parts of water, but this may vary with the type of grain). The contents of the pot are brought to a boil and reduced to a simmer and then cooked covered until the water is absorbed, and the grains are cooked. The amount of water may vary with the type of grain and is determined by the grain's moisture starch contents and the desired finished texture in terms of moistness and the degree to which the grains have been cooked. The precise amount of water to be added is difficult to determine. It is preferable to add extra water because excess water can be either absorbed by the grains if they stay in the covered pot after cooking or drained if excess is still present. Too little water will prevent the grains to be cooked to their desired texture. Detailed cooking methods and recipes are included in the recipe appendix (Appendix A). Overall, whole grains require longer cooking times than their refined counterparts. For instance, white rice usually takes 20 minutes to cook, whereas brown rice, triticale, spelt, and wild rice require 40–50 minutes to cook, depending on the variety and grain size. A standard recipe to cook one cup of brown rice using the simmering method includes washing the rice by submerging it in about one quart of water followed by stirring and draining; repeat two more times or until water is not cloudy. Add the rice to a pot with 2.5 cups of water, bring to a boil, and then reduce the heat to medium. Let the rice cook for about 30–40 minutes, stirring occasionally. Once cooked, keep the covered pot with the rice in it for about 10–15 minutes to allow all the water to be absorbed.

The same procedure outlined for brown rice can be used for wheat berries, triticale, and Kamut; each require about 45–60 minutes of cook time. Soaking the grains in water overnight helps hydrate the starch and decrease cooking times. Pearled barley usually requires about 35 minutes to cook because some of the bran is lost in the polishing process. Smaller grains such as quinoa, amaranth, teff and millet require less time – about 20–25 minutes – to cook using the simmering method. Always verify whether the grain has been precooked because this will decrease the time required to achieve the desired texture. In this case, follow the manufacturer's instructions. Farro can be cooked by adding the grains to boiling water and returning the water to a boil and cook for about 20–25 minutes giving time for the grain to absorb some of the water and to soften. The resulting texture is like cooked rice.

The pilaf method consists of two steps. In the first one, the grains are cooked in fat. The choice of cooking fat depends on the desired flavor. For instance, oils such as corn or canola transfer little flavor to the grains, whereas olive oil and sesame seed oil impart their characteristic flavor profiles to the finished dish. Fat helps keep the individual kernels separated, which allows them to cook more uniformly to attain a fluffy texture, preventing the grains from sticking to each other. Cooking in oil also produces more flavor and allows other aromatics such as onions to be cooked in oil together with the grain. The second step consists of cooking them in liquid until the grain is fully cooked and the liquid is absorbed. This second step is usually carried out in the oven for uniform heating. The typical water-to-grain ratio is 2:1 measured by volume, and this is remarkably consistent for different grains and applies to both refined and whole grains. Detailed cooking instructions can be found in the recipe appendix (Appendix A).

The main steps of the pilaf method include heating the fat source in a heavy pan and adding onions until they become light but not browned. Then the grains are added until they are coated with the fat source and lightly toasted. The proper amount of liquid is then added and brought to a simmer. Finally, the pot is covered where it can cook on the stovetop or transferred to the oven. All these steps can be carried out in the same pan. A Dutch oven-style pot that can be tightly covered and transferred into the oven produces the best results. This method produces fully cooked grains that are separated from each other. As with the simmering method, whole grains take longer to cook than refined grains. White rice usually takes 30 minutes to cook using the pilaf method. In contrast, brown rice and whole grains such as farro, wheat berries, triticale, and Kamut require about 45–60 minutes to cook. Pearled barley usually takes about 35 minutes to cook, whereas smaller grains such as quinoa, amaranth, and millet require about 25–30 minutes.

The risotto method involves initially sautéing the grains followed by the addition of small amounts of liquid while stirring until the liquid is absorbed. This process

TABLE 4.2
Cooking Time (in minutes) for Various Grains Using the Simmering or Pilaf Methods

Grain	Simmering Method	Pilaf Method
White rice	20	30
Quinoa, amaranth, teff, and millet	20–25	25–30
Pearled barley	35	35
Brown rice, triticale, spelt, and wild rice	40–50	45–60
Wheat berries, triticale, and Kamut	45–60	45–60

is repeated until the desired cooked texture is developed. During the initial sautéing step, onions maybe added to enhance flavor. This method develops a grain with creamy consistency because the stirring step brings some of the starch out of the grain, which makes grains stick to each other. Whole grains usually require longer to cook than refined grains using this method, and doneness is usually determined by reaching the desired texture (Table 4.2).

LEGUMES

Legumes are a large group of plants that produce seed pods that split along two opposite sides when they ripen. Legumes include beans (including kidney beans, cannellini beans, navy beans, fava beans, pinto beans, and black-eyed peas), peas, lentils, green beans, soybeans, chickpeas, broad beans, alfalfa, clover, and lupine (Polak, Phillips, & Campbell, 2015; Tang et al., 2020). Some legumes are consumed fresh such as peas, soybeans, green beans, and dried beans, also referred to as pulses, and represent several varieties of seeds, normally left in the pod until they mature and are subsequently shelled and dried (Figure 4.5).

Beans and legumes are sources of plant protein and are rich in dietary fiber, vitamins, and minerals (Polak et al., 2015). For instance, one half cup serving of legumes, about 115 calories, provides 20 g of carbohydrate – 7 or 8 g of which are fiber – and 8 g of protein (Polak et al., 2015). Of note, beans contribute a substantial amount of lysine, an essential amino acid for human metabolism (Messina, 2014). Most cereal grains contribute low amounts of lysine to the diet, and thus, plant-based diets may fall short of meeting the lysine needs if legumes are not included in the diet. Furthermore, beans and legumes have a low GI, which is important for T2D prevention (Tang et al., 2020). Beans contribute high amounts of resistant starch (between 1.7 and 4.2 g per 100 g of cooked beans). Resistant starch includes complex carbohydrates that are not digested in the small intestine and together with their fiber content are responsible for their low GI (Messina, 2014). Moreover, dietary fiber and resistant starch help with elimination, provide a feeling of satiety, and improve glycemic control (Zanovec, O' Neil, & Nicklas, 2011). Dried beans contain oligosaccharides including raffinose, stachyose, and verbascose in levels ranging from 1% to 12% of their dry weight (Rebello et al., 2014). Humans lack alpha-galactosidase enzymes

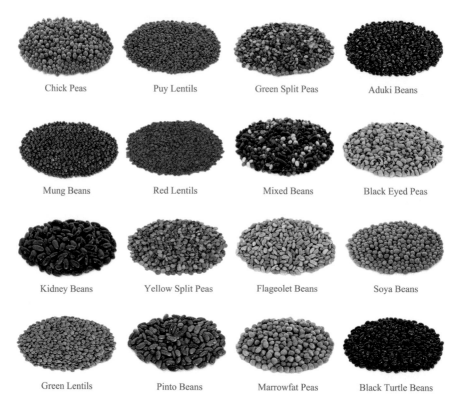

FIGURE 4.5   Beans and legumes.

in the upper gastrointestinal tract required to break them down, which results in fermentation in the lower tract where they produce gases that produce bloating and flatulence (Rebello et al., 2014). This may pose a barrier to consumption, which can be overcome by introducing small amounts into the diet to develop resistance and by soaking and rinsing dried beans prior to cooking to remove some of these oligosaccharides. In addition to their macronutrient contribution, beans contain substantial amounts of iron, zinc, calcium, potassium, magnesium, and folate (Messina, 2014; Rebello et al., 2014). Finally, due to their low cost, legumes are a cost-effective source of many of these nutrients (Zanovec et al., 2011).

EPIDEMIOLOGY

Evidence from large observational studies points to a suggestive inverse association of total legume consumption and risk of T2D (Schwingshackl et al., 2017; Tang et al., 2020). Significant associations have been observed for consumption of soy products including soy milk, tofu, soy protein, and soy isoflavones with reduced risk of T2D (Tang et al., 2020). Legumes are an important source of plant-based protein (Polak et al., 2015), which has shown to be significantly associated with decreased risk of T2D when consumed in place of other sources of animal protein including red meat, processed red meat, poultry, eggs, and fish (Malik, Li, Tobias, Pan, & Hu, 2016). In terms of T2D patient evidence, results from clinical trials show that diets rich in legumes lead to decreases in blood glucose and HbA1c levels compared to control diets without legumes (Hosseinpour-Niazi, Mirmiran, Hedayati, & Azizi, 2015; D. J. A. Jenkins et al., 2012).

TYPES OF LEGUMES

Fresh beans are picked when immature as green beans, string beans, or snap beans and normally consumed in their edible pod. The most common categories include American green beans, French haricot vert, and yellow wax. Before cooking, the strings along the seams must be removed. The pods may be cooked whole or cut into various shapes and sizes and cooked by steaming, sautéing, or simmering. When simmering, place the cleaned green beans into boiling water and adjust heat to a simmer. Cook for 3–5 minutes, drain, and run under cold water to chill. Green beans may be seasoned or dressed or used in soups or salads. Sugar snap peas can be sautéed uncovered for 1–2 minutes under medium heat and then finished covered under low heat for 3–5 more minutes.

Dried beans include varieties that are left to ripen on the vine until they reach maturity and are ready for harvest. After harvest, they are shelled and dried in air dryers. Dried beans have been used for thousands of years in several cultures and are an important part of diets today. The most commonly used types of dried legumes are kidney beans, peas, and lentils.

- Adzuki beans are small, oval-shaped beans with a thick red skin.
- Anasazi beans are popular in the U.S. Southwest and can be used in recipes that call for pinto beans.
- Black-eyed peas are a variety of cowpeas beans, despite their name. They are oval shaped with a white color and are used in traditional recipes in the U.S. south.
- Fava beans are flat beans of creamy-brown color. They have a tough skin and starchy texture.
- Green and yellow peas are left on the vine until they become mature and dry. They are available in whole or split form without the hull to ease the cooking process. Soaking them in water before cooking speeds up the process.
- Garbanzo beans or chickpeas are round and yellow-brown in color, about twice the size as peas. They are a central ingredient in Mediterranean dishes. They can be cooked whole and ground into flour and are the main ingredient in hummus.
- Kidney beans as a category encompass many varieties of beans including red and pink kidney beans, pinto beans, black beans, cranberry beans, Calypso beans, and Appaloosa beans.
- Lentils are small lens-shaped legumes. They usually cook faster than kidney beans, and they do not require soaking before cooking, but doing so may reduce cooking time. Green and brown lentils are most commonly used in most Western countries, whereas red lentils are most commonly used across South Asia. Yellow lentils are less commonly used.

- Lima beans are flat, broad beans that come in a wide range of colors from white to green in color. They have a starchy texture and are usually harvested when immature and consumed as a vegetable rather than in the dry form. They are used in soups and salads.
- Lupini beans are a member of the pea family and common in Spanish and Italian cuisine. They have a flat shape and high protein content. They need extensive soaking to remove bitterness.
- Mung beans are small, round beans with a green skin and white interior. They are available in their dried form either whole or hulled and split (requiring less cooking time). Mung beans do not require presoaking and can be cooked into a puree.
- Pinto beans are a brown-color bean with color speckles. They are used in the U.S. Southwest whole or refried.
- Soybeans are one of the world's most important bean varieties with high protein and oil content. The fresh version is prepared as a vegetable, whereas the dry variety requires long cooking times and are consumed directly in salads or prepared into other foods such as soybean paste, tofu, and tempeh.

COOKING METHODS

Most legumes are dry and hard and must be rehydrated to make them edible. Beans must be cleaned and sorted to discard shriveled beans, dirt, and pebbles. Before soaking, beans must be rinsed by covering them in water, discarding any skins that may float to the top, and then draining and rinsing again under cold water. The preferred soaking method includes placing them overnight in room-temperature water that is equivalent to three times the volume of legumes. Soaking helps soften the beans and remove some of the indigestible simple oligosaccharides, which is an important step to decrease the gastrointestinal distress some people experience when consuming beans (Nyombaire, Siddiq, & Dolan, 2002). Soaking has the additional benefit of decreasing levels of lectins and oxalate, which are present in beans and legumes and can interfere with the absorption of some minerals such as calcium, iron, phosphorus, and zinc (Shi, Arntfield, & Nickerson, 2018). A small amount of salt may be added (although not required) to the soaking liquid to improve flavor and help soften the beans as some of the sodium ions replace the calcium and magnesium ions, allowing the water to permeate through the skin: for 450 g (1 pound) of dried beans, dissolve three tablespoons of salt in 4 liters of water ("Salty Soak for Beans," 2020). The soaking liquid must be drained before cooking and followed by rinsing with fresh water prior to cooking. Split peas and lentils usually do not require soaking. An alternative method for quick-soaking dried beans begins with cleaning and rinsing the beans followed by placing the beans under cold water until covered by about 5 cm (2 inches). Then, bring them to a boil, and reduce to a 2-minute simmer. To finish, remove the beans from the heat source, and let them stand for 1 hour before draining and proceeding with cooking.

After soaking, the beans are ready for cooking. The preferred method is to simmer them in water, enough to cover them by 3–5 cm (1 or 2 inches). To start, bring the water to a boil, add spices and flavorings, and reduce to a simmer and cook covered until tender. Avoid cooking beans and legumes at boiling temperature as the finished bean may become tough; keep in mind that some legumes require up to 3 hours of cooking. During cooking, foam will form and float to the top, which may be skimmed as it forms. The exact cooking time will vary with each type of legume since size and the hardness of the shell will determine how quickly they become tender, but it will range from 1 to 3 hours. The ideal target texture is soft and creamy, and the shape of the bean should remain intact, unless a puree is desired. Once the legumes are cooked, they can be used in a variety of ways including finishing them in flavored liquid such as with baked beans, finishing them in oil or fat such as refried beans, or using them in salads, soups, and stews. The steps listed above work for most dried beans and chickpeas. In contrast, lentils are relatively quick to cook. The preparation steps are similar to those required to cook dried beans. Begin by placing lentils in three times their volume of water, bring the water to a boil, reduce to a simmer, and cook uncovered. Lentils normally require about 20 minutes to develop a tender texture. Drain, chill with cold water, and use in soups, salads, or side dishes. Split peas require less time to cook completely (5–8 minutes). Detailed recipes can be found in Appendix A.

A quick preparation alternative to cooking beans from their dried form is to use canned beans. Their nutritional value is comparable to their dried forms, except that sodium tends to be much higher (Zanovec et al., 2011). To help decrease sodium, choose lower sodium brands, and before preparation, drain and rinse the beans. Some studies show that these steps can result in ~40% sodium reduction (Duyff, Mount, & Jones, 2011). For someone just beginning to include legumes in their diet, smaller beans and portions are recommended. As beans become a part of the diet, tolerance can improve due to the gut microbiota. Moreover, the healthy microbes of the microbiota help to control weight and decrease the risk of T2D (Physicians Committee for Responsible Medicine, 2016). A recommendation of just ½ cup a day of legumes can be a step toward a more nutrient-dense food intake, which can become a frequently eaten food for improved health.

FRUITS AND VEGETABLES

Consumption of fruits and vegetables is modestly associated with reduced risk of T2D, independent of overall dietary patterns and adiposity. A meta-analysis of observational studies found that for every 100 g/day increment, fruit and vegetable consumption was associated with a 2% decrease of T2D risk (Schwingshackl et al., 2017). Fiber intake and the rich antioxidant content of many fruits and vegetables are believed to be responsible for their beneficial properties (Weickert & Pfeiffer, 2018). Habitual fruit consumption has been associated with favorable profiles of anthropometric indices, particularly decreased weight changes and waist circumference (Schwingshackl, Hoffmann, et al., 2015). A separate cross-sectional study found that participants who regularly consumed fruits and leafy vegetables had lower levels of Hb1Ac than those who reported not consuming fruits and vegetables (Sargeant et al., 2001). Cooking and preparation methods for most vegetables can be found in Chapter 2, Effects of Food Processing, Storage, and Manufacturing on Nutrients.

NUTS AND SEEDS

Nuts are the edible seed of a fruit surrounded by a hard shell consisting of a single kernel. The term is usually extended to include any seed or fruit with an outer shell such as peanuts and walnuts, which have two kernels (peanuts are legumes that grow underground). Nuts contain substantial amounts of fat that are susceptible to oxidation, and because of this, they should be stored in nonmetal airtight containers and away from light. Nuts can be used as ingredients in many dishes including salads and baked goods. The most commonly used nuts in everyday dishes include almonds, brazil nuts, cashews, hazelnuts, macadamia nuts, peanuts, pecans, pine nuts, pistachios, and walnuts (Figure 4.6).

Nuts contain important micronutrients, including carotenoids, vitamins B3, B9, and E in addition to minerals such as magnesium, potassium, calcium, and/or phosphorus and phenolic compounds (Hernández-Alonso, Camacho-Barcia, Bulló, & Salas-Salvadó, 2017). In particular, pistachios contain beta-carotenes, lutein, and zeaxanthin (Hernández-Alonso et al., 2017). In terms of macronutrient content, nuts contain high amounts of fat, ranging from 44% to 79%; most of this fat is in the form of mono-unsaturated fatty acids (9%–60%) or poly-unsaturated fatty acids (1.5%–47%) and lower amounts of protein (8%–26%) and carbohydrates (12%–30%) with some of it in the form of fiber (3.4%–12.5%) (Hernández-Alonso et al., 2017).

Frequent consumption of nuts and seeds may play a role in improving insulin sensitivity and slow down the development of T2D. Whereas the findings of a recent meta-analysis did not find a significant association between daily consumption of one serving of nuts (considered to be 1 ounce or 28 g), the analysis showed benefits in Asian populations where nut consumption is higher than in Western populations (Schwingshackl et al., 2017). Other studies observed benefits for specific types of nuts. For instance, findings from the Nurses' Health Study showed that consuming of walnuts at least twice a week compared to never or rarely was associated with lower risk of T2D (Pan, Sun, Manson, Willett, & Hu, 2013). A separate meta-analysis of clinical trials observed that consumption of peanuts or tree nuts (about 52 g/day) for up to 3 months had favorable effects on markers of insulin resistance and fasting insulin but not effect on fasting glucose or HbA1c levels (Tindall, Johnston, Kris-Etherton, & Petersen, 2019). The beneficial effect of most trials seems limited

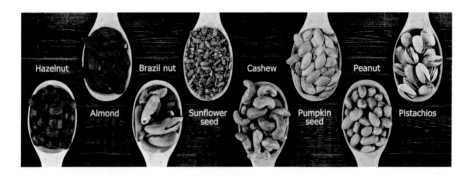

FIGURE 4.6   Nuts.

to shorter follow-up studies, which is consistent with evidence from other studies that observed a role of almonds, pistachios, or mixed nuts in the reduction of postprandial glucose levels compared with a meal with starchy components (Hernández-Alonso et al., 2017). More details regarding using nuts and seeds in culinary preparations can be found in Chapter 5, Hypertension and Hypercholesterolemia.

COFFEE AND TEA

Coffee is the fruit of a group of plants of the genus *Coffea*, *C. arabica* and *C. canephora*, which are cultivated in many tropical regions of the world. The fruit is referred to as the cherry, and the seeds are the coffee beans. Coffee is made from the roasted ground roasted beans. The two most widely used are arabica, which accounts for about 60% of the coffee trade volume and makes coffee with more commercially prized flavor profiles, and robusta, which is a more resilient variety than arabica and accounts for the remaining 40% and contains higher concentrations of caffeine and antioxidants (Ludwig, Clifford, Lean, Ashiharad, & Crozier, 2014). Coffee contains several classes of antioxidant compounds with a variety of bioactive properties of which the main categories are chlorogenic acids (CGAs), caffeine, cafestol, kahweol, trigonelline, and melanoidins (Ludwig et al., 2014) in addition to other components such as tannins, lignans, and anthocyanins (Grosso, Godos, Galvano, & Giovannucci, 2017). CGAs represent the higher proportion of phenolic compounds in green coffee beans and have known antioxidant and anti-inflammatory effects (Grosso et al., 2017). Many of these compounds are responsible for the wide-ranging health benefits of coffee intake including cardiovascular health outcomes to T2D, some forms of cancer, and Parkinson's disease (Grosso et al., 2017).

Several observational studies have shown a link between coffee intake and lower risk of T2D. A meta-analysis that included results from 26 different studies observed that coffee intake, measured as an increment of two servings per day, was significantly associated with lower risk of T2D (X. Jiang, Zhang, & Jiang, 2014). The results were very similar for regular and decaffeinated coffee intake; the study estimated that for every two cups of coffee per day increment, the risk of T2D decreased by 11% whereas for decaffeinated coffee, the risk reduction was 14% (X. Jiang et al., 2014). Both short-term and long-term clinical trials have found that regular coffee may improve glucose metabolism, particularly by reducing the increases in plasma glucose and increasing insulin response (Reis, Dórea, & da Costa, 2019). The same review noted that these improvements were observed despite acute increases in plasma glucose 1–3 hours after coffee consumption (Reis et al., 2019). A separate meta-analysis of green coffee extract supplementation reported reductions of fasting blood glucose but not insulin levels and a reduction in measures of insulin resistance only among participants who consumed the highest level of extracts, suggesting that coffee antioxidants maybe partially responsible for the associations observed in large observational studies (Nikpayam et al., 2019). Of interest, habitual coffee consumption has been associated with lower incidence of obesity, measured either as BMI for overall adiposity or waist circumference, for central adiposity (Lee et al., 2019). Excess body weight is one of the most important modifiable risk factors of T2D, and thus, it is possible that the link between coffee consumption and T2D prevention is multi-pronged with a portion of its potential effects coming through weight control and other through the action of the antioxidants it contains.

The link between tea intake and onset of T2D is less conclusive than the evidence for coffee; a previous meta-analysis observed that regular tea consumption is associated with lower T2D risk with an average 18% reduction in risk for those consuming 3–4 cups per day vs. nondrinkers (Huxley et al., 2009). A meta-analysis of clinical trials has shown a potential benefit of regular tea consumption in the reduction of fasting blood glucose levels (Kondo et al., 2019).

RED MEAT

Red meat and processed red meat have consistently been linked with increased risk of T2D in epidemiological literature. A recent meta-analysis of observational studies found that every 100 g increase per day in red meat intake was associated with a 17% increase in risk of T2D and for each additional daily 50 g increase in processed red meats was associated with 37% higher T2D risk (Schwingshackl et al., 2017). A separate study that pooled data from 14 different populations found that red meat was linked to higher fasting blood glucose concentrations, and red and processed red meat intake was associated with increased fasting blood glucose and fasting insulin concentrations (Fretts et al., 2015). The associations were partially explained by adiposity (measured as BMI in these studies), which is independently associated with insulin resistance and incidence of T2D. However, red meats contain heme iron and amino acids that can influence beta-cell function and insulin secretion, which in turn contribute to the development of T2D (Fretts et al., 2015). This hypothesis is supported by the fact that total iron consumption is not associated with risk of T2D; however, heme iron from red meat is associated with higher risk of T2D in U.S. populations (R. Jiang et al., 2004; Rajpathak, Ma, Manson, Willett, & Hu, 2006). Furthermore, processed red meats such as hot dogs, ham, bacon and sausage contain nitrosamines, which are the products of nitrate additives used during manufacturing with the amino acids present in meat. Nitrosamines have been hypothesized to have their own independent toxic effects on beta-cell function (Fretts et al., 2015).

With regard to cooking methods, a recent study observed that frequently cooking meat including red meat, poultry, and fish using open flame or high-temperature methods such as grilling, barbecuing, broiling, or roasting was associated with higher risk of T2D compared with using this method more sparingly (2–4 per month). The results persisted even after taking into account total meat consumption and are thought to be related to the production of heterocyclic aromatic amines, polycyclic aromatic hydrocarbons, and advanced glycation end products, which can influence chronic inflammation and decrease insulin sensitivity (G. Liu, Zong, et al., 2018).

SUGAR-SWEETENED BEVERAGES

Sugar-sweetened beverages are any liquids that are sweetened with various forms of added sugars such as sugar, corn sweetener, corn syrup, dextrose, fructose, glucose, high-fructose corn syrup, honey, lactose, malt syrup, maltose, molasses, raw sugar, and sucrose. These beverages include soda, sports drinks, energy drinks, sweetened waters, and coffee and tea beverages with added sugars (U.S. Department of Health and Human Services and U.S. Department of Agriculture, 2015). There is a well-established link between sugar-sweetened beverage consumption and increased T2D risk. A meta-analysis of observational studies observed that for every daily 250 ml consumption increase, there was a 21% increase in T2D risk (Schwingshackl et al., 2017). Evidence from a separate study showed that these associations seemed to be relevant mostly for consumption of sugar-sweetened beverages and artificially sweetened beverages but inconclusive for fruit juice intake (Imamura et al., 2016). Consumption of sugary drinks is a risk factor of weight gain and obesity, but these associations persist after accounting for adiposity (Malik & Hu, 2019). There are various mechanisms linking sugar intake through sugary beverages including elevations of blood glucose levels and dysregulation of chronic inflammation that may lead to the development of insulin resistance (Malik & Hu, 2019; Schwingshackl et al., 2017). Furthermore, consuming fructose in the form of high-fructose corn syrup may have its own independent effects when consumed in excess as it may lead to increase in hepatic de novo lipogenesis and insulin resistance (Malik & Hu, 2019).

CONCLUSIONS

Food choices can play an important role in the prevention and management of T2D, especially if paired with healthy lifestyle habits such as maintaining a healthy weight, avoiding smoking, and engaging in regular physical activity. This chapter reviewed the available nutrition evidence for many food groups relevant to the development of T2D.

Consuming whole grains, legumes, nuts, fruits, and vegetables can be a valuable way to make positive contributions to our cardiometabolic health. The sections outlined in the chapter described the available range of ingredients with special emphasis on whole grains and legumes and provided general guidelines for preparation and cooking to help incorporate them into everyday cooking. The cooking techniques used to prepare whole grains are similar to those already in use to cook refined grains, except that they require small changes to cooking times or preparation steps with the positive consequence of increasing the range of cereal grains available to our diets and with a much-improved nutrient profile.

Beans and legumes are important sources of dietary fiber, plant protein, and micronutrients. This chapter included a list of the most commonly available ingredients and outlined the main preparation and cooking steps with alternatives to make these products more efficient. This chapter also covers the evidence to support that the consumption of nuts, seeds, fruits, and vegetables as well as coffee and tea relates to T2D management. Finally, this chapter covers a small list of food groups to limit or avoid including sugar-sweetened beverages and red and processed red meat, which have consistently been linked with higher risk of T2D. Throughout the chapter, we aimed at presenting the profound effects that diet has on health by reviewing the most important food groups related to T2D prevention and management as well as simple preparation methods that allow their inclusion into everyday cooking.

REFERENCES

Abdullah, A., Peeters, A., de Courten, M., & Stoelwinder, J. (2010). The magnitude of association between overweight and obesity and the risk of diabetes: A meta-analysis of
prospective cohort studies. *Diabetes Research and Clinical Practice, 89*(3), 309–319.
doi:10.1016/j.diabres.2010.04.012.

American Diabetes Association. (2017). Cardiovascular disease and risk management.
Diabetes Care, 40(January), S75–S87. doi:10.2337/dc17-S012.

American Diabetes Association. (2019). Classification and diagnosis of diabetes: Standards
of medical care in diabetes-2019. *Diabetes Care, 42*(January), S13–S28. doi:10.2337/
dc19-S002.

Ardisson Korat, A. V, Willett, W. C., & Hu, F. B. (2014). Diet, lifestyle, and genetic risk factors for type 2 diabetes: A review from the Nurses Health Study, Nurses Health Study
2, and Health Professionals Follow-up Study. *Current Nutrition Reports, 3*(4), 345–354.
Retrieved from http://www.embase.com/search/results?subaction=viewrecord&from=
export&id=L601038396.

Buse, J. B., Ginsberg, H. N., Bakris, G. L., Clark, N. G., Costa, F., Eckel, R., … Stone, N. J. (2007).
Primary prevention of cardiovascular diseases in people with diabetes mellitus: A scientific statement from the American Heart Association and the American Diabetes
Association. *Circulation, 115*(1), 114–126. doi:10.1161/CIRCULATIONAHA.106.
179294.

Călinoiu, L. F., & Vodnar, D. C. (2018). Whole grains and phenolic acids: A review on bioactivity, functionality, health benefits and bioavailability. *Nutrients, 10,* 1615. doi:10.3390/
nu10111615.

Centers for Disease Control and Prevention. (2014). National Diabetes Statistics Report:
Estimates of Diabetes and Its Burden in the United States, 2014. US Department of
Health and Human Services.

Centers for Disease Control and Prevention. (2019). On Your Way to Preventing Type 2
Diabetes. United States Department of Health and Human Services. Retrieved from
https://www.cdc.gov/diabetes/pdfs/prevent/On-your-way-to-preventing-type-2-
diabetes.pdf.

Centers for Disease Control and Prevention. (2020). National Diabetes Statistics Report:
Estimates of Diabetes and Its Burden in the United States, 2020. US Department of
Health and Human Services.

Chiuve, S. E., Fung, T. T., Rimm, E. B., Hu, F. B., McCullough, M. L., Wang, M., … Willett,
W. C. (2012). Alternative Dietary Indices Both Strongly Predict Risk of Chronic
Disease. *Journal of Nutrition, 142*(6), 1009–1018. doi:10.3945/jn.111.157222.

de Koning, L., Chiuve, S. E., Fung, T. T., Willett, W. C., Rimm, E. B., & Hu, F. B. (2011). Diet-
Quality Scores and the Risk of Type 2 Diabetes in Men. *Diabetes Care, 34,* 1150–1156.
doi:10.2337/dc10-2352.

Della Pepa, G., Vetrani, C., Vitale, M., & Riccardi, G. (2018). Wholegrain intake and risk of
type 2 diabetes: Evidence from epidemiological and intervention studies. *Nutrients,
10*(9). doi:10.3390/nu10091288.

Duyff, R. L., Mount, J. R., & Jones, J. B. (2011). No sodium reduction in canned beans after
draining, rinsing. *Journal of Culinary Science & Technology, 9*(2), 106–112.

Evert, A. B., Boucher, J. L., Cypress, M., Dunbar, S. A., Franz, M. J., Mayer-Davis, E. J., …
Yancy, W. S. (2014). Nutrition therapy recommendations for the management of adults
with diabetes. *Diabetes Care, 37*(SUPPL.1), 120–143. doi:10.2337/dc14-S120.

Fretts, A. M., Follis, J. L., Nettleton, J. A., Lemaitre, R. N., Ngwa, J. S., Wojczynski, M. K.,
… Siscovick, D. S. (2015). Consumption of meat is associated with higher fasting glucose and insulin concentrations regardless of glucose and insulin genetic risk scores:
A meta-analysis of 50,345 Caucasians. *American Journal of Clinical Nutrition, 102,*
1266–1278. doi:10.3945/ajcn.114.101238.

Grøntved, A., Pan, A., Mekary, R. A., Stampfer, M., Willett, W. C., Manson, J. E., & Hu, F. B. (2014). Muscle-strengthening and conditioning activities and risk of type 2 diabetes: A prospective study in two cohorts of US women. *PLoS Medicine, 11*(1), e1001587. doi:10.1371/journal.pmed.1001587.

Grøntved, A., Rimm, E. B., Willett, W. C., Andersen, L. B., & Hu, F. B. (2014). A prospective study of weight training and risk of type 2 diabetes mellitus in men. *Archives of Internal Medicine, 172*(17), 1306–1312. doi:10.1001/archinternmed.2012.3138.

Grosso, G., Godos, J., Galvano, F., & Giovannucci, E. L. (2017). Coffee, caffeine, and health outcomes: An umbrella review. *Annual Review of Nutrition, 37*(1), 131–156. doi:10.1146/annurev-nutr-071816-064941.

He, M., Van Dam, R. M., Rimm, E., Hu, F. B., & Qi, L. (2010). Whole-grain, cereal fiber, bran, and germ intake and the risks of all-cause and cardiovascular disease-specific mortality among women with type 2 diabetes mellitus. *Circulation, 121*(20), 2162–2168. doi:10.1161/CIRCULATIONAHA.109.907360.

Hernández-Alonso, P., Camacho-Barcia, L., Bulló, M., & Salas-Salvadó, J. (2017). Nuts and dried fruits: An update of their beneficial effects on type 2 diabetes. *Nutrients, 9*, 673. doi:10.3390/nu9070673.

Hosseinpour-Niazi, S., Mirmiran, P., Hedayati, M., & Azizi, F. (2015). Substitution of red meat with legumes in the therapeutic lifestyle change diet based on dietary advice improves cardiometabolic risk factors in overweight type 2 diabetes patients: A cross-over randomized clinical trial. *European Journal of Clinical Nutrition, 69*(5), 592–597. doi:10.1038/ejcn.2014.228.

Hu, E. A., Pan, A., Malik, V., & Sun, Q. (2012). White rice consumption and risk of type 2 diabetes: Meta-analysis and systematic review. *BMJ, 344*(March), e1454. doi:10.1136/bmj.e1454.

Hu, F. B., Li, T. Y., Colditz, G. A., Willett, W. C., & Manson, J. E. (2014). Television watching and other sedentary behaviors in relation to risk of obesity and type 2 diabetes mellitus in women. *Journal of the American Medical Association, 289*(14), 1785–1791.

Hu, Y., Zong, G., Liu, G., Wang, M., Rosner, B., Pan, A., … Sun, Q. (2018). Smoking cessation, weight change, type 2 diabetes, and mortality. *New England Journal of Medicine, 379*(7), 623–632.

Huxley, R., Man, C., Lee, Y., Barzi, F., Timmermeister, L., Czernichow, S., … Woodward, M. (2009). Coffee, decaffeinated coffee, and tea consumption in relation to incident type 2 diabetes mellitus. A systematic review with meta-analysis. *Archives of Internal Medicine, 169*(22), 2053–2063.

Imamura, F., O'Connor, L., Ye, Z., Mursu, J., Hayashino, Y., Bhupathiraju, S. N., & Forouhi, N. G. (2016). Consumption of sugar sweetened beverages, artificially sweetened beverages, and fruit juice and incidence of type 2 diabetes: Systematic review, meta-analysis, and estimation of population attributable fraction. *British Journal of Sports Medicine, 50*, 496–504. doi:10.1136/bjsports-2016-h3576rep.

International Diabetes Federation. (2013). *IDF Diabetes Atlas*, 6th edition. Retrieved from http://www.idf.org/diabetesatlas (accessed June 16, 2014).

International Diabetes Federation. (2019). *IDF Diabetes Atlas 2019*, 9th edition. Retrieved from http://www.idf.org/about-diabetes/facts-figures.

Jannasch, F., Kroger, J., & Schulze, M. B. (2017). Dietary patterns and type 2 diabetes: A systematic literature review and meta- analysis of prospective studies. *The Journal of Nutrition, 147*, 1174–1182. doi:10.3945/jn.116.242552.as.

Jenkins, D. J. (1981). Glycemic index of foods: A physiological basis for carbohydrate exchange. *American Journal of Clinical Nutrition, 34*(3), 363–366.

Jenkins, D. J. A., Kendall, C. W. C., Augustin, L. S. A., Mitchell, S., Sahye-Pudaruth, S., Blanco Mejia, S., … Josse, R. G. (2012). Effect of legumes as part of a low glycemic index diet on glycemic control and cardiovascular risk factors in type 2 diabetes mellitus: A randomized controlled trial. *Archives of Internal Medicine, 172*(21), 1653–1660. doi:10.1001/2013.jamainternmed.70.

Jiang, R., Ma, J., Ascherio, A., Stampfer, M. J., Willett, W. C., & Hu, F. B. (2004). Dietary iron intake and blood donations in relation to risk of type 2 diabetes in men: A prospective cohort study. *The American Journal of Clinical Nutrition, 79*, 70–75.

Jiang, X., Zhang, D., & Jiang, W. (2014). Coffee and caffeine intake and incidence of type 2 diabetes mellitus: A meta-analysis of prospective studies. *European Journal of Nutrition, 53*(1), 25–38. doi:10.1007/s00394-013-0603-x.

Kahn, C. R., Ferris, H. A., & O'neill, B. T. (2020). Pathophysiology of Type 2 Diabetes Mellitus. In S. Melmed, R. Auchus, A. Goldfine, R. Koenig, C. Rosen, & R. Williams (Eds.), *Williams Textbook of Endocrinology* (14th edition, pp. 1349–1370). Philadelphia, PA: Elsevier.

Knowler, W. C., Barrett-Connor, E., Fowler, S. E., Hamman, R. F., Lachin, J. M., Walker, E. A, & Nathan, D. M. (2002). Reduction in the incidence of type 2 diabetes with lifestyle intervention or metformin. *The New England Journal of Medicine, 346*(6), 393–403. doi:10.1056/NEJMoa012512.

Kondo, Y., Goto, A., Noma, H., Iso, H., Hayashi, K., & Noda, M. (2019). Effects of coffee and tea consumption on glucose metabolism: A systematic review and network meta-analysis. *Nutrients, 11*(1), 1–16. doi:10.3390/nu11010048.

Lee, A., Lim, W., Kim, S., Khil, H., Cheon, E., An, S., ... Hsieh, C. (2019). Coffee intake and obesity: A meta-analysis. *Nutrients, 11*, 1274–.

Ley, S. H., Hamdy, O., Mohan, V., & Hu, F. B. (2014a). Prevention and management of type 2 diabetes: Dietary components and nutritional strategies. *The Lancet, 383*, 1999–2007. doi:10.1016/S0140-6736(14)60613-9.

Ley, S. H., Hamdy, O., Mohan, V., & Hu, F. B. (2014b). Prevention and management of type 2 diabetes: Dietary components and nutritional strategies. *The Lancet, 383*(9933), 1999–2007. doi:10.1016/S0140-6736(14)60613-9.

Liu, G., Li, Y. L., Hu, Y. H., Zong, G., Li, S., Rimm, E. B., ... Sun, Q. (2018). Influence of lifestyle on incident cardiovascular disease and mortality in patients with diabetes mellitus. *Journal of the American College of Cardiology, 71*(25), 2867–2876.

Liu, G., Zong, G., Wu, K., Hu, Y., Li, Y., Willett, W. C., ... Sun, Q. (2018). Meat cooking methods and risk of type 2 diabetes: Results from three prospective cohort studies. *Diabetes Care, 41*, 1049–1060. doi:10.2337/dc17-1992.

Liu, S., Willett, W. C., Stampfer, M. J., Hu, F. B., Franz, M., Sampson, L., ... Manson, J. E. (2000). A prospective study of dietary glycemic load, carbohydrate intake, and risk of coronary heart disease in US women. *The American Journal of Clinical Nutrition, 71*(April), 1455–1461.

Livesey, G., Taylor, R., Livesey, H. F., Buyken, A. E., Jenkins, D. J. A., Augustin, L. S. A., ... Miller, J. C. B. (2019). Dietary glycemic index and load and the risk of type 2 diabetes: A systematic review and updated meta-analyses of prospective cohort studies. *Nutrients, 11*(6). doi:10.3390/nu11061280.

Ludwig, I. A., Clifford, M. N., Lean, M. E. J., Ashiharad, H., & Crozier, A. (2014). Coffee: Biochemistry and potential impact on health. *Food & Function, 5*, 1695–1717. doi:10.1039/c4ja00138a.

Malik, V. S., & Hu, F. B. (2019). Sugar-sweetened beverages and cardiometabolic health: An update of the evidence. *Nutrients, 11*(1840), 1–17.

Malik, V. S., Li, Y., Tobias, D. K., Pan, A., & Hu, F. B. (2016). Dietary protein intake and risk of type 2 diabetes in US men and women. *American Journal of Epidemiology, 183*(8), 715–728. doi:10.1093/aje/kwv268.

Medina-Remón, A., Kirwan, R., Lamuela-Raventós, R. M., & Estruch, R. (2018). Dietary patterns and the risk of obesity, type 2 diabetes mellitus, cardiovascular diseases, asthma, and neurodegenerative diseases. *Critical Reviews in Food Science and Nutrition, 58*(2), 262–296. doi:10.1080/10408398.2016.1158690.

Messina, V. (2014). Nutritional and health benefits of dried beans. *The American Journal of Clinical Nutrition, 100*(suppl_1), 437s–442s. doi:10.3945/ajcn.113.071472.2.

Nikpayam, O., Najafi, M., Ghaffari, S., Jafarabadi, M. A., Sohrab, G., & Roshanravan, N. (2019). Effects of green coffee extract on fasting blood glucose, insulin concentration and homeostatic model assessment of insulin resistance (HOMA-IR): A systematic review and meta-analysis of interventional studies. *Diabetology and Metabolic Syndrome, 11*(1), 1–8. doi:10.1186/s13098-019-0489-8.

Nyombaire, G., Siddiq, M., & Dolan, K. (2002). Effect of soaking and cooking on the oligosaccharides and lectins in red kidney beans. *USDA*, 31–32.

Pan, A., Sun, Q., Manson, J. E., Willett, W. C., & Hu, F. B. (2013). Walnut consumption is associated with lower risk of type 2 diabetes in women. *The Journal of Nutrition, 143*, 512–518. doi:10.3945/jn.112.172171.questionnaires.

Physicians Committee for Responsible Medicine. (2016). The Physicians Committee Releases Seven Dietary Guidelines for a Healthy Microbiota. Retrieved April 8, 2020, from https://www.pcrm.org/news/news-releases/physicians-committee-releases-seven-dietary-guidelines-healthy-microbiota.

Polak, R., Phillips, E. M., & Campbell, A. (2015). Legumes: Health benefits and culinary approaches to increase intake. *Clinical Diabetes, 33*(4), 198–205. doi:10.2337/diaclin.33.4.198.

Pop-Busui, R., Boulton, A. J. M., Feldman, E. L., Bril, V., Freeman, R., Malik, R. A., ... Ziegler, D. (2017). Diabetic neuropathy: A position statement by the American diabetes association. *Diabetes Care, 40*(1), 136–154. doi:10.2337/dc16-2042.

Qian, F., Ardisson Korat, A., Malik, V., & Hu, F. B. (2016). Metabolic effects of monounsaturated fatty acid-enriched diets compared with carbohydrate or polyunsaturated fatty acid-enriched diets in patients with type 2 diabetes: A systematic review and meta-analysis of randomized controlled trials. *Diabetes Care, 39*(8), 1448–1457. doi:10.2337/dc16-0513.

Qian, F., Liu, G., Hu, F. B., Bhupathiraju, S. N., & Sun, Q. (2019). Association between plant-based dietary patterns and risk of type 2 diabetes: A systematic review and meta-analysis. *JAMA Internal Medicine, 179*(10), 1335–1344. doi:10.1001/jamainternmed.2019.2195.

Rajpathak, S., Ma, J., Manson, J., Willett, W., & Hu, F. B. (2006). Iron intake and the risk of type 2 diabetes in women. *Diabetes Care, 29*, 1370–1376. doi:10.2337/dc06-0119.

Rebello, C. J., Greenway, F. L., & Finley, J. W. (2014). Whole grains and pulses: A comparison of the nutritional and health benefits. *Journal of Agricultural and Food Chemistry, 62*(29), 7029–7049. doi:10.1021/jf500932z.

Reis, C. E. G., Dórea, J. G., & da Costa, T. H. M. (2019). Effects of coffee consumption on glucose metabolism: A systematic review of clinical trials. *Journal of Traditional and Complementary Medicine, 9*(3), 184–191. doi:10.1016/j.jtcme.2018.01.001.

Ross, A. B., van der Kamp, J. W., King, R., Lê, K. A., Mejborn, H., Seal, C. J., & Thielecke, F. (2017). Perspective: A definition for whole-grain food products - Recommendations from the Healthgrain Forum. *Advances in Nutrition, 8*, 525–531. doi:10.3945/an.116.014001.

Salas-Salvadó, J., Becerra-Tomás, N., Papandreou, C., & Bulló, M. (2019). Dietary patterns emphasizing the consumption of plant foods in the management of type 2 diabetes: A narrative review. *Advances in Nutrition, 10*, S320–S331. doi:10.1093/advances/nmy102.

Salas-Salvado, J., Bullo, M., Estruch, R., Ros, E., Covas, M. I., Ibarrola-Jurado, N., ... Martinez-Gonzalez, M. A. (2014). Original research prevention of diabetes with Mediterranean diets. *Annal, 160*, 1–11.

Salas-Salvado, J., Bullo, M., Martinez-Gonzalez, M. A., Ibarrola-Jurado, N., Basora, J., Estruch, R., ... Ruiz-Gutierrez, V. (2011). Reduction in the incidence of type 2 diabetes with the Mediterranean diet. *Dabetes Care, 34*(1), 14–19. doi:10.2337/dc10-1288.

Salmeron, J., Manson, J. E., Stampfer, M. J., Colditz, G. A., Wing, A. L., & Willett, W. C. (1997). Dietary fiber, glycemic load, and risk of non-insulin-dependent diabetes mellitus in women. *Diet and Diabetes, 277*(6), 472–477.

Salty Soak for Beans. (2020). Retrieved April 8, 2020, from https://www.cooksillustrated.com/how_tos/5803-salty-soak-for-beans.

Sargeant, L. A., Khaw, K. T., Bingham, S., Day, N. E., Luben, R. N., Oakes, S., ... Wareham, N. J. (2001). Fruit and vegetable intake and population glycosylated haemoglobin levels: The EPIC-Norfolk study. *European Journal of Clinical Nutrition, 55*(5), 342–348. doi:10.1038/sj.ejcn.1601162.

Schwingshackl, L., Hoffmann, G., Kalle-Uhlmann, T., Arregui, M., Buijsse, B., & Boeing, H. (2015). Fruit and vegetable consumption and changes in anthropometric variables in adult populations: A systematic review and meta-analysis of prospective cohort studies. *PLoS One, 10*(10), e0140846. doi:10.1371/journal.pone.0140846.

Schwingshackl, L., Hoffmann, G., Lampousi, A. M., Knüppel, S., Iqbal, K., Schwedhelm, C., ... Boeing, H. (2017). Food groups and risk of type 2 diabetes mellitus: A systematic review and meta-analysis of prospective studies. *European Journal of Epidemiology, 32*(5), 363–375. doi:10.1007/s10654-017-0246-y.

Schwingshackl, L., Missbach, B., König, J., & Hoffmann, G. (2015). Adherence to a Mediterranean diet and risk of diabetes: A systematic review and meta-analysis. *Public Health Nutrition, 18*(7), 1292–1299. doi:10.1017/S1368980014001542.

Shi, L., Arntfield, S., & Nickerson, M. (2018). Changes in levels of phytic acid, lectins and oxalates during soaking and cooking of Canadian pulses. *Food Research International, 107*, 660–668.

Sun, Q., Spiegelman, D., van Dam, R. M., Holmes, M. D., Malik, V. S., Willett, W. C., & Hu, F. B. (2010). White rice, brown rice, and risk of type 2 diabetes in US men and women. *Archives of Internal Medicine, 170*(11), 961–970.

Tang, J., Wan, Y., Zhao, M., Zhong, H., Zheng, J.-S., & Feng, F. (2020). Legume and soy intake and risk of type 2 diabetes: A systematic review and meta-analysis of prospective cohort studies. *The American Journal of Clinical Nutrition*, 1–12. doi:10.1093/ajcn/nqz338.

The expert committee on the diagnosis and classification of diabetes mellitus. (1997). Report of the expert committee on the diagnosis and classification of diabetes mellitus. *Diabetes Care, 20*(January), 1183–1197. doi:10.2337/diacare.25.2007.S5.

Tindall, A. M., Johnston, E. A., Kris-Etherton, P. M., & Petersen, K. S. (2019). The effect of nuts on markers of glycemic control: A systematic review and meta-Analysis of randomized controlled trials. *American Journal of Clinical Nutrition, 109*(2), 297–314. doi:10.1093/ajcn/nqy236.

U.S. Department of Health and Human Services and U.S. Department of Agriculture. *2015–2020 Dietary Guidelines for Americans*. 8th Edition. December 2015. Available at http://health.gov/dietaryguidelines/2015/guidelines.

van der Kamp, J. W., Poutanen, K., Seal, C. J., & Richardson, D. P. (2014). The HEALTHGRAIN definition of 'whole grain.' *Food & Nutrition Research, 58*(22100), 1–8. doi:10.32388/4ycwaw.

Vazquez, G., Duval, S., Jacobs, D. R., & Silventoinen, K. (2007). Comparison of body mass index, waist circumference, and waist/hip ratio in predicting incident diabetes: A meta-analysis. *Epidemiologic Reviews, 29*, 115–128. doi:10.1093/epirev/mxm008.

Willett, W. C., Sacks, F., Trichopoulou, A., Drescher, G., Ferro-Luzzi, A., Helsing, E., & Trichopoulos, D. (1995). Mediterranean diet pyramid: A cultural model for healthy eating. *The American Journal of Clinical Nutrition, 61*(6), 1402S–1406S.

Weickert, M. O., & Pfeiffer, A. F. (2018). Impact of dietary fiber consumption on insulin resistance and the prevention of type 2 diabetes. *The Journal of Nutrition, 148*(1), 7–12. doi:10.1093/jn/nxx008.

Willett, W., Manson, J., & Liu, S. (2002). Glycemic index, glycemic load, and risk of type 2 diabetes. *The American Journal of Clinical Nutrition*, *76*, 274S–280S.

Yaribeygi, H., Farrokhi, F. R., Butler, A. E., & Sahebkar, A. (2019). Insulin resistance: Review of the underlying molecular mechanisms. *Journal of Cellular Physiology*, *234*, 8152–8161. doi:10.1002/jcp.27603.

Zaccardi, F., Dhalwani, N. N., Papamargaritis, D., Webb, D. R., Murphy, G. J., Davies, M. J., & Khunti, K. (2017). Nonlinear association of BMI with all-cause and cardiovascular mortality in type 2 diabetes mellitus: A systematic review and meta-analysis of 414,587 participants in prospective studies. *Diabetologia*, *60*(2), 240–248. doi:10.1007/s00125-016-4162-6.

Zanovec, M., O' Neil, C. E., & Nicklas, T. A. (2011). Comparison of nutrient density and nutrient-to-cost between cooked and canned beans. *Food and Nutrition Sciences*, *02*(02), 66–73. doi:10.4236/fns.2011.22009.

Zhang, L., Curhan, G. C., Hu, F. B., Rimm, E. B., & Forman, J. P. (2011). Association between passive an active smoking and incident type 2 diabetes in women. *Diabetes Care*, *34*(January), 892–897. doi:10.2337/dc10-2087.

5 Cardiovascular Risk Factors

Hypertension and Hyperlipidemia

Nicole M. Farmer
National Institutes of Health, Clinical Center

CONTENTS

DOI: 10.1201/b22377-5

BACKGROUND

Cardiovascular disease (CVD) remains the leading cause of morbidity and mortality in the world. Globally, CVD represents 31% of all global deaths. In 2016, 17.9 million people died from CVD (WHO, 2021). Among US adults in 2015, the prevalence of CVD in adults is 49.2% and increases with age in both males and females (Virani et al., 2021).

CVD consists of multiple disorders including atherosclerosis, cerebrovascular disease, and heart failure, among other conditions. Established risk factors for CVD include diabetes, inflammation, metabolic syndrome, hypercholesterolemia, dementia, atherosclerosis, and hypertension (Virani et al., 2021).

Dietary intake and nutritional status, primarily over nutrition, are underlying issues in the prevention and management of CVD risk factors. Diet and lifestyle intervention studies have provided substantial evidence for a role of diet and nutrition in reduction of risk factors (Estruch et al., 2018; Ornish et al., 1998, 1999). This chapter will focus on the use of nutrition and dietary strategies to reduce these principle risk factors, with a focus on hypertension due to the depth of the evidence on use of diet for prevention and management. An important component of this chapter is the exploration of culinary methods that preserve specific nutrients and foods that play a significant role in pathophysiology of hypertension and other CVD risk factors.

HYPERTENSION

Hypertension is an important CVD risk factor to address as it is a major contributor to the pathogenesis of CVD and associated mortality (Virani et al., 2021). According to the 2017 guidelines by the American College of Cardiology and American Heart Association (ACC/AHA, 2017), hypertension is defined as a systolic blood pressure (SBP) greater than 120 mmHg and/or a diastolic blood pressure (DBP) greater than

80 mmHg. Hypertension is a multifactorial disease and can be classified as secondary or essential. Secondary hypertension occurs in 5%–10% of all diagnosed cases and is associated with various renal, endocrine, neurological, and CVD. Essential hypertension represents 90% of all diagnosed cases. Although the mechanisms involved in its pathogenesis are less clear, a multitude of factors, including lifestyle, are associated with essential hypertension. Antihypertensive drugs are the common approach employed to treat essential hypertension. These drugs include diuretics, angiotensin-converting enzyme (ACE) inhibitors, vasodilators, as well as blockers of β-adrenoceptors, calcium channels, and α-adrenoceptors. These drugs play an important role in the management of hypertension, but management and especially prevention can be mitigated though various lifestyle factors, including diet.

PATHOPHYSIOLOGY

One of the key advances in understanding the pathophysiology, or development, of CVD and hypertension is elucidating the interaction between contributory factors of genetics and environment. This interaction is principally driven by environmental daily life exposures, such as nutritional status and exposure to nutrients, which then cause downstream disturbances of gene expression patterns involved in vascular responses. The initial vascular responses include inflammation, oxidative stress, and vascular immune dysfunction, which then propagate endothelial and vascular smooth muscle dysfunction and lead to vasoconstriction and hypertension (Houston, 2013). These responses are augmented by changes in the renal system involving renin-angiotensin-angiotensinogen-system (RAAS). The next section will cover the multiple responses and systems involved in hypertension development in order to provide a framework for understanding the role of nutrition and nutrients.

RENIN-ANGIOTENSIN-ALDOSTERONE SYSTEM

RAAS is an essential part of blood pressure regulation. The system consists of enzymes and chemical messengers and involves multiple organs. The first step in RAAS is the liver's production of angiotensinogen, which is converted by the enzyme renin into angiotensin I. This is the rate-limiting step in the RAAS system. Angiotensin I is then converted mostly in the lungs into angiotensin II by ACE. Angiotensin II has biological effects on blood pressure, including constriction of blood vessels, sodium and water retention by kidneys, and atherosclerotic changes to the vessels. The actions from angiotensin II stimulate the production of aldosterone in the adrenal glands. Aldosterone in turn also has blood pressure-related effects as it increases sodium and water retention by the kidneys. In addition to functioning at a multiorgan level, the RAAS system can also function at local organ levels, such as blood vessels and the heart.

As the enzyme involved in the rate-limiting step of the RAAS, renin plays an integral part in regulating blood pressure. The kidneys play a key role in regulating the production of renin. Within each nephron of the kidney, there is a point where the incoming arteriole from the body (afferent arteriole) comes into contact with the distal tubule that takes the filtrated blood to collecting ducts and then to the bladder. This area is called the juxtaglomerular apparatus and is where renin is produced and secreted. The location of the apparatus allows it to receive information about the body's blood pressure need within the afferent arteriole and receive information about the components of the tubule infiltrate. Lastly, the apparatus receives information from the central nervous system via nerve endings within the apparatus, thus allowing the production of renin to be connected to increased sympathetic nervous activity.

ANTIOXIDANTS AND INFLAMMATION

Antioxidant deficiency and excess free-radical production have been implicated in human hypertension in numerous epidemiologic, observational, and interventional studies (Houston, 2014). Activation of the RAAS system and sympathetic activity in the setting of imbalance in sodium and potassium can lead to downstream effects within the vasculature that further lead to blood pressure and risk for CVD (Figure 5.1).

A decrease in potassium and increase in sodium can have direct effects on available antioxidants and oxidation of lipids, especially within cell membranes.

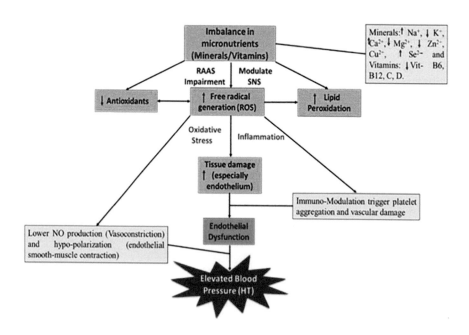

FIGURE 5.1 Sequential impact of imbalanced micronutrients on blood pressure and hypertension. (From Chiu et al. 2021.)

Both RAAS and SNS activity can increase free-radical generation, which further decreases available antioxidants and lipid peroxidation. Collectively, these steps create oxidative stress within the body.

A crucial effect of oxidative stress is a decrease in antioxidant availability, which can limit inflammation and lead to tissue damage within the cells that line blood vessels (endothelial cells). Upon initiation of tissue damage, the body responds with platelet aggregation and further vascular damage, which involves the activating molecule, tissue factor.

Additionally, the production of free radicals leads to a decrease in the availability of nitric oxide. Nitric oxide is a compound that causes vasodilation, relaxation of muscles along blood vessels. Dietary nitrate content may help to improve cardiometabolic outcomes due to the potential for increased nitric oxide production. Approximately 60%–80% inorganic nitrate exposure in the human diet is contributed by vegetable consumption (Menni et al., 2021). Nitric oxide is a major signaling molecule in the human body and has a key role in maintaining vascular tone, smooth muscle cell proliferation, platelet activity, and inflammation. Biological plausibility for the cardioprotective and blood pressure-lowering effect of vegetables has been linked to their inorganic nitrate (NO_3^-)/nitrite (NO_2^-). In fact, nitrate-rich green leafy vegetables and vitamin C-rich fruits and vegetables contribute to the apparent cardiovascular protective effect of total fruit and vegetable intake (Menni et al., 2021). Evidence-based diets shown to reduce blood pressure and CVD risk factors, including the DASH, Mediterranean, and traditional Japanese diets, naturally contain higher quantities of inorganic nitrate (147–1,222 mg/day) relative to a typical Western-style diet (about 75 mg/day) (Hord et al., 2009). One serving of nitrate-rich vegetables (such as beetroot) has been estimated to produce more NO under specific conditions than can be endogenously formed by the classical L-arginine–nitric oxide synthase (NOS) pathway (Hord, 2011).

GLUCOSE AND INSULIN RESISTANCE

Insulin, the hormone responsible for regulating blood glucose levels, plays a role in sodium regulation. At the site of the kidney tubules, insulin can increase sodium reabsorption, thus increasing blood volume and blood pressure. Insulin resistance is a condition in which the body's cells become resistant to the effects of insulin. As a result, the pancreas has to secrete higher levels of insulin in order decrease blood glucose levels. Insulin resistance can be a risk factor for hypertension. For instance, when insulin resistance is present, there is serine phosphorylation of the insulin-receptor substrate-1 which then leads to reduced nitric oxide bioavailability and impaired vascular relaxation (Muniyappa & Sowers, 2013). Insulin resistance is also a key factor in the development of obesity as higher insulin levels promote weight gain through multiple pathways. Given the relationship with insulin and sodium within the kidney tubules, interventions that improve insulin sensitivity and thus decrease insulin levels could help reduce blood pressure.

Consumption of foods with a lower glycemic index (GI) may improve insulin sensitivity, and thus reduce insulin resistance. Intake of carbohydrates that have lower GI, such as fiber, can lead to a reduction in SBP and DBP (Evans et al., 2017).

In addition to glucose, other dietary sugars may be involved in regulating factors that can affect blood pressure, specifically fructose consumption. Between 1970 and 2006, fructose consumption drastically increased, amounting to approximately 50% of all per capita added sugar consumption. Today, fructose consumption occurs as a result of use of high fructose corn syrup (HFCS) in food production and manufacturing mainly through consumption of HFCS, as opposed to other sources of fructose such as fruits (Harvard Health, 2011). The issue of dietary fructose and health is linked to the quantity consumed. It has been considered that moderate fructose consumption of ≤50 g/day or ~10% of energy has no deleterious effect on lipid and glucose control (Rizkalla, 2010). However, a study utilizing euglycemic-hyperinsulinemic clamps with glucose labeling reported that consumption of 40 g/day for 3 weeks in young healthy men can alter hepatic insulin sensitivity and lipid metabolism (Aeberli et al., 2013). To date, current estimates of daily consumption range from an average daily intake of fructose of 49 g (Komnenov et al., 2019) to 54.7g/day, with the latter representing 10.2% of total caloric intake (Vos et al., 2008).

Fructose is metabolized primarily in the liver. After absorption in the liver, ATP decreases rapidly as the phosphate is transferred to fructose. This transfer makes conversion to lipid precursors occur more easily, thus enhancing lipogenesis and production of uric acid (Bray, 2013). For individuals with already present CVD risk factors of obesity and diabetes, this can make fructose consumption hazardous. Epidemiological cross-sectional studies suggest that these direct effects of fructose are pertinent to the consumption of the fructose-containing sugars, sucrose, and HFCS (Stanhope, 2016). Outside of hepatic effects, fructose consumption may cause increased energy intake through failure to stimulate production of the appetite suppressant hormone, leptin. In addition, functional magnetic resonance imaging of the brain demonstrates that the reward systems in the brain may respond differently to fructose or fructose-containing sugars compared with glucose or aspartame (Stanhope, 2016).

Dietary fructose intake in conjunction with high salt intake can contribute to hypertension. Fructose can impair insulin signaling in insulin-responsive tissues and can contribute to insulin resistance (Baena et al., 2016). In the setting of insulin resistance, more circulating insulin is present which can lead to increased sympathetic response that further elevates blood pressure (Figure 5.2). Fructose can also influence intestinal sodium absorption leading to increase expression of sodium and hydrogen transport proteins, and rat models demonstrate that fructose can increase reabsorption within the kidney proximal tubule, the site of sodium reabsorption. In fact, rat models have shown that at a fructose consumption of 40% of daily caloric intake led to an increased tail cuff blood pressure reading. A renal proximal tubule mechanism was suggested by increased proximal tubule expression of sodium transporters compared to control rats in the study (Gonzalez-Vicente, et al. 2018).

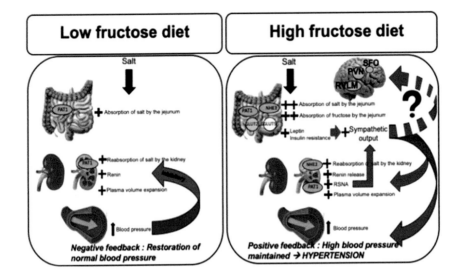

FIGURE 5.2 Multilevel role of fructose in regulation of blood pressure. Left panel shows conditions under low-fructose diet. The right panel shows increased sodium reabsorption in the jejunum and renal distal tubular, as well as the role of fructose in insulin resistance and resultant sympathetic activity. (From Komnenov et al., 2019.)

DIETARY PATTERNS FOR CVD RISK FACTORS

DIETARY APPROACHES TO STOP HYPERTENSION

The Dietary Approaches to Stop Hypertension (DASH) I and II diet trials have demonstrated significant reductions in blood pressure for prehypertensive and stage I hypertensive patients. In DASH I, untreated hypertensive subjects with SBP < 160 mmHg and DBP 80–95 mmHg were placed on one of three diets for 4 weeks (Appel et al., 1997). The diets were control diet, fruit and vegetable diet (F + V), and combined diet that added F + V and low-fat dairy. The DASH II trial added progressive sodium restriction in each group. Both DASH I and DASH II led to significant decreases in SBP by 10.7/5.2 mmHg in the hypertensive patients in DASH I and 11.5/6.8 mmHg in the hypertensive patients in DASH II. These reductions persisted as long as the patients were on the diet. In connection with the role of oxidative stress and hypertension, the low sodium DASH diet decreased oxidative stress as measured by urine F2-isoprostanes, and plasma nitrite levels also increased.

MEDITERRANEAN DIET

Consumption of a Mediterranean diet is associated with a lower risk of CVD. The PREDIMED trial involved the randomization of 7,447 participants between 55 and 80 years of age who were at high cardiovascular risk to one of three diets: a Mediterranean diet supplemented with extra-virgin olive oil, a Mediterranean diet supplemented with mixed nuts, or a control diet (advice to reduce dietary fat).

Participants received quarterly educational sessions and, depending on group assignment, free provision of extra-virgin olive oil, mixed nuts, or small nonfood gifts. After a median follow-up of 4.8 years, the PREDIMED study found that consumption of the intervention diets led to a significant reduction in cardiovascular-related events (stroke) (Estruch et al., 2018). However, all three diets led to a decrease in SBP, with the Mediterranean diets leading to further decrease in DBP than the low-fat control diet (Toledo et al., 2013).

Results of the PREDIMED (Prevención con Dieta Mediterránea) trial suggest that in addition to nut consumption, consumption of extra-virgin olive oil (EVOO) may have been beneficial. The components of EVOO that may confer CVD-related benefits are many and include monounsaturated fats (MUFA), the fatty acid oleic acid and polyphenols. The CVD-related effects of EVOO include inflammation, positive effect on cholesterol, and antioxidative properties. A further impact of the Mediterranean diet on blood pressure and endothelial function was shown through the MedDiet study conducted in 166 older (age > 64) healthy Australians who were randomized to consume either a Mediterreanan diet ($n = 85$) or their habitual diet ($n = 81$). The MedDiet resulted in lower SBP at 3 and 6 months (Courtney et al., 2017).

SPECIFIC NUTRIENTS AND FOODS FROM DIETARY PATTERNS FOR CVD RISK FACTORS

OLIVE OIL

Olives are small fruits that are rich in oil; about 30% oil is present in the pulp layer that surround the centrally placed seed. Olives are also enriched with bitter phenolic compounds. These compounds help protect the fruit from microbes and mammals. The color of a fully ripe olive is purple due to the flavonoid anthocyanin in the outer layer. But olives are picked for production of olive oil just before turning purple, while they are still green in color. Chlorophyll and the carotenoids (lutein and beta-carotene) cause the greenish color to occur. This green color is responsible for the greenish hue present in olive oil.

The process of making olive oil consists of first creating a paste made from finely grinding the olives and pits into a paste to break the fruit cells open and free the oil (McGee, p. 340). The paste is then mixed and then pressed to squeeze both oil and watery liquid from the solids. Oil extracted in the first press is called EVOO. Subsequent steps extract the remaining oil through repeatedly pressing and heating of the paste. Within the oil is mostly monounsaturated fat (oleic acid) that is considered less vulnerable to oxidation than polyunsaturated fats (PUFA).

Olive oil also contains polyphenols, but the content can differ dramatically between olive oil products. EVOO has the highest content of polyphenols with four main groups of phenol compounds: simple phenols (hydroxytyrosol), flavonoids, secoiridoids, and lignans. Of interest, the greatest source of the polyphenol, lignans, in the PREDIMED cohort was EVOO. Lignans were one of the polyphenols associated with the greatest all-cause mortality reduction within the study (Tresserra-Rimbau et al., 2014). Further analysis demonstrated a potential ability of the polyphenols present in EVOO to downregulate the expression of pro-atherosclerosis genes and related inflammatory and lipid oxidative markers. Hydroxytyrosol is the polyphenol that often has the highest content in EVOO, and it can be measured through urinary excretion to mark adherence with consumption.

Olive Oil: Culinary Strategies

Due to the presence of chlorophyll, olive oil is susceptible to light. Photooxidation from light can lead to change in aroma or taste. To prevent photooxidation, olive oil should be stored in dark containers and in cool conditions. Propensity for oxidation with olive oil occurs not only with light, but also with heat application. However, in traditional cooking, olive oil is not just used at the end of cooking but is used throughout cooking and using several different cooking methods including roasting, sautéing, and stir-frying. Therefore, there are reports that cooking with olive oil can cause oxidation and prevent receipt of benefits from polyphenols within olive oil. Some studies in which olive oil is exposed to high heat under long time periods have shown that oxidation occurs, but these studies do not replicate everyday life cooking times (Attya et al., 2010; Cerretani et al., 2009). In theory, these cooking methods could diminish polyphenols by causing them to leach into the cooking medium or through degradation and transformation of polyphenol content (Lozano-Castellón et al., 2020).

There is an obvious need to reconcile the everyday use of olive oil, evidence from studies such as PREDIMED and Seven Countries study suggest a CVD-related benefit despite the potential change from thermal processes. Lozano-Castellón et al. (2020) conducted a study to replicate home cooking practices and measure resultant olive oil-specific polyphenols. To replicate home practices, the researchers used the EVOO and sauté method in which EVOO was heated at moderate and high temperature. Foods used were 200 g of potatoes and 100 g of chicken pan-fried at both temperatures: 120°C for 20 and 60 minutes and 170°C at 15 and 30 minutes. In the study, there was a loss of 40% at 120°C and 70% at 170°C for the most common polyphenol, secoiridoids. The 40% reduction level maintains the European Union-established health benefits from olive oil. Interestingly, there was an increase in the lignan concentration. Although lignan is found in a smaller amount in olive oil compared to other polyphenols, the finding from this food science study may assist in explaining in the PREDIMED sub study trial finding that lignin was the polyphenol linked with cholesterol improvement.

WHOLE GRAINS

Reduction of CVD risk factors, such as total and LDL cholesterol and fasting glucose, due to whole-grain consumption has been reported through several meta-analyses of prospective cohort studies (Mellen, et al., 2008; deMunter et al., 2007; Ye et al., 2012). When comparing intervention trials, Marshall et al. (2020) found evidence for CVD risk factor reduction, but not enough evidence among intervention studies to support use of whole grains for CVD prevention and management. This may have been due to heterogeneity of whole grains among the 22 studies reviewed in the meta-analyses. Interestingly, despite this heterogeneity, consumption of all types of whole grains did lead to an improvement in hemoglobin A1c and C-reactive protein.

Culinary strategies for whole grains are covered in Chapter 2 Effects of Food Processing, Storage, and Cooking on nutrients in plant-based foods: Fruits, Vegetables, Cereals, and Grains.

NUTS

Clinical studies have evaluated the effects of many different nuts and peanuts on lipids, lipoproteins, and various CHD risk factors, including oxidation, inflammation, and vascular reactivity. Nuts often contain various levels of fatty acids and thus fat types. Nuts can be 50% or more oil and 10%–25% protein (McGee, p. 502). Most fats in nuts are more monounsaturated, then saturated or polyunsaturated. However, walnuts and pecans are primarily polyunsaturated. With respect to cholesterol reduction, the effects of nut consumption may not be completely explained by just the fatty acid profile of nuts (Degirolamo and Rudel, 2010). Thus, other nutritional components of nuts, such as plant protein (macronutrient) or fiber (macronutrient) may play a role. Additionally, nuts can be sources of micronutrients such as potassium, calcium, and magnesium and phytochemicals such as polyphenols, phytosterols, and amino acids like arginine (Kris-Etherton et al., 2008).

In terms of gluco-metabolic-related CVD risk factors, nuts have the ability to lower postprandial glucose response when consumed with high GI foods (Kendall et al., 2010). Within the PREDIMED study, there was a significant role for the nut diet compared to the control diet with respect to reduction in the risk of stroke.

Nuts: Culinary Strategies

Nuts are often consumed uncooked with minimal processing such as soaking. Nuts are also components in cooked meals and can be enjoyed roasted or fried. Therefore, it is important to understand the effects of these cooking methods on the health benefits of nuts.

Nuts are high in polyphenol antioxidants that have the ability to bind lipoproteins and inhibit oxidative processes that lead to atherosclerosis *in vivo*. Multiple studies have shown that both roasting and frying nuts do not lower polyphenol amounts nor antioxidant activity content (Ghazzawi & Al-Ismail, 2017; Vinson & Cai, 2012). Examples of cooking times used in studies include roasting at 110°C for 16 minutes and frying at 175°C for 2.5 minutes. Walnuts in particular maintained the highest lipoprotein-bound antioxidant activity. With regard to fat content, cooking also does not lead to changes in fatty acid profile of MUFA when roasted or fried, particularly for cashew nuts.

LEGUMES

The intake of legumes (which include dietary pulses, soybeans, peanuts, fresh peas, and beans) is recommended for lowering LDL cholesterol and blood pressure (Viguiliouk et al., 2019). Mechanisms for how legumes may have this effect include fiber content of legumes. A study of a sample of US adults found that on an average day, only 7.9% of adults consume dry beans and peas (Mitchell et al., 2009). In this sample, daily consumption of ½ a cup of pulses (dry beans or peas) was associated with higher intakes of fiber, protein, folate, zinc, iron, and magnesium. Perhaps also important was the association with lower intakes of saturated fat and total fat.

Culinary strategies for whole grains are covered in Chapter 2 Effects of Food Processing, Storage, and Manufacturing on Nutrients.

SPECIFIC NUTRIENTS AND CVD RISK FACTORS

The next section of this chapter will discuss specific nutrients and foods involved in the pathophysiology of hypertension and where applicable, other CVD risk factors. After each nutrient or food, culinary strategies are discussed.

ADVANCED GLYCATION END-PRODUCTS

Advanced glycation end-products (AGEs) occur as a result of oxidation. These end-products can cause damage to blood vessels, specifically causing inflammation, and are suspected to contribute to arterial inflammation and stiffness. The formation of AGEs occurs in three phases: Maillard reaction; oxidation of glucose; and peroxidation of lipids and through the polyol pathway (Figure 5.3). All of the pathways are led by blood levels of glucose, thus showing the role of AGEs in CVD risk factors related to glucometabolic conditions, such as obesity and metabolic syndrome. In the first

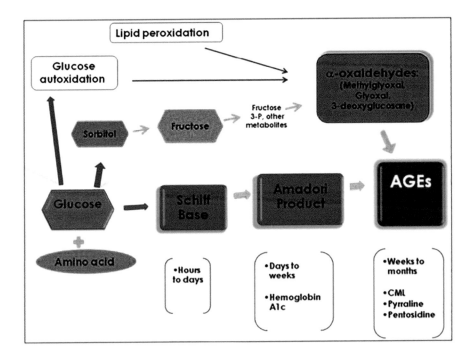

FIGURE 5.3. Formation of AGEs. (From Luevano-Contreras and Chapman-Novakofski 2010.)

pathway, glucose attaches to a free amino acid, usually lysine and arginine, of a protein, lipid, or DNA in a nonenzymatic way to form a Schiff base. This nonenzymatic first step depends on glucose concentration and occurs within hours. Importantly, during this time, if glucose concentration decreases, then the reaction involving the Schiff base is reversible. The second phase of AGE formation involves the Schiff base undergoing chemical rearrangement over a period of days. This phase forms Amadori products which are stable compounds, of which the test for measuring glucose levels over a period of time hemoglobin A1c is one. Accumulation of Amadori products will undergo chemical rearrangements to form crosslinked proteins. This process is irreversible and occurs over weeks to months (Luevano-Contreras and Chapman-Novakofski, 2010).

AGEs can also form non-Maillard reactions. The second formation pathway occurs from the autooxidation of glucose and the peroxidation of lipids, known an α-oxaldehydes (Figure 5.3). And the third pathway for formation of AGEs involves the polyol pathway, where glucose is converted to sorbitol by the enzyme aldose reductase and then to fructose through enzymatic action of sorbitol dehydrogenase (Figure 5.3). Fructose metabolites (as fructose 3-phosphate) then are converted into α-oxaldehydes and interact with monoacids to form AGEs. The formation of AGEs leads to several biomarkers for in vivo formation. The most widely known AGEs are carboxymethyl-lysine (CML) (found in Maillard reactions), pentosidine and pyrraline (found in Maillard reactions), and methylglyoxal (an α-oxaldehyde).

AGEs: Culinary Strategies

AGEs are naturally present in uncooked animal-derived foods and processed foods such as fruit and carbonated drinks. However, a wide variety of foods in modern diets are exposed to cooking or thermal processing for reasons of safety and convenience as well as to enhance flavor, color, and appearance. These processing steps can become a source of dietary AGEs. Recent studies using the oral administration of a single AGE-rich meal to human beings as well as labeled single protein-AGEs or diets enriched with specific AGEs to mice clearly show that dietary AGEs are absorbed and contribute significantly to the body's AGE pool. Culinary strategies to reduce AGEs can include alternative cooking methods as cooking can result in the formation of new AGEs. In particular, grilling, broiling, roasting, searing, and frying can increase and accelerate new AGE formation. High heat cooking has received the most attention for culinary reduction of AGEs.

Plant extracts are known to inhibit protein glycation that occurs during the AGE process. Polyphenols are thought to play a role in inhibiting protein glycation. Experimental studies using herbs and spices have identified particular spices and herbs that can inhibit AGE formation. In a study comparing common culinary herbs and spices, phenolics from spices were found to inhibit AGE, measured by index of albumin glycation, formation more than herbs (Dearlove et al., 2008). The most potent inhibitors included extracts of cloves, ground Jamaican allspice, and cinnamon. Potent herbs tested included sage, marjoram, tarragon, and rosemary. Overall, the concentration of phenolics that inhibited glycation by 50% was typically 4–12 g/mL.

In a similar study, however, involving the herbs thyme and parsley, the phenolic content and antioxidant potential of these ingredients were not related to the inhibition of advanced glycation products (Ramkissoon et al., 2012). This result suggests that for some herbs, substances other than phenolic compounds may be involved in inhibiting AGEs. Of note, these studies did not utilize cooking methods in the experiments to mimic home cooking conditions.

MICRONUTRIENTS

Our physiological response to sodium and potassium provides insight into the role of nutritional environments and blood pressure. Minimally processed foods contain very little sodium. Therefore, it was advantageous for the body to develop mechanisms that can promote retention of sodium, especially during stressful or threatening times when elevated blood pressure is needed to deliver oxygen to skeletal muscles. This regulation is found in the RAAS system in which low sodium levels in the kidney's filtrate or low pressure in the incoming blood vessel to the kidney's nephron lead to increased production of renin and the RAAS system.

In contrast to sodium, minimally processed foods largely contain the nutrient, potassium. Potassium regulation within the body thus is not as important for physiologic responses as the body's physiology system would have relied on steady intake through the diet. Interestingly, potassium supplementation or high dietary intake can promote natriuresis, loss of sodium within urine.

Sodium

Sodium is a required micronutrient of the body and is needed to maintain homeostasis by regulating the membrane potential, fluid volume, acid–base balance, and nervous system. Excessive dietary sodium is a major contributor to hypertension, with almost 1 in 3 Americans (Sacks et al., 2001; Aburto et al., 2013; Institute of Medicine, 2013). The Dietary Guidelines for Americans 2020 (USDA) recommend a maximum dietary sodium intake of 2300 mg/day for the general population and 1,500 mg/day for CVD at-risk groups, persons aged 51 years and above, and persons of any age with hypertension, diabetes, or chronic kidney disease, whereas the World Health Organization (WHO) (World Health Organization, 2012) recommends adults consume less than 2,000 mg of sodium or 5 g of salt.

Within the US diet, most exposure to sodium occurs through salt (sodium chloride (NaCl)) added to foods during food processing, as a food ingredient, a processing aid for food-safety reasons (IOM, 2013). Packaged foods and restaurant foods contribute more than 75% of dietary sodium in the US diet with about 10% sodium consumption occurring naturally in foods and 5%–10% from added salt during cooking or at a meal as discretionary salt (USDA, 2020). Two food categories contribute about 2/3rd of total sodium intake: "grain products" and "meat, poultry, fish, and mixtures" (Agarwal et al., 2015). One global study found that in European and Northern American countries, sodium intake is primarily from sodium added in manufactured foods (approximately 75% of intake) (Brown et al., 2009). Overall sodium intake across all population subgroups exceeds the Dietary Guidelines 2010 recommendations. However, sodium intake measured as a function of food intake has decreased significantly during the last decade for all US ethnicities (Fulgoni, 2014).

International guidelines recommend that all people consume less than 2.0 g of sodium per day. However, no randomized trials have demonstrated that reducing sodium leads to a reduction in CVD. In their absence, the next option is to examine the association between sodium consumption and CVD in observational studies. Several recent prospective cohort studies have indicated that while high intake of sodium (>6 g/day) is associated with higher risk of CVD compared to those with moderate intake (3–5 g/day), lower intake (<3 g/day) is also associated with a higher risk (despite lower blood pressure levels) (O'Donnell et al., 2014). However, most of these studies were conducted in populations at increased risk of CVD. Current epidemiologic evidence supports that an optimal level of sodium intake is in the range of about 3–5 g/day, as this range is associated with the lowest risk of CVD in prospective cohort studies. Interestingly, epidemiologic studies show that there is a J-shaped relationship for the relationship of sodium intake with mortality risk (Alderman & Cohen, 2012; Stolarz-Skrzypek et al., 2011). And one meta-analysis identified that sodium restriction is associated with higher cholesterol (LDL) and triglyceride (Graudal et al., 2020).

Salt: Types of Salt and CVD Risk Factors

Salt, sodium chloride (NaCl), is an inorganic mineral produced from salt mines or found in oceans and ultimately from the rocks that erode into the oceans. NaCl dissolves in water into separate single atoms that carry electrical charge (sodium ions positively charged and chloride ions negatively charged). These single atoms readily enter our foods, reacting with proteins and plant cell walls to generate flavor. There are several types of salt (sodium complexed with chloride) products available for consumer use (Table 5.1). The most commonly used salt is table salt, which is mined from underground salt deposits. It is then processed to give it a fine

---

TABLE 5.1

Types of Cooking Salt

Type of Salt	Description	Specified Culinary Use
Table salt	Most common salt. Usually from salt mines and mixed with trace amount of anticaking agents (e.g., calcium silicate) to prevent clumping.	Preferred in baking because of fine-grained texture and ability to provide accurate measurements.
Iodized table salt	Iodine added to table salt to prevent iodine deficiency.	
Sea salt	Unrefined salt derived from an ocean or sea. Harvested by channeling ocean water into large clay trays and allowing the sun and wind to evaporate the water naturally. Due to minimal processing, contains traces of minerals: iron, magnesium, calcium, potassium, manganese, zinc, iodine.	Coarse salt is a larger grained sea salt crystal. Resists caking because it is less moisture-sensitive.

(Continued)

TABLE 5.1 (*Continued*)
Types of Cooking Salt

Type of Salt	Description	Specified Culinary Use
Coarse salt	Coarse salt is a larger grained sea salt crystal.	Resists caking because it is less moisture-sensitive.
Kosher salt	Kosher salt is made of crystals that are larger and rougher than other salt crystals. The larger crystals are ideal for curing meat, a step in the koshering process.	Flakes dissolve easily and have less pungent flavor than table salt. Salt of choice for making seasoning mixes. Diamond Crystal Kosher salt has crystals that are hollow and therefore has half the sodium of regular table salt for the same volume: ! teaspoon contains 1,120 mg of sodium.
Pickling salt	Table salt without anticaking agents.	Anticaking agents are removed as they do not dissolve as readily as salt and therefore can cloud brines.
Celtic salt	Naturally moist salt harvested from Atlantic seawater off the coast of Brittany, France. Hand harvesting process in traditional Celtic manner using wooden rakes instead of metal ones.	Because of moisture and no caking agents, clumping may occur.
Fleur de Sel (flower of salt)	Artisan sea salt composed of young crystals that naturally form on the surface of salt evaporation ponds. Harvested by hand under specific weather conditions. Usually comes from salt beds of west-central France. Characteristic aroma occurs from traces of algae.	Due to the expense of the labor-intensive salt, used as last-minute condiment when cooking with salt.
Hawaiian red sea salt	Natural mineral volcanic red clay is added to enrich natural salt with iron oxide.	Clay imparts subtler flavor than other salts.
Himalayan sea salt	Natural salt mined from salt rocks in the Himalayan region. The salt rock imparts the pink color.	
Encapsulated salt	Salt crystals encased in fat.	Can block ability of salt to bind to protein and provide juicing texture with meat.
Salt substitutes	Salts made from potassium chloride.	Impart salty, bitter or metallic taste.
Light salt	Blend of salt substitute and salt.	May lessen adverse tastes present in salt substitutes.

Source: Information in table adapted from Powers and Hess (2010, pp. 229–230); McGee (2004, pp. 641–644).

texture, but the processing steps remove minerals from the salt. During processing, additives are also added to prevent clumping. Sea salt is produced by the evaporation of seawater which naturally contains sodium and other minerals. There is expected variation in the amount of minerals within sea water depending on the environment in which the minerals are precipitated. Studies evaluating the sodium content between table and sea salt have varied minimally, consistently showing similar sodium amounts of one teaspoon equating to approximately 2,300 mg of sodium. However, differences in minerals due to processing step differences are expected. For instance, Fayet-Moore et al (2020) found that among 31 different Himalayan pink sea salt brands (salt made from rock salt located close to the Himalayas) available in Australia, one teaspoon (5 g) of pink salt contained minerals including potassium, calcium, and magnesium. However, the amounts of minerals were trace and were not expected to make a clinically significant contribution to nutrient intake. In addition to nutritive minerals, there may also be concerns about nonnutritive minerals among pink salt in particular. Although the study found levels of cadmium and lead in the salt products, at least for cadmium, the levels did not surpass recommended levels.

Despite the trace amounts of beneficial micronutrients in sea salt, there may be biological effects of sea salt and iodized salt to consider. In mouse models, mice given iodized salt had an increase in the incidence of obesity when compared to mice given naturally manufactured salt. Conversely, sea salt has been previously reported to help prevent obesity in high-fat diet-induced obese mice (Ju et al., 2016). Park et al. found a significant decrease in body weight in a group of mice fed a high-fat diet and given cube sea salt versus iodized (NaCl) salt after 12–16 weeks. Furthermore, the high-fat diet and iodized salt group had more accumulated lipid droplets and increased number of liver inflammatory cells than the cube seal salt group (Park et al., 2020). It is important to note that these studies provide interesting hypotheses about the role of iodine in obesity. However, to date, these findings are reported in mouse models, and the effects of sea salt and iodized salt on body weight in humans remain to be determined.

Sodium and Salt: Culinary Strategies

In cooking, salt increases the water-binding capacity of proteins, thus increasing the juiciness of meat and poultry (Powers and Hess, 2010, p.228). Salt also helps to stabilize batter and extends shelf life through its antimicrobial effects. Therefore, salt is often used in professional culinary settings, such as restaurants, but many menu items exceed the total daily recommendation for sodium intake. For example, a three-course meal of an appetizer, an entrée, and a dessert in some restaurants averages 4,545 mg sodium, or 198% of the recommended daily dietary intake (Monlezun et al., 2015). With Americans eating more outside of the home in recent years, finding ways to decrease sodium intake within restaurant foods becomes important. In a study of 105 individuals, Monlezun et al. found that a 15% reduction in sodium in restaurant-prepared recipes was undetected by participants in comparison to a recipe that had 0% reduction in sodium (Monlezun et al., 2015). Similarly, studies involving taste acceptability of the DASH diet found that both the intermediate and lower sodium levels of each diet are at least as acceptable as the higher sodium level in persons with or at risk for hypertension (Karanja et al., 2007).

Food-based strategies to reduce sodium but still maintain enhancement of taste intensity is shown through modulating spatial distribution of tastants (ingredients that register taste). This strategy shows the potential to avoid undesirable changes in sensory properties and is based on the contrast between areas with high and low concentration or the presence of a high concentration of tastants on the surface of the food, and how the location can determine an improvement in taste perception. Greater degree in the heterogeneity of spatial aroma distribution could reportedly increase perceived intensity and duration of oral processing.

Cross-modal perception is perception that involves interactions between two or more different sensory modalities. Flavor is a cerebral construction resulting from the integration in the brain of chemosensory signals derived from food, such as smell, colors, texture, temperature, sound, and trigeminal sensations (i.e., mouth dryness with tannins). Studies show that cross-modal odor-taste interactions can aid in sodium reduction (Thomas-Danguin et al., 2019). The interaction is hypothesized to occur because olfactory cues might enhance perception of the salty taste. Taste-odor interactions are also reported to result in sweet taste. The use of aromas could be an efficient strategy and known as odor-induced saltiness enhancement (OISE). Several salt-associated odors/aromas have been observed to induce saltiness enhancement, such as cheese, soy sauce, sardine, ham, and bacon (Lawrence et al., 2009). An aroma could be used to enhance salty taste in foods containing a small amount of NaCl and may compensate for up to a 20% decrease in the food salt content (Thomas-Danguin et al., 2019). Of note, if the salt concentration is already high, the aroma-taste interaction has a weaker effect (Ponzo, et al., 2021).

Salt is not only an ingredient, but it is also the only food that represents the taste, salt. Taste signifies the connection of the tongue and taste buds in the mouth to recognize the basic tastes of sweet, sour, bitter, salty, and umami. In sodium-reduced cooking, involving the balance of tastes is crucial to maintaining intended tastes and pleasure from ingredient compounds. Taste-to-taste interactions occur at the level of epithelial cells on the tongue but also have cognitive mechanism involving messaging of taste to the brain. In relation to reduction of salt, these taste-to-taste interactions can be leveraged while cooking. For example, salt and sour mixtures symmetrically affect intensity of the other, with enhancement at low concentrations and suppression or no effect at high intensities/concentration (Breslin and Beauchamp, 1997). Moreover, sweetness suppresses salty taste at moderate intensities. Salt also potentiates flavor through concentration-dependent suppression of bitterness and the release of sweetness (Breslin and Beauchamp, 1997). In fact, it is hypothesized the preference for salt may stem from the ability of salt to suppress unpleasant flavors, like bitterness.

Utilization of herbs and spices can also be useful to help reduce sodium intake while preserving taste and flavor. It is possible that use of additional herbs increases the intensity of certain aromas and flavors in a cross-modal interaction, and this leads to the increased saltiness perception. In a controlled taste study, the addition of oregano, basil, marjoram, thyme, and bay leaf leads to maintenance of flavor in the presence of sodium reduction in both tomato and chicken noodle soup (Wang et al., 2014). A blend of the herbs and spices cumin, ginger, paprika, and turmeric maintained flavor in legume dishes as tested with 94 participants in a randomized cross-over study despite a 50% reduction in sodium from the control dishes (Dougkas et al., 2019). There is a potential application for this approach in the home setting. In a multifactorial behavioral intervention among adults at risk for CVD

(Anderson et al., 2015), culinary education sessions including the utilization of herbs in home cooking settings led to a reduction of sodium measured by urinary sodium excretion.

A potential strategy for salt reduction is based on the position of salt in food matrices. This strategy is based on the contrast between areas with high and low concentration or the presence of a high concentration of taste on the surface of the food. The overall effect is on taste perception. A greater degree in the heterogeneity of spatial aroma distribution can increase perceived intensity, duration of oral processing, and the saliva content in the bolus (Konitzer et al., 2013; Ponzo et al., 2021). The increase in heterogeneity distribution of tastes in various salt containing food products, such as sausages, can significantly increase the intensity of taste. In home cooking situations, this strategy could be done by salting food after cooking, just before the consumption, so that the NaCl crystals remain on the surface (Ponzo et al., 2021).

Reduction of sodium intake can also occur through use of salt substitutes. These substitutes are often made from potassium chloride. Although reduced exposure to sodium occurs with these substitutes, there may be increased salty taste that occurs with cooking. Other tastes associated with the use of KCl include bitter or metallic (Sinopoli and Lawless, 2012). Moreover, use of potassium chloride for seasoning may not be recommended for individuals with chronic kidney conditions, a condition in which sodium reduction is often optimal. For these individuals, use of other sodium reduction strategies may be useful.

POTASSIUM

Potassium decreases intravascular volume on a short-term basis, partly through decreased sodium reabsorption, i.e., increased urinary sodium excretion. Other putative mechanisms of action for potassium including alterations in baroreflex sensitivity and sensitivity to receptors and hormones that influence vascular smooth muscle and sympathetic nervous system cell function have been postulated (Houston, 2011). These effects may be important to lowering blood pressure in addition to the natriuretic effects of potassium.

The average US dietary intake of potassium (K+) is 45 mEq per day, which is equivalent to a potassium to sodium (K+/Na+) ratio of less than 1:2 (Houston and Harper, 2008). However, the recommended intake of K+ is 650 mEq per day with a K+/Na+ ratio of over 5:1. To date, meta-analyses have found inconsistent results in multiple studies (Weaver, 2013). However, through an analysis of four meta-analyses, Houston (2011) suggests that there is a dose-response effect with potassium that should be considered.

Potassium intake decreased with the agricultural revolution when energy intake shifted from a variety of plants including potassium-rich tubers to cereals. Potassium intake then further decreased with a shift to highly refined processed foods (Weaver, 2013). Naturally, potassium is found mostly in fruits and vegetables. Potatoes are a high source of potassium (300 mg/100 g). But for Americans, the top dietary potassium sources are milk, coffee, chicken and beef dishes, orange and grapefruit juice, and potatoes. Potassium in foods is present with phosphate, sulfate, citrate, and many organic anions including proteins.

Although potassium is advantageous for blood pressure, it is important to note some medical conditions in which increased potassium intake is not recommended. These can include chronic kidney disease and renal conditions that occur more often with diabetes, such as type 4 renal tubular acidosis.

Potassium: Culinary Strategies

Like other minerals, potassium is reduced with cooking. However, culinary methods can be used to prevent the loss of potassium and other minerals. These methods include the following (Kimura and Itokawa, 1990):

- Consuming the boiled food with the liquid
- Addition of a small amount of salt (about 1% NaCl) in boiling water
- Avoid excess boiling
- Select mineral protective cooking methods, such as stewing

Cookware may also be a factor in preventing loss of minerals such as potassium. Water-free cooking using muti-ply cookware that allows for water-free cooking was assessed in comparison with traditional cookware in a study of 57 participants by Mori et al. (2012). Biomarkers of 24-hour urinary potassium and vitamin C were used to determine vegetable intake. Participants in the cookware experimental group were provided vegetables daily for 2 weeks and instructed to consume 350 g of vegetables daily. Photographs of food during cooking, serving plates, and post eating were provided to research staff. Participants in the water-free cookware group had significantly higher potassium levels after 2 weeks compared to their baseline and compared to the traditional cookware group and control group.

For individuals on a potassium-restricted diet, loss of potassium with cooking is advantageous. As mentioned earlier, within minimally processed foods, white potatoes are high sources of potassium. Retention or loss of potassium in white potatoes is particularly sensitive to preparation and cooking methods. Methods that retain minerals within white potatoes include boiling potatoes whole, bake potatoes once, roast potatoes, or microwave potatoes (Bethke and Jansky, 2008). While cutting or shredding potatoes into small pieces and then boiling the small pieces for 10 minutes can decrease potassium levels by 50%–75% (Bethke and Jansky, 2008). Additionally, double boiling small pieces of potatoes can reduce potassium levels among a variety of potatoes including Idaho, red bliss, Yukon, purple, and fingerling (Burrowes and Ramer, 2008).

MAGNESIUM

A high dietary intake of magnesium of at least 500–1,000 mg/day is associated with decreases in BP in most of the reported epidemiologic, observational, and clinical trials, but the results are less consistent than those seen with Na+ and K+ (Houston and Harper, 2008). In most epidemiologic studies, there is an inverse relationship between dietary magnesium intake and BP (Laurant and Touyz, 2000). A study of 60 essential hypertensive subjects given magnesium supplements showed a significant reduction in BP over an 8-week period documented by 24-hour ambulatory BP, home, and office BP. Magnesium competes with Na+ for binding sites on vascular smooth muscle and acts like a calcium channel blocker, increases prostaglandin E (PGE), and binds in a necessary-cooperative manner with potassium, inducing vasodilation and BP reduction. Magnesium may also have a role to play in other CVD risk factors, as it helps to regulate insulin sensitivity. Interestingly, magnesium is an essential cofactor for the delta6-desaturase enzyme that is the rate-limiting step for conversion of linoleic acid (omega-6) to gamma-linolenic acid. In terms of CVD, GLA elongates to form dihomogamma-linoleic acid (DGLA), the precursor of prostaglandin E1, a vasodilator and platelet inhibitor (Sergeant et al., 2016).

ZINC

Low serum zinc levels in observational studies correlate with hypertension as well as in type II diabetes, hyperlipidemia, elevated lipoprotein (a), 2-hour postprandial plasma insulin levels, and insulin resistance (Garcia Zozaya and Padilla Viloria, 1997). In addition, zinc plays a role in insulin resistance, membrane ion exchange, RAAS, and SNS effects. Zinc is also a factor in the enzyme-based elongation of linoleic acid (omega-6) to GLA and to DGLA, as animal models have shown that the desaturase enzymes key for this elongation are dependent on zinc availability (Knez et al., 2017).

Magnesium and Zinc: Culinary Strategies

As discussed earlier in this chapter, vegetables are a source of nutrients, including fiber, vitamins, and polyphenols that are protective for CVD. Particular vegetables, such as green leafy vegetables contain significant amounts of these nutrients, and consumption can aid in protection from CVD. Understanding cooking methods which can preserve some these nutrients is thus important. Further explanations on cooking methods to preserve minerals, such as magnesium, within vegetables can be found in Chapter 2, Effects of Food Processing, Storage, and Manufacturing on Nutrients.

MACRONUTRIENTS

Higher intakes of total fat, saturated fatty acids, and carbohydrates are associated with higher blood pressure, whereas higher protein intake is reportedly associated with lower blood pressure. Replacement of saturated fatty acids with carbohydrates was associated with the most adverse effects on lipids, whereas replacement of saturated fatty acids with unsaturated fats improved some risk markers (LDL cholesterol and blood pressure) but seemed to worsen others (HDL cholesterol and triglycerides). The observed associations between saturated fatty acids and CVD events were approximated by the simulated associations mediated through the effects on the ApoB-to-ApoA1 ratio but not with other lipid markers including LDL cholesterol (Mente et al., 2017).

PROTEIN

Protein can have both protective and contributory effects on blood pressure. Proteins are comprised of amino acids. Amino acids can potentially influence the cardiovascular system through the microbiome, brain, and vascular biology. Short-term, strictly controlled, randomized clinical trials show a BP-lowering effect of increased protein intake, but longer and less controlled trials show inconsistent results. In addition, most controlled feeding trials with protein have exchanged carbohydrates for proteins. The primary macronutrient component of pulses is protein. Data from the prospective study INTER-SALT (International Study of Sodium, Potassium and Blood Pressure) indicated that 37 g/day of protein leads to a decrease in SBP (by 3 mmHg) and DBP (by 2.5 mmHg).

Investigations of specific amino acids have identified several amino acids involved in blood pressure regulation. These include branched chain amino acids (BCAA), arginine, methionine, and the aromatic amino acids, including tryptophan. Of these amino acids, the most consistent evidence in the literature is from studies on dietary supplementation of arginine for lowering blood pressure. However, studies using dietary sources for arginine have not shown consistent results.

The type of protein source may be an important factor in the BP effect, animal protein being less effective than nonanimal protein (Appel, 2003). However, lean or wild animal protein with less saturated fat and more essential omega-3 and omega-6 fatty acids may reduce BP, lipids, and CHD risk. When compared to animal proteins, plant proteins have a reduced content of key amino acids, such as methionine, lysine, and tryptophan. Among population-based studies evaluating plant versus animal protein, plant protein is found to have the stronger association with lower blood pressure. However, vegetarians have a significantly higher intake of the nonessential amino acids arginine, glycine, alanine, and serine. And vegetarians are also more likely to be exposed to a low content of other putative metabolic stressors, such as saturated fats and certain lipid-derived compounds present in protein sources of animal origin. The specific amino acids from plant proteins that relate to blood pressure remain mostly unknown; however, soy protein studies with blood pressure as an endpoint suggest that soy may be a plant protein of interest. Hemp protein is a plant-based source of the amino acid arginine, and studies involving spontaneous hypertensive rats show blood pressure-lowering response with hemp seed administration.

Animal and plant protein sources may also contain peptides, short chain of amino acids, that can influence blood pressure. Bioactive peptides remain inactive when bonded to other amino acids within the primary structure of a food protein, but after release via hydrolysis, the free forms of these peptides can affect biological processes. Bioactive peptides have been shown to act as antihypertensive agents by inhibiting renin, ACE, and angiotensin-II receptor activities and enhancing blood NO levels. Different types of bioactive peptides, derived from numerous sources including dairy, meat, fish, poultry, canola, buckwheat, algae, and hemp, have shown hypotensive effects in animal models (Samsamikor et al., 2020).

Protein: Culinary Strategies

Protein structure is affected by cooking methods. This is especially relevant for sources of animal protein cooking contributes to the oxidative cleavage of the porphyrin ring, and in turn heme-iron can be released and accelerate oxidative deterioration. Furthermore, oxidation in meat induced by cooking can be partly attributed to the fact that the meat loses its natural antioxidant properties when heated. Heat can also cause damage to the cellular structure of meat, making it more exposed to oxygen, and triggering reactive oxygen species (ROS). The ROS can subsequently attack lipid and protein molecules producing lipid and protein oxidation. Other considerations with cooking and protein extend beyond animal sources. Those include the fact that cooking methods can increase absolute amino acid concentrations and availability.

ALLIUM VEGETABLES: GARLIC AND ONION

The allium vegetables, onion (*Allium cepa*) and garlic (*Allium sativum*), are recognized as antiplatelet agents that may contribute to the prevention of CVD. When fresh Allium tissues are crushed, then cytoplasmic precursors called S-alk(en)yl-L-cysteine sulfoxides (ACSOs) are cleaved by the enzyme alliinase, which converts ACSOs to sulfenic acids. Ultimately, the unstable sulfenic acids condense into pairs and form thiosulfinates. Due to the presence of thiosulfinates, garlic has both blood pressure-lowering and cholesterol-lowering properties. Studies have found that garlic has antioxidant, antithrombotic, antimicrobial, antitumor, and anti-inflammatory activities. Components of garlic that relate to these properties include at least 100 volatile and nonvolatile sulfur-containing bioactive compounds. These components include S-allylcysteine, saponins, ajoene, flavonoids, and phenolics. The pungent smell of garlic hails from thiosulfinates of which allicin makes up 70%–80% within garlic (Shouk et al., 2014). Not all garlic preparations are processed similarly and are not comparable in antihypertensive potency (Houston, 2011). In addition, cultivated garlic (*Allium sativum*), wild uncultivated garlic, or bear garlic (*Allium ursinum*) and aged or fresh garlic and long-acting garlic preparations will have variable effects. Approximately 10,000 mg of allicin (one of the active ingredients in garlic) per day, the amount contained in four cloves of garlic (4 g), is required to achieve a significant BP-lowering effect.

Onions differ in their thiosulfinate content from garlic. Onions contain lachrymatory factor (LF) synthase enzymes, which convert sulfenic acids into the LF responsible for inducing tearing when raw onions are chopped (Cavagnaro and Galmarini, 2012). With regard to CVD health, the reaction between the LF and sulfenic acids leads to the antiplatelet cepaenes and other sulfur compounds within onions.

Garlic and Onion: Culinary Strategies

Allium vegetables are not consumed raw, and the bioactive compounds are relatively unstable. Thus, it is important to determine how cooking methods may disrupt the CVD protective properties from garlic. In a study of the antiplatelet effect of allicin, heating garlic at 200°C for under 6 minutes led to a reduction in the antiplatelet effect for garlic that was uncrushed prior to heating (Cavagnaro et al., 2007). However, garlic that was crushed did not lose the effect completely. Most importantly, the partial loss of antithrombotic effect for crushed garlic was compensated through increasing the amount of garlic.

For onions, the effects of cooking are not as straightforward as for garlic. Similar to garlic, studies find that crushing onion prior to cooking can lead to contrasting results depending on cooking times. To provide a comparison with garlic, Cavagnaro et al. evaluated effects of microwave (t 500 W for 0.75, 1.5, and 3.0 s/g of fresh weight) and convection gas oven (heated to 200°C) heating on the antiplatelet activity of onions. Crushed onions lost all antiplatelet activity after 10 minutes of convection oven heating comparable to raw onions. In comparison, whole onions lost theirs after 30 minutes. When microwaved, both whole and crushed onions lost entire activity after less than 4 minutes, with whole onions losing activity before crushed ones. The difference between crushed and whole onions is important to highlight. In crushed onions, the alliinase enzyme action has already started and the antiplatelet activity depends on loss of thiosulfinates. In comparison, in whole onions, antiplatelet activity depends on the effect of heat on alliinase activity. Lastly, this study observed a proaggregatory effect for crushed onions after 20–30 minutes of convection oven heating. This finding may be explained by presence of more heat tolerant platelet stimulating compounds present in onions. Other studies have reported similar results of proaggregatory effects of onions with extensive heating, such as boiling (Chen et al., 1999). This potential pro-platelet activity with extensively cooked onions might be offset with inclusion of other antiplatelet action, such as flavonoids, in a meal or dish.

POLYPHENOLS

TEA

All types of tea: black, green, white, and oolong, are made from the leaves of the *Camellia sinensis* plant. The plant grows indigenously in tepid climates within China, Japan, India, and Thailand. To make green tea, freshly picked leaves are immediately steamed and parched (Matthews, 2010). This processing time and step leads green tea to contain more of the polyphenols, catechins. In comparison, black tea is made through fermentation of the tea leaves, and this processing leads to a different polyphenol profile, theaflavins.

The effects of long-term green or black tea ingestion on BP in humans have not been studied extensively, and the results are inconsistent (Hodgson et al. 1999). However, green tea and black tea contain extracts of active components, catechins, that have demonstrated reduction in BP. The catechin epigallocatechin gallate (EGCG) in green tea is one example. A meta-analysis of nine observational and intervention studies with CVD events and outcome found that individuals who did not consume green tea had higher risks of CVD, intracerebral hemorrhage, and cerebral infarction compared to <1 cup green tea per day (Pang et al., 2016). While individuals who drank 1–3 cups per day or ≥4 cups/day had a reduced risk of myocardial infarction and stroke compared to those who drank <1 cup per day.

GREEN TEA: CULINARY METHODS

Brewing temperature and time can have a significant effect on the amount of catechins present in green tea (Saklar et al., 2015; Vuong et al., 2011). Brewing at a temperature of 85°C leads to the highest retention of EGCG compared to 75°C or 95°C. This temperature corresponds to water that is not yet boiling. Steeping times that maximize the concentration of EGCG are no more than 3 minutes. Prolonged steeping can lead to significant loss of EGCG. Additionally, the amount of caffeine in green tea is maximized at temperatures and time optimal for EGCG retention.

LYCOPENE

Lycopene is a lipophile carotenoid polyphenol found in tomato and tomato products. Lycopene has antihypertensive effects due to the ability to inhibit ACE and due to its antioxidant effect, reducing oxidative stress induced by angiotensin-II and indirectly enhancing production of nitric oxide in the endothelium (Li and Xu, 2013; Khan et al., 2016; Paran et al., 2009, Ren et al., 2017). A study including 8,556 adult overweight and obese participants demonstrated association of lycopene and lycopene/uric acid ratio with lower prevalence of hypertension (Han and Liu, 2017). Paran et al. reported a decrease in both systolic and DBP in 54 patients with moderate hypertension, treated with ACE inhibitors or calcium channel blockers, after 6 weeks of tomato extract supplementation, suggesting a cause-effect relationship (Paran et al., 2009). Li and Xu concluded, in a metanalysis, that lycopene supplementation (more than 12 mg/day) might significantly reduce systolic, but not DBP, in prehypertensive or hypertensive patients (Li and Xu, 2013).

Lycopene: Culinary Strategies

Since lycopene is lipid-soluble, consuming lycopene-rich foods like tomato or watermelon with fat increases its bioavailability. For example, consuming salads with full-fat dressing results in higher blood carotenoid levels than eating salads with reduced fat dressing. However, when salads were consumed without fat in the same study, no measurable lycopene uptake occurred. The consumption of tomato salsa with avocado (as lipid source) can led to a 4.4-fold increase in lycopene absorption as compared with salsa without avocado (Arballo et al., 2021).

Several lycopene isomers (different arrangement of atoms within the molecule) are present in nature. About 90% of the lycopene in dietary sources is found in the linear, all-trans conformation. This conformation is not easily absorbed into human tissues. The cis-isomers of lycopene which have a shorter length are better absorbed due to better solubility in micelles and lower tendency to aggregate (Boileau et al., 2002). A particular cis-isomer of lycopene is the Z (cis)-lycopene, especially because of its antioxidant capacity. Recent studies have focused on producing ingredients and products with a high content of Z-lycopene isomers, using organic solvents and vegetable oils (Honda et al., 2019). Ingredients such as EVOO and the components of the Mediterranean-based sofrito may provide higher content of Z-lycopene. In one study of home ingredients used for sofrito, EVOO, garlic, and onion, the use of onion improved the bioavailability of lycopene in the tomato products when cooked by the traditional method of heating EVOO for 1 minute at low to medium heat (4 on range), sautéing chopped onions and garlic for 1 minute, and then adding chopped tomatoes and lowering heat (2 on range). The findings of this study may explain that of Hurtado-Barraso et al. who found that a single dose of 240 g (~1 cup)/70 kg tomato sofrito in the presence of a low-antioxidant diet decreased both TNF-α and C-reactive protein levels after 24 hours.

Because Z-isomer lycopene exhibits greater bioavailability and antioxidant activity, and most recently exhibited equal or higher antiobesity activity than the all-E-isomers, it is important to identify foods that increase the content of Z-isomers when cooking tomato-based ingredients. One study by Honda et al. evaluated 131 kids of food ingredients on the Z-isomer content of tomato puree (lycopene content, 12 mg/100 g; Z-isomer content, 9.2%) lycopene under the heat conditions of 80°C (126°F) for 1 hour (Honda et al., 2019). The top five ingredients that promoted Z-isomerization of lycopene were dried Kurome (21.6%), dried kombu (20.9%), fresh wild arugula, (20.2%), fresh arugula, (20.1%), fresh wasabi, and dried hijiki (20.0%). Other foods identified as important for Z-isomerization included onion, garlic and leek, as found in other studies. Brassica species, such as mustard seed, and the Raphanus species, such as daikon radish, were also identified, as well as shitake mushrooms. The authors hypothesize that polysulfides (shitake mushrooms), isothiocyanates (*Brassica* and *Raphanus* species; wasabi), carbon disulfide (arugula), and iodine (seaweed) are the major causative food compounds that promote Z-isomerization. Interestingly, polysulfides, carbon disulfide, and iodine display electrophilic properties. Moreover, the attention to electrophilic properties of foods is also supported by studies that show that ferrous iron, an electrophilic metal, promotes Z-isomerization of carotenoids (Honda et al., 2015).

Fiber

Within vegetables, two types of fiber exist: soluble and insoluble. Insoluble fiber includes plant cellulose and lignans, while soluble fiber includes guar gum, beta-glucans, pectins, and psyllium.

Relevant to CVD risk factor reduction, soluble fibers can lower cholesterol through binding of bile acids. The available bile acid pool is related to levels of cholesterol as a function of the enterohepatic system, which regulates the production of cholesterol in relation to absorption of intestinal bile acids. When the available bile acid pool is decreased, then cholesterol production is decreased. Medications that bind intestinal bile acids deplete the endogenous bile acid pool by approximately 40%. This binding can increase bile acid synthesis from cholesterol, thus reducing low-lipoprotein cholesterol (LDL-C) by 15%–26% (Insull, 2006).

Fiber: Culinary Methods

The ability of vegetables, in particular green leafy vegetables, to bind bile acids and decrease the available pool is influenced by cooking methods. To study the ability of cooked vegetables to bind bile acids, in vitro digestion models are used to mimic the mouth, stomach, and duodenal environments. Water-based cooking methods that involve minimal cooking of kale greens, microwaving at 3 minutes and steaming at 8 minutes, showed preservation of bile acid-binding capacity in comparison to the cholestyramine, a bile acid-binding cholesterol-lowering medicine (Yang et al., 2017; Kahlon et al., 2008). Kahlon et al. (2008) found that under steaming conditions, differences in bile acid-binding capacity of vegetables occurred: collard greens = kale = mustard greens > broccoli > Brussels sprouts = spinach = green bell pepper > cabbage.

TURMERIC AND CURCUMIN

Curcumin is a major phenolic component of the spice turmeric. Curcumin has multiple functions that can affect CVD, including anti-inflammatory, antioxidant, and lipid-modifying. Several human trials have reported reduction of blood pressure levels with curcumin/turmeric administration (Hadi et al., 2019). However, the results from trials have provided conflicting evidence with some trials reporting no significant changes (Hadi et al., 2019). A meta-synthesis of 11 studies equating to 748 patients found that the duration of curcumin ($\geq$12-weeks) is a significant factor in lowering SBP, a significant reduction in SBP with mean reduction of about 1.24 mmHg (Hadi et al., 2019). Possible mechanisms for the role of curcumin in blood pressure include increase bioavailability of nitric oxide (Santos-Parker et al., 2017) and downregulation of angiotensin-II receptor-1 (Yao et al., 2016).

Turmeric and Curcumin: Culinary Strategies

Turmeric is widely used in certain traditional cuisines, and its health-promoting benefits through use in cooking have been widely reported. Because it is fat-soluble, the bioavailability of curcumin is increased in the presence of fats (Stohs et al., 2020). In addition, black pepper (piperine) in small amounts can stimulate the gastrointestinal system, thus preventing efflux of curcumin (Stohs et al., 2020). However, curcumin's overall poor systemic bioavailability fails to explain the reported effects. Studies that have investigated this quandary find that the degradation products from curcumin in fact maintain oxygen scavenging activity than the curcumin parent compound (Shen et al., 2016). Food processing can help to regulate biological activity of plant bioactive substances. Therefore, the next logical line of investigation is to identify whether processing that may occur during cooking may affect the activity of these degradation products. A series of experiments have been reported in which turmeric (1mg/mL) is boiled (heated for 1 hour in water at 100°C), roasted (200°C for 1 hour with an electric heating pan dryer), and fried (150°C for 10 minutes in blended edible oils) and then applied to rat neuronal cells in addition to measuring antioxidant activity using total antioxidant capacity (Sun et al., 2019). When comparing these three cooking methods, boiling and roasting were found to maintain antioxidant activity more than frying. However, all cooking methods had lower activity than the uncooked curcumin. Thus, with an average amount of 200 mg curcumin within one teaspoon of turmeric (Tayyem et al., 2006), cooking with turmeric may indeed preserve the function of curcumin needed to maintain antioxidant properties and CVD protection.

CARDIOVASCULAR KEY POINTS

- Dietary patterns such as the Mediterranean diet can be helpful particularly with use of EVOO and regular physical activity. Avoiding dietary patterns that increase uric acid may also be helpful.
- To date, nutrition-based prevention of CVD has focused on reduction of risk factors, such as hypertension.
- Relevant cooking methods to maintain cardiovascular protective nutrients include the following:
  - EVOO – heating under moderate heat can increase the amount of polyphenol lignan, found to be a significant polyphenol for CVD protection
  - Allium vegetables (onions and garlic) – crushing garlic prior to heating prevents the heat-induced loss of antiplatelet activity chemicals, thiosulfinates
  - SOFRITO – use of onions in combination with tomatoes in SOFRITO increases availability of the polyphenol lycopene

Edible blended oils are made with different vegetable fats and contain different nutrition qualities and prices. Different manufacturers in the blended oil market produce many different brands of blended oils. Studies evaluating the main ingredients of general blended oils have found sunflower oil, soybean, corn germ, and cottonseed oils might be added. Cost and price are also a factor in determining the ingredients used in blended oils. The main ingredient in low-cost blended oils is rapeseed oil, to which soybean oil is often added (Xu et al., 2016).

REFERENCES

Aburto NJ, Ziolkovska A, Hooper L, Elliott P, Meerpohl JJ. Effect of lower sodium intake on health: systematic review and meta-analyses. *Br Med J.* 2013;346:f1326.

Aeberli I, Hochuli M, Gerber PA, Sze L, Murer SB, Tappy L, Spinas GA, Berneis K. Moderate amounts of fructose consumption impair insulin sensitivity in healthy young men: a randomized controlled trial. *Diabetes Care.* 2013 Jan;36(1):150–6.

Agarwal S, Fulgoni VL 3rd, Spence L, Samuel P. Sodium intake status in United States and potential reduction modeling: an NHANES 2007–2010 analysis. *Food Sci Nutr.* 2015;3(6):577–85. Published 2015 Jun 9. doi:10.1002/fsn3.248.

Alderman MH, Cohen HW. Dietary sodium intake and cardiovascular mortality: controversy resolved? *Am J Hypertens.* 2012;25:727–34.

American College of Cardiology and American Heart Association Hypertension Guidelines. https://www.acc.org/latest-in-cardiology/articles/2017/11/08/11/47/mon-5pm-bp-guideline-aha-2017.

Anderson CA, Cobb LK, Miller ER 3rd, et al. Effects of a behavioral intervention that emphasizes spices and herbs on adherence to recommended sodium intake: results of the SPICE randomized clinical trial. *Am J Clin Nutr.* 2015;102(3):671–9.

Appel LJ. The effects of protein intake on blood pressure and cardiovascular disease. *Curr Opin Lipidol.* 2003 Feb;14(1):55–9.

Appel LJ, Moore TJ, Obarzanek E, Vollmer WM, Svetkey LP, Sacks FM, Bray GA, Vogt TM, Cutler JA, Windhauser MM, Lin PH, Karanja N. A clinical trial of the effects of dietary patterns on blood pressure. DASH Collaborative Research Group. *N Engl J Med.* 1997 Apr 17;336(16):1117–24.

Arballo J, Amengual J, Erdman JW Jr. Lycopene: a critical review of digestion, absorption, metabolism, and excretion. *Antioxidants (Basel).* 2021 Feb 25;10(3):342.

Attya M, Benabdelkamel H, Perri E, Russo A, Sindona G. Effects of conventional heating on the stability of major olive oil phenolic compounds by tandem mass spectrometry and isotope dilution assay. *Molecules.* 2010;15:8734–46.

Baena M, Sangüesa G, Dávalos A, Latasa MJ, Sala-Vila A, Sánchez RM, Roglans N, Laguna JC, Alegret M. Fructose, but not glucose, impairs insulin signaling in the three major insulin-sensitive tissues. *Sci Rep.* 2016 May 19;6:26149.

Bethke PC, Jansky SH. The effects of boiling and leaching on the content of potassium and other minerals in potatoes. *J Food Sci.* 2008 Jun;73(5):H80–5.

Boileau TW, Boileau AC, Erdman JW Jr. Bioavailability of all-trans and cis-isomers of lycopene. *Exp Biol Med (Maywood).* 2002 Nov;227(10):914–9.

Bray GA. Energy and fructose from beverages sweetened with sugar or high-fructose corn syrup pose a health risk for some people. *Adv Nutr.* 2013 Mar 1;4(2):220–5.

Breslin P, Beauchamp G. Salt enhances flavour by suppressing bitterness. *Nature.* 1997;387:563.

Brown IJ, Tzoulaki I, Candeias V, Elliott P. Salt intakes around the world: implications for public health. *Int J Epidemiol.* 2009 Jun;38(3):791–813.

Burrowes JD, Ramer NJ. Changes in potassium content of different potato varieties after cooking. *J Ren Nutr.* 2008 Nov;18(6):530–4.

Cavagnaro PF, Galmarini CR. Effect of processing and cooking conditions on onion (Allium cepa L.) induced antiplatelet activity and thiosulfinate content. *J Agric Food Chem.* 2012;60(35):8731–7.

Cavagnaro PF, Camargo A, Galmarini CR, Simon PW. Effect of cooking on garlic (Allium sativum L.) antiplatelet activity and thiosulfinates content. *J Agric Food Chem.* 2007 Feb 21;55(4):1280–8.

Cerretani L, Bendini A, Rodriguez-Estrada MT, Vittadini E, Chiavaro E. Microwave heating of different commercial categories of olive oil: part I. Effect on chemical oxidative stability indices and phenolic compounds. *Food Chem.* 2009;115:1381–8.

Chen JH, Tsai SJ, Chen HI. Welsh onion (Allium fistulosum L.) extracts alter vascular responses in rat aortae. *J Cardiovasc Pharmacol.* 1999 Apr;33(4):515–20.

Chiu HF, Venkatakrishnan K, Golovinskaia O, Wang CK. Impact of micronutrients on hypertension: evidence from Clinical Trials with a Special Focus on Meta-Analysis. *Nutrients.* 2021 Feb 10;13(2):588.

Dearlove RP, Greenspan P, Hartle DK, Swanson RB, Hargrove JL. Inhibition of protein glycation by extracts of culinary herbs and spices. *J Med Food.* 2008 Jun;11(2):275–81.

Degirolamo C, Rudel LL. Dietary monounsaturated fatty acids appear not to provide cardioprotection. *Curr Atheroscler Rep.* 2010;12(6):391–6.

de Munter JS, Hu FB, Spiegelman D, Franz M, van Dam RM. Whole grain, bran, and germ intake and risk of type 2 diabetes: a prospective cohort study and systematic review. *PLoS Med.* 2007;4(8):e261. doi: 10.1371/journal.pmed.0040261

Dougkas A, Vannereux M, Giboreau A. The impact of herbs and spices on increasing the appreciation and intake of low-salt legume-based meals. *Nutrients.* 2019;11(12):2901. Published 2019 Dec 1.

Estruch R, Ros E, Salas-Salvadó J, Covas MI, Corella D, Arós F, Gómez-Gracia E, Ruiz-Gutiérrez V, Fiol M, Lapetra J, Lamuela-Raventos RM, Serra-Majem L, Pintó X, Basora J, Muñoz MA, Sorlí JV, Martínez JA, Martínez-González MA; PREDIMED Study Investigators. Primary prevention of cardiovascular disease with a Mediterranean diet.

N Engl J Med. 2013 Apr 4;368(14):1279–90. doi: 10.1056/NEJMoa1200303. Epub 2013 Feb 25. Retraction in: N Engl J Med. 2018 Jun 21;378(25):2441–2442. Erratum in: N Engl J Med. 2014 Feb 27;370(9):886. Corrected and republished in: N Engl J Med. 2018 Jun 21;378(25):e34.

Evans CE, Greenwood DC, Threapleton DE, Gale CP, Cleghorn CL, Burley VJ. Glycemic index, glycemic load, and blood pressure: a systematic review and meta-analysis of randomized controlled trials. *Am J Clin Nutr.* 2017 May;105(5):1176–90.

Fayet-Moore F, Wibisono C, Carr P, Duve E, Petocz P, Lancaster G, McMillan J, Marshall S, Blumfield M. An analysis of the mineral composition of pink salt available in Australia. *Foods.* 2020 Oct 19;9(10):1490. doi: 10.3390/foods9101490.

Fulgoni VL 3rd, Agarwal S, Spence L, Samuel P. Sodium intake in US ethnic subgroups and potential impact of a new sodium reduction technology: NHANES Dietary Modeling. *Nutr J.* 2014 Dec 18;13(1):120.

García Zozaya JL, Padilla Viloria M. Alterations of calcium, magnesium, and zinc in essential hypertension: their relation to the renin-angiotensin-aldosterone system]. *Invest Clin.* 1997 Nov;38(Suppl 2):27–40.

Ghazzawi HA, Al-Ismail K. A comprehensive study on the effect of roasting and frying on fatty acids profiles and antioxidant capacity of almonds, pine, cashew, and pistachio. *J Food Qual.* 2017;2017:9038257.

Gonzalez-Vicente A, Hong NJ, Yang N, Cabral PD, Berthiaume JM, Dominici FP, Garvin JL. Dietary fructose increases the sensitivity of proximal tubules to angiotensin II in rats fed high-salt diets. *Nutrients.* 2018;10:1244.

Graudal NA, Hubeck-Graudal T, Jurgens G. Effects of low sodium diet versus high sodium diet on blood pressure, renin, aldosterone, catecholamines, cholesterol, and triglyceride. *Cochrane Database Syst Rev.* 2020 Dec 12;12:CD004022.

Hadi A, Pourmasoumi M, Ghaedi E, Sahebkar A. The effect of Curcumin/Turmeric on blood pressure modulation: a systematic review and meta-analysis. *Pharmacol Res.* 2019 Dec;150:104505. doi: 10.1016/j.phrs.2019.104505. Epub 2019 Oct 21.

Han GM, Liu P. Higher serum lycopene is associated with reduced prevalence of hypertension in overweight or obese adults. *Eur J Integr Med.* 2017;13:34–40.

Harvard Health. 2011. https://www.health.harvard.edu/blog/is-fructose-bad-for-you-201104262 425#:~:text=In%20the%201800s%20and%20early, (73%20grams%20for%20adolescents). Accessed: May 2021.

Hodgson JM, Puddey IB, Burke V, Beilin LJ, Jordan N. Effects on blood pressure of drinking green and black tea. *J Hypertens.* 1999 Apr;17(4):457–63.

Honda M, Kawana T, Takehara M, Inoue Y. Enhanced E/Z isomerization of (all-E)-lycopene by employing iron(III) chloride as a catalyst. *J Food Sci.* 2015;80:C1453–9.

Honda M, Kageyama H, Hibino T. et al. Enhanced Z-isomerization of tomato lycopene through the optimal combination of food ingredients. *Sci Rep.* 2019;9:7979.

Hord NG. Dietary nitrates, nitrites, and cardiovascular disease. *Curr Atheroscler Rep.* 2011 Dec;13(6):484–92.

Hord NG, Tang Y, Bryan NS. Food sources of nitrates and nitrites: the physiologic context for potential health benefits. *Am J Clin Nutr.* 2009;90:1–10.

Houston M. The role of nutrition and nutraceutical supplements in the treatment of hypertension. *World J Cardiol.* 2014;6(2):38–66. doi:10.4330/wjc.v6.i2.38.

Houston MC. The importance of potassium in managing hypertension. *Curr Hypertens Rep.* 2011 Aug;13(4):309–17.

Houston M. Nutrition and nutraceutical supplements for the treatment of hypertension: part III. *J Clin Hypertens (Greenwich).* 2013 Dec;15(12):931–7.

Houston MC, Harper KJ. Potassium, magnesium, and calcium: their role in both the cause and treatment of hypertension. *J Clin Hypertens (Greenwich).* 2008 Jul;10(7 Suppl 2):3–11.

Hurtado-Barroso S, Martínez-Huélamo M, Rinaldi de Alvarenga JF, et al. Acute Effect of a Single Dose of Tomato *Sofrito* on Plasmatic Inflammatory Biomarkers in Healthy Men. *Nutrients.* 2019;11(4):851. doi:10.3390/nu11040851

Institute of Medicine. 2013. *Sodium intake in populations: assessment of evidence.* Washington, DC: The National Academies Press. p. 210.

Insull W Jr. Clinical utility of bile acid sequestrants in the treatment of dyslipidemia: a scientific review. *South Med J.* 2006 Mar;99(3):257–73.

Ju J, Song JL, Park ES, Do MS, Park KY. Korean solar salts reduce obesity and alter its related markers in diet-induced obese mice. *Nutr Res Pract.* 2016;10:629–34.

Kahlon TS, Chiu MC, Chapman MH. Steam cooking significantly improves in vitro bile acid binding of collard greens, kale, mustard greens, broccoli, green bell pepper, and cabbage. *Nutr Res.* 2008 Jun;28(6):351–7.

Karanja N, Lancaster KJ, Vollmer WM, Lin PH, Most MM, Ard JD, Swain JF, Sacks FM, Obarzanek E. Acceptability of sodium-reduced research diets, including the Dietary Approaches To Stop Hypertension diet, among adults with prehypertension and stage 1 hypertension. *J Am Diet Assoc.* 2007 Sep;107(9):1530–8.

Kendall CWC, Josse AR, Esfahani A, Jenkins DJA. Nuts, metabolic syndrome and diabetes. *Br J Nutr.* 2010;104:465–73.

Khan NI, Noori S, Mahboob T. Efficacy of lycopene on modulation of renal antioxidant enzymes, ACE and ACE gene expression in hyperlipidaemic rats. *J Renin Angiotensin Aldosterone Syst.* 2016 Sep 27;17(3):1470320316664611.

Kimura M, Itokawa Y. Cooking losses of minerals in foods and its nutritional significance. *J Nutr Sci Vitaminol (Tokyo).* 1990;36(Suppl 1):S25–32; discussion S33. PMID: 2081985.

Knez M, Stangoulis JCR, Glibetic M, Tako E. The linoleic acid: Dihomo-γ-Linolenic acid ratio (LA:DGLA)—An emerging biomarker of Zn status. *Nutrients.* 2017;9(8):825. doi: 10.3390/nu9080825.

Komnenov D, Levanovich PE, Rossi NF. Hypertension associated with fructose and high salt: renal and sympathetic mechanisms. *Nutrients.* 2019;11(3):569. Published 2019 Mar 7. doi: 10.3390/nu11030569.

Konitzer K, Pflaum T, Oliveira P, Arendt E, Koehler P, Hofmann T. Kinetics of sodium release from wheat bread crumb as affected by sodium distribution. *J Agric Food Chem.* 2013 Nov 13;61(45):10659–69.

Kris-Etherton PM, Hu F, Ros E, Sabate J. The role of tree nuts and peanuts in the prevention of coronary heart disease: multiple potential mechanisms. *J Nutr.* 2008;138:1746S–51S.

Laurant P, Touyz RM. Physiological and pathophysiological role of magnesium in the cardiovascular system: implications in hypertension. *J Hypertens.* 2000 Sep;18(9):1177–91.

Lawrence G, Salles C, Septier C, Busch J, Thomas-Danguin T. Odour–taste interactions: a way to enhance saltiness in low-salt content solutions. *Food Qual Prefer.* 2009;20:241–8. doi: 10.1016/j.foodqual.2008.10.004.

Li X, Xu J. Lycopene supplement and blood pressure: an updated meta-analysis of intervention trials. *Nutrients.* 2013 Sep 18;5(9):3696–712.

Lozano-Castellón J, Vallverdú-Queralt A, Rinaldi de Alvarenga JF, Illán M, Torrado-Prat X, Lamuela-Raventós RM. Domestic sautéing with EVOO: change in the phenolic profile. *Antioxidants.* 2020;9(1):77.

Luevano-Contreras C, Chapman-Novakofski K. Dietary advanced glycation end products and aging. *Nutrients.* 2010;2(12):1247–65. doi: 10.3390/nu2121247.

Marshall S, Petocz P, Duve E, Abbott K, Cassettari T, Blumfield M, Fayet-Moore F. The effect of replacing refined grains with whole grains on cardiovascular risk factors: a systematic review and meta-analysis of randomized controlled trials with GRADE clinical recommendation. *J Acad Nutr Diet.* 2020 Nov;120(11):1859–1883.e31.

Matthews CM. Steep your genes in health: drink tea. *Proc (Bayl Univ Med Cent).* 2010;23(2):142–4.

McGee H. 2004. *On food and cooking: the science and lore of the kitchen.* New York: Scribner. p. 340.

McGee H. 2004. *On food and cooking: the science and lore of the kitchen.* New York: Scribner. p. 502.

Mellen PB, Walsh TF, Herrington DM. Whole grain intake and cardiovascular disease: a meta-analysis. *Nutr Metab Cardiovasc Dis.* 2008;18:283–90.

Menni, C., Louca, P., Berry, S.E. et al. High intake of vegetables is linked to lower white blood cell profile and the effect is mediated by the gut microbiome. *BMC Med.* 2021; 19:37.

Mente A, Dehghan M, Rangarajan S, McQueen M, Dagenais G, Wielgosz A, Lear S, Li W, Chen H, Yi S, Wang Y, Diaz R, Avezum A, Lopez-Jaramillo P, Seron P, Kumar R, Gupta R, Mohan V, Swaminathan S, Kutty R, Zatonska K, Iqbal R, Yusuf R, Mohammadifard N, Khatib R, Nasir NM, Ismail N, Oguz A, Rosengren A, Yusufali A, Wentzel-Viljoen E, Puoane T, Chifamba J, Teo K, Anand SS, Yusuf S; Prospective Urban Rural Epidemiology (PURE) study investigators. Association of dietary nutrients with blood lipids and blood pressure in 18 countries: a cross-sectional analysis from the PURE study. *Lancet Diabetes Endocrinol.* 2017 Oct;5(10):774–87. doi: 10.1016/S2213-8587(17)30283-8.

Mitchell DC, Lawrence FR, Hartman TJ, Curran JM. Consumption of dry beans, peas, and lentils could improve diet quality in the US population. *J Am Diet Assoc* 2009;109(5):909–13.

Monlezun DJ, Matamoros N, Huggins C. et al. Biting into integrated quality improvement: medical student and staff blinded taste test for sodium reduction improving medical education and care? *J Med Pers.* 2015;13:112–7.

Mori M, Hamada A, Mori H, Yamori Y, Tsuda K. Effects of cooking using multi-ply cookware on absorption of potassium and vitamins: a randomized double-blind placebo control study. *Int J Food Sci Nutr.* 2012;63(5):530–6. doi: 10.3109/09637486.2011. 642342.

Muniyappa R, Sowers JR. Role of insulin resistance in endothelial dysfunction. *Rev Endocr Metab Disord.* 2013; 14:5–12.

O'Donnell M, Mente A, Yusuf S. Evidence relating sodium intake to blood pressure and CVD. *Curr Cardiol Rep.* 2014;16(10):529. doi: 10.1007/s11886-014-0529-9.

Ornish D, Scherwitz LW, Billings JH, et al. Intensive lifestyle changes for reversal of coronary heart disease. *JAMA.* 1998 Dec 16;280(23):2001–7. doi: 10.1001/jama.280.23.2001. Erratum in: JAMA 1999 Apr 21;281(15):1380. DOI: http://dx.doi.org/10.1001/jama.281.15.1380.

Pang J, Zhang Z, Zheng TZ, Bassig BA, Mao C, Liu X, Zhu Y, Shi K, Ge J, Yang YJ, Bai M, Peng Y. Green tea consumption and risk of cardiovascular and ischemic related diseases: a meta-analysis. *Int J Cardiol.* 2016 Jan 1;202:967–74.

Paran E, Novack V, Engelhard YN, Hazan-Halevy I. The effects of natural antioxidants from tomato extract in treated but uncontrolled hypertensive patients. *Cardiovasc Drugs Ther.* 2009 Apr;23(2):145–51.

Park ES, Yu T, Yang K. et al. Cube natural sea salt ameliorates obesity in high fat diet-induced obese mice and 3T3-L1 adipocytes. *Sci Rep.* 2020;10:3407.

Ponzo V, Pellegrini M, Costelli P, et al. Strategies for reducing salt and sugar intakes in individuals at increased cardiometabolic risk. *Nutrients.* 2021;13(1):279. Published 2021 Jan 19.

Powers C, Hess MA. 2010. *Essentials of nutrition for chefs.* Chicago, IL: Culinary Nutrition Publishing.

Ramkissoon JS, Mahomoodally MF, Ahmed N, Subratty AH. Relationship between total phenolic content, antioxidant potential, and antiglycation abilities of common culinary herbs and spices. *J Med Food.* 2012 Dec;15(12):1116–23.

Ren XS, Tong Y, Ling L, Chen D, Sun HJ, Zhou H, Qi XH, Chen Q, Li YH, Kang YM, Zhu GQ. NLRP3 gene deletion attenuates angiotensin II-induced phenotypic transformation of vascular smooth muscle cells and vascular remodeling. *Cell Physiol Biochem.* 2017;44(6):2269–80.

Rizkalla SW. Health implications of fructose consumption: a review of recent data. *Nutr Metab (Lond).* 2010;7:82. Published 2010 Nov 4. doi:10.1186/1743-7075-7-82.

Sacks FM, Svetkey LP, Vollmer WM, Appel LJ, Bray GA, Harsha D, and DASH-Sodium Collaborative Research Group. Effects on blood pressure of reduced dietary sodium and the Dietary Approaches to Stop Hypertension (DASH) diet. *N Engl J Med.* 2001;344:3–10.

Saklar S, Ertas E, Ozdemir IS, Karadeniz B. Effects of different brewing conditions on catechin content and sensory acceptance in Turkish green tea infusions. *J Food Sci Technol.* 2015;52(10):6639–46. doi: 10.1007/s13197-015-1746-y.

Samsamikor M, Mackay D, Mollard RC, et al. A double-blind, randomized, crossover trial protocol of whole hemp seed protein and hemp seed protein hydrolysate consumption for hypertension. *Trials.* 2020;21:354.

Santos-Parker JR, Strahler TR, Bassett CJ, Bispham NZ, Chonchol MB, Seals DR. Curcumin supplementation improves vascular endothelial function in healthy middle-aged and older adults by increasing nitric oxide bioavailability and reducing oxidative stress. *Aging (Albany NY).* 2017;9(1):187–208.

Sergeant S, Rahbar E, Chilton FH. Gamma-linolenic acid, Dihommo-gamma linolenic, eicosanoids and inflammatory processes. *Eur J Pharmacol.* 2016;785:77–86.

Shen L, Liu CC, An CY, Ji HF. How does curcumin work with poor bioavailability? Clues from experimental and theoretical studies. *Sci Rep.* 2016 Feb 18;6:20872.

Shouk R, Abdou A, Shetty K, Sarkar D, Eid AH. Mechanisms underlying the antihypertensive effects of garlic bioactives. *Nutr Res.* 2014;34(2):106–15.

Sinopoli DA, Lawless HT. Taste properties of potassium chloride alone and in mixtures with sodium chloride using a check-all-that-apply method. *J Food Sci.* 2012 Sep;77(9):S319–22.

Stanhope KL. Sugar consumption, metabolic disease and obesity: the state of the controversy. *Crit Rev Clin Lab Sci.* 2016;53(1):52–67.

Stohs SJ, Chen O, Ray SD, Ji J, Bucci LR, Preuss HG. Highly bioavailable forms of curcumin and promising avenues for curcumin-based research and application: a review. *Molecules.* 2020;25(6):1397. Published 2020 Mar 19. doi: 10.3390/molecules25061397.

Stolarz-Skrzypek K, Kuznetsova T, Thijs L, Tikhonoff V, Seidlerová J, Richart T, Jin Y, Olszanecka A, Malyutina S, Casiglia E, et al. Fatal and nonfatal outcomes, incidence of hypertension, and blood pressure changes in relation to urinary sodium excretion. *JAMA.* 2011;305:1777–85.

Sun JL, Ji HF, Shen L. Impact of cooking on the antioxidant activity of spice turmeric. *Food Nutr Res.* 2019;63 Published 2019 May 31. doi: 10.29219/fnr.v63.3451.

Tayyem RF, Heath DD, Al-Delaimy WK, Rock CL. Curcumin content of turmeric and curry powders. *Nutr Cancer.* 2006;55(2):126–31.

Thomas-Danguin T, Guichard E, Salles C. Cross-modal interactions as a strategy to enhance salty taste and to maintain liking of low-salt food: a review. *Food Funct.* 2019 Sep 1;10(9):5269–81.

Toledo E, Hu FB, Estruch R. et al. Effect of the Mediterranean diet on blood pressure in the PREDIMED trial: results from a randomized controlled trial. *BMC Med.* 2013;11:207. doi: 10.1186/1741-7015-11-207.

Tresserra-Rimbau A, Rimm EB, Medina-Remón A, Martínez-González MA, de la Torre R, Corella D, Salas-Salvadó J, Gómez-Gracia E, Lapetra J, Arós F, et al. Inverse association between habitual polyphenol intake and incidence of cardiovascular events in the PREDIMED study. *Nutr Metab Cardiovasc Dis.* 2014;24:639–47.

USDA. 2020. Dietary Guidelines for Americans. https://www.dietaryguidelines.gov/sites/default/files/2020-12/Dietary_Guidelines_for_Americans_2020-2025.pdf.

Viguiliouk E, Glenn AJ, Nishi SK, et al. Associations between dietary pulses alone or with other legumes and cardiometabolic disease outcomes: an umbrella review and updated systematic review and meta-analysis of prospective cohort studies. *Adv Nutr.* 2019;10(Suppl_4):S308–19. doi: 10.1093/advances/nmz113.

Vinson JA, Cai Y. Nuts, especially walnuts, have both antioxidant quantity and efficacy and exhibit significant potential health benefits. *Food Funct.* 2012 Feb;3(2):134–40.

Virani SS, Alonso A, Aparicio HJ, Benjamin EJ, Bittencourt MS, Callaway CW, Carson AP, Chamberlain AM, Cheng S, Delling FN, Elkind MSV, Evenson KR, Ferguson JF, Gupta DK, Khan SS, Kissela BM, Knutson KL, Lee CD, Lewis TT, Liu J, Loop MS, Lutsey PL, Ma J, Mackey J, Martin SS, Matchar DB, Mussolino ME, Navaneethan SD, Perak AM, Roth GA, Samad Z, Satou GM, Schroeder EB, Shah SH, Shay CM, Stokes A, VanWagner LB, Wang NY, Tsao CW; American Heart Association Council on Epidemiology and Prevention Statistics Committee and Stroke Statistics Subcommittee. Heart disease and stroke statistics-2021 update: a report from the American Heart Association. *Circulation.* 2021 Feb 23;143(8):e254–e743.

Vos MB, Kimmons JE, Gillespie C, Welsh J, Blanck HM. Dietary fructose consumption among US children and adults: the Third National Health and Nutrition Examination Survey. *Medscape J Med.* 2008 Jul 9;10(7):160.

Vuong QV, Golding JB, Stathopoulos CE, Nguyen MH, Roach PD. Optimizing conditions for the extraction of catechins from green tea using hot water. *J Sep Sci.* 2011 Nov;34(21):3099–106.

Wang C, Lee Y, Lee SY. Consumer acceptance of model soup system with varying levels of herbs and salt. *J food Sci.* 2014;79(10):S2098–106.

Weaver CM. Potassium and health. *Adv Nutr.* 2013;4(3):368S–77S. Published 2013 May 1.

World Health Organization. 2012. *Guideline: sodium intake for adults and children.* Geneva: World Health Organization (WHO). p. 56.

World Health Organization. https://www.who.int/news-room/fact-sheets/detail/cardiovascular-diseases-(cvds) Accessed: May 2021.

Xu J, Liu XF, Wang YT. A detection method of vegetable oils in edible blended oil based on three-dimensional fluorescence spectroscopy technique. *Food Chem.* 2016 Dec;212:72–7.

Yang IF, Jayaprakasha GK, Patil BS. In vitro bile acid binding capacities of red leaf lettuce and cruciferous vegetables. *J Agric Food Chem.* 2017 Sep 13;65(36):8054–62.

Yao Y, Wang W, Li M, et al. Curcumin exerts its anti-hypertensive effect by down-regulating the AT1 receptor in vascular smooth muscle cells. *Sci Rep.* 2016;6:25579. Published 2016 May 5.

Ye EQ, Chacko SA, Chou EL, Kugizaki M, Liu S. Greater whole-grain intake is associated with lower risk of type 2 diabetes, cardiovascular disease, and weight gain. *J Nutr.* 2012;142:1304–13.

6 Nonalcoholic Fatty Liver Disease

Xonna M. Clark
Xonna M. Clark LLC

CONTENTS

DOI: 10.1201/b22377-6

INTRODUCTION

Nonalcoholic fatty liver disease (NAFLD) or hepatic steatosis is a condition characterized by an excessive amount of fat accumulating in the liver. NAFLD is a common disease found in industrialized nations such as the United States. In fact, it is estimated that up to 25% of Americans have developed NAFLD (Perumpail et al. 2017). This condition is often comorbid with other metabolic problems such as high triglycerides, low HDL cholesterol, blood sugar dysregulation, insulin resistance, high blood pressure, gout, metabolic syndrome, and obesity. Nonalcoholic steatohepatitis (NASH) is a subcategory of NAFLD that results in inflammation and cellular damage in the liver along with the excessive accumulation of fat and is considered the more serious form of NAFLD (LaBrecque et al. 2014). If left untreated, NAFLD can lead to the development of NASH, which creates a risk of progression to other disease states such as fibrosis, cirrhosis of the liver, and other complications (Iser and Ryan 2013).

NASH is also more common for those 50 years and older as the prevalence of the more progressive forms (NASH and Cirrhosis) tends to increase with age (Iser and Ryan 2013).

PATHOPHYSIOLOGY

NAFLD occurs due to excessive amounts of fat being deposited within the liver. In addition to metabolic comorbidities, this can result from the use of certain drugs and genetic metabolic errors (Jensen et al. 2018). From a nutritional perspective, hepatic fat accumulation is a result of the excessive consumption of fats (particularly trans and saturated fats) and refined carbohydrates (Mirmiran, Amirhamidi, Ejtahed, Bahadoran, and Azizi 2017). Excessive caloric intake is also a major contributing factor (Yasutake et al. 2014). Each of these variables (trans and saturated fats, refined carbohydrates, and excessive caloric intake) dysregulate blood sugar levels and result in the increased storage of fat, including within the liver.

Fructose also plays a key role in the development of NAFLD, specifically in its processed form as high-fructose corn syrup. Human clinical trials have shown that reducing excess or processed fructose consumption for patients with NAFLD results in the improvement of inflammatory markers associated with the progression of this disease (Jin et al. 2014). In its unprocessed form, fructose is a simple sugar that occurs naturally in fruit, vegetables, and many syrups or sweeteners such as honey. It is also found in sucrose or common table sugar. There has been a strong correlation with excess fructose consumption and increased risk of metabolic syndrome, diabetes, cardiovascular disease, obesity, and NAFLD (Tetri, Basaranoqlu, Brunt, Yerian, and Neuschwander-Tetri 2008). Figure 6.1 illustrates the impact of excess fructose on mediating factors and its progression to NAFLD.

However, there is a suggestion of fructose intake from fruits actually having a protective effect. A study done by Kanerva, Sandboge, Kaartinen, Männistö, and Eriksson (2014) showed an inverse association between a high amount of fructose consumption from fruit and risk of developing NAFLD (Kanerva et al. 2014). In this study, 54%–80% of study participants consumed fructose as whole fruits, and 0%–8% consumed fructose as soft drinks (Kanerva et al. 2014). Fructose from fruit may be less likely to contribute to NAFLD when compared to sugar or high-fructose

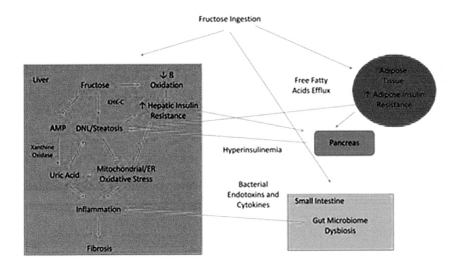

FIGURE 6.1 Fructose mechanism mediating development and progression of NAFLD (Jensen, et al. 2018).

corn syrup sweetened beverages due to fruit containing hepatic protective nutrients such as vitamins E and C and antioxidants such as flavanols, epicatechin, and ascorbate (Jensen et al. 2018; Vasdev, Gill, Parai, Longerich, and Gadag 2002). Thus, moderate consumption of fruit (1–2 servings/day) appears to be protective.

In its unnatural form as high-fructose corn syrup, fructose has been used heavily in many processed foods and drinks. High-fructose corn syrup is thought specifically to contribute to the development of NAFLD. Both excessive intake and regular consumption of this form of fructose in beverages, condiments, and other processed foods can be easily converted to fat and leads to insulin resistance even more so than other forms of sugar (Lim, Mietus-Snyder, Valente, Schwarz, and Lustiq 2010). In healthy rodents, both NAFLD and NASH have been induced with the addition of high-fructose corn syrup into the rodent's diet (Tetri et al. 2008; Kawasaki et al. 2009).

High-fructose corn syrup differs from other sugars in contributing to NAFLD because of the metabolism difference in the liver between it and glucose. Glucose metabolism uses glucokinase and hexokinase, where in fructose metabolism, fructokinase, principally fructokinase C, is used (Jensen et al. 2018). This creates the difference between the metabolism of the two sugars. While both produce glucose, glycogen, and triglycerides, fructose metabolism reduces intercellular phosphate and ATP levels due to an increase in nucleotide turnover and uric acid accumulation, where glucose metabolism does not (Jensen et al. 2018). This leads to temporary blocking of protein synthesis and increases in oxidative stress and mitochondrial dysfunction, which are key factors in the development of NAFLD and its comorbidities (Jensen et al. 2018).

The gut and immune system are also impacted by fructokinase. Fructokinase C is readily expressed in the small intestine. Excessive intake of fructose allows for fructose metabolism in the small intestine, which can lead to disruption of the tight junctions (Jensen et al. 2018). This may result in gut permeability, allowing for endotoxins to move through the system and alter the microbiome, triggering fat accumulation in the liver (Jensen et al. 2018). The endotoxins present in the system also can activate the innate immune system in response to inflammation (Jensen et al. 2018).

In addition to fructokinase, a second mechanism by which fructose may contribute to NAFLD is that fructose metabolism may raise uric acid levels (Lanaspa et al. 2012). Foods high in fructose can increase uric acid levels in the liver, increasing oxidative stress, which may lead to gout, kidney disease, and metabolic disease. Uric acid levels are a predictor of NAFLD. Reducing the amount of fructose has shown to reduce uric acid levels and the impact on the body (Jensen et al. 2018).

Fat accumulation in the liver also can be stimulated by fructose consumption inducing oxidative stress in the mitochondria. Acontinase-2 and enoyl CoA hydrase are enzymes found in the mitochondria that are sensitive to oxidative stress (Jensen et al. 2018). Fructose and uric acid decrease acontinase-2 activity, leading to the accumulation of citrate, which moves into the cytoplasm, stimulates ATP citrate lyase, and activates lipogenesis (Jensen et al. 2018). This can also impair fatty acid oxidation by decreasing enoyl CoA hydratase-1 activity, which stimulates AMP Deaminase-2 and reduces AMP-activated protein kinase, which regulates enoyl CoA hydratase-1. This results in accumulation of fat and stimulation of gluconeogenesis (Jensen et al. 2018).

Comparable to fructose, consumption of ultra-processed foods, which are usually high in trans-fat, saturated fat, salt, and processed sugar, may also lead to NAFLD by way of increasing oxidative stress in the body. Pathways for oxidative stress contributing to NAFLD overlap with that of fructose and uric acid. Prevention or mitigation of oxidative stress load by dietary approaches, such as reducing fructose and ultra-processed foods, thus offers mechanisms for prevention.

THERAPEUTIC APPROACHES FOR TREATING NONALCOHOLIC FATTY LIVER DISEASE

LIFESTYLE MODIFICATIONS

Lifestyle modifications can be a first-line therapy to preventing and treating NAFLD since there is such a strong association between NAFLD and insulin resistance. These modifications include reduction of a sedentary lifestyle via dietary changes, frequent physical exercise, and long-term, sustainable weight loss. These therapeutic measures should be taken in all patients with NAFLD, regardless of the severity of their liver disease. However, for those who are overweight and have insulin resistance in particular, the need to make lifestyle modifications is critical to prevent the progression of NAFLD into NASH and its complications. The efficacy of these measures should be assessed every 6 months by a licensed healthcare provider.

DIETARY MODIFICATIONS: REDUCING INTAKE OF ULTRA-PROCESSED FOODS WHILE EATING A WHOLE-FOOD DIET

Eating ultra-processed food contributes to metabolic conditions that can progress to NAFLD or serve as comorbidities, primarily due to its high content of trans-fats, saturated fats, salt, and processed sugar.

These ultra-processed food components have found their way into countless foods and drinks readily available in our society. When walking into a grocery store, 68% of the food items will have a form of added sugar in them (Popkin and Hawkes 2016). Heavily ultra-processed foods such as breads, soft drinks, frozen or canned foods, snacks, pizzas, cookies, and cakes account for more than 50% of our caloric intake as a nation. More than 20% of the calories in these ultra-processed foods come in the form of added sugar (Martínez Steele et al. 2016). The fact that these foods are very cheap and easily available to most means that we as a society are consuming more sugar than ever before (Drewnowski and Darmon 2005). Considering that sugar converts easily to fat and can be stored in the liver, reducing the intake of processed foods and eating more whole foods are important for the treatment of fatty liver disease (Fan and Cao 2013). The consumption of soft drinks, processed foods, and rich sources of high-fructose corn syrup should be eliminated or, at least, kept to a minimum depending on the health status of the individual. Healthcare providers should encourage consumption of foods like low glycemic fruits such as avocado, berries, and citrus, vegetables, sustainably caught seafood, and healthy meats as they contain beneficial nutrients that help prevent and/or treat NAFLD.

The following tables outline foods to avoid, foods to include, and how to make substitutions to create a more health-promotive diet to prevent or reverse NAFLD and NASH. Tables 6.1–6.6 provide a list of sweeteners, which people at risk of or with NAFLD should avoid.

TABLE 6.1
Processed Foods to Avoid

Processed foods are manufactured foods that have been modified from natural unprocessed whole food sources. Such modification of whole foods occurs in varying degrees depending on the types of additives and processing techniques used. Such degree and style of processing dictates the processed food nutritive quality and impact on human health.

It is recommended to opt for whole food options when eating. Consumption of only the most minimally processed foods is recommended while avoiding processed and ultra-processed foods all together.

Whole or Minimally Processed Foods
- Fresh, dry, or frozen foods in their "whole" form without any additives or processing
- Fresh fruits and vegetables from produce sections of grocery store, farmers market, or garden
- Dried whole grains, legumes, nuts, and seeds such as brown rice, lentils, chickpeas, and almonds
- Frozen or refrigerated items without added sugar or other ingredients such as fish, meat, eggs, and plain dairy products
- Root vegetables such as potatoes, sweet potatoes, carrots, parsnips, radishes, turnips, etc.

Processed Foods
- Foods manufactured with added salt, sugar, or other substances (oils, fat, and other food extracts)
- Cheese, vegetables preserved in brine solutions, salted/smoked/canned meat, fish, or other foods

Ultra-Processed Foods
- Formulated using multiple ingredients including the addition of substances not required for culinary purposes (flavoring, coloring, sweeteners, emulsifiers, and other sensory enhancing chemicals)
- Bread, breakfast cereal, cake, snacks, frozen premade meals, soda, sauces, pizza, desserts, candy, instant-meals

TABLE 6.2
Whole Foods to Include

Whole foods are described as "unprocessed" or "minimally" processed as mentioned in the above table. They are foods consumed in the form nature provides. They are most optimally consumed fresh without any preservation. Healthy cooking techniques may be utilized such as grilling, boiling, roasting, or sautéing, and some whole foods may be eaten raw, sprouted, or dehydrated

Vegetables
- Dark leafy greens, root vegetables, cucumbers, squash, peppers, mushrooms, broccoli

Grains (dried)
- Brown/wild/red/black/basmati rice, spelt, barely, fenugreek, whole oats

Nuts and Seeds
- Almonds, brazil nuts, cashews, pistachios, walnuts, pumpkin seeds, sunflower seeds

Meat and Poultry
- Fresh beef, pork, chicken, lamb, duck, wild game, etc.

Fish and Shellfish
- Fresh trout, salmon, tilapia, carb, lobster, shrimp, etc.

Optimal Whole Food Forms to Buy

Fresh, frozen, dried, raw
- Fresh > Frozen

Select organic produce when possible

Meat and Poultry
- Local/grass-fed/pasture raised are optimal quality when buying
- Local butchers or the meat and poultry department of the grocery store are sources of such quality; online resources are also available

Fish and Shellfish
- Fresh/wild-caught are optimal quality when buying
- The seafood section at grocery store is a source of such quality; online resources are also available

TABLE 6.3
Swapping Processed Foods for Whole Foods

Pantry and Fridge Reset: Slow Transition

This option allows for more ease in transitioning to a whole-food diet by swapping groups of processed foods one at a time for whole food alternatives. It allows time to get to know the process of prepping and cooking whole foods for meals one at a time.

How to Start:

Processed Snacks for Whole Food Snacks
- **Remove:** cookies, chips, pretzels, cakes, frozen deserts
- **Add:** apples, carrots, nut butters, avocados, citrus, nuts, seeds, berries

Refined Carbohydrates to Complex Carbohydrates
- **Remove:** pastas, breads, cereals
- **Add:** sweet potatoes, apples, carrots, celery, whole oats, legumes, lentils

(Continued)

TABLE 6.3 (*Continued*)
Swapping Processed Foods for Whole Foods

Pantry and Fridge Reset: Hard Reset

Some people prefer to go all-in at once, revamping the food items in their household. If this is the case, there are some good tips on how to make this quick transition.

How to Start:
- Plan your meals for the coming week
- Eliminate all the processed food items out of the fridge and pantry
- Go to the grocery store and stock up on whole food items
- Dedicate one day a week for meal prep for the week
- Reserve time during the week for quick meal prep

REDUCING INTAKE OF FRUCTOSE

TABLE 6.4
Foods High in Fructose to Avoid[a]

Dairy:

Dairy food items commonly have added sugar as an ingredient. Be sure to read labels and consume only those free of sweeteners. Dairy-free alternatives commonly contain added sugar as well. Be sure to buy unsweetened items regardless of dairy content.
- Flavored milks
- Flavored or sweetened yogurts
- Condensed milk
- Coffee creamers
- Ice cream

Drinks:

Most flavored soft drinks contain high sugar particularly in the form of added sweeteners such as high-fructose corn syrup. The drinks listed below are best eliminated from the diet for optimal treatment.
- Alcohol: beer, wine, sherry, mixed drinks
- Carbonated soft drinks
- Fruit juices
- Lemonade
- Sweetened dairy drinks: milk shakes, flavored milk
- Vegetable juices
- Protein drinks

(Continued)

TABLE 6.4 (*Continued*)
Foods High in Fructose to Avoid[a]

Sauces:
- Barbeque sauces
- Brown sauces
- Chutneys
- Ketchups
- Relishes
- Soy-based sauces
- Sweet and sour sauces
- Tomato sauces

Prepacked and Processed Foods:
- For these food items, it is best to avoid them when possible considering the increased likelihood of such products having added fructose as a sweetening agent while also having high sugar content as well.
- See Table 6.1 *Processed Foods to Avoid* for a complete list of processed foods to avoid.

[a] UW Health. 2015. Fructose-restricted diet [PDF file]. Retrieved from: https://www.uwhealth.org/healthfacts/nutrition/376.pdf.

TABLE 6.5
Foods Low in Fructose to Include[a]

Fruits:
- Avocado
- Berries (fresh)
- Grapefruit
- Jack fruit
- Lemons
- Limes
- Rhubarb

Meat and Seafood:
Make sure such foods are free of added sweeteners. Processed meat products containing sweeteners commonly include jerky, deli items, cured meats, canned meats, or fish, especially previously breaded and seasoned meat or fish. It is recommended to avoid processed meats.
- Eggs
- Fish
- Shellfish
- Poultry
- Wild game
- Beef
- Lamb

(*Continued*)

TABLE 6.5 (*Continued*)

Foods Low in Fructose to Include[a]

Vegetables:

Most vegetables have lower fructose levels when compared to fruits.

- Asparagus
- Broccoli
- Cauliflower
- Celery
- Cucumbers
- Dark leafy greens
- Green peppers
- Root vegetables
- Squash

[a] UW Health. 2015. Fructose-restricted diet [PDF file]. Retrieved from: https://www.uwhealth.org/healthfacts/nutrition/376.pdf.

TABLE 6.6

Fructose Sweeteners to Avoid[a]

For optimal treatment, it is best to avoid ALL sweeteners regardless of fructose content

- Agave syrup
- Corn syrup/high-fructose corn syrup
- Carmel
- Fructose
- Fruit juice concentrates
- Fruit juice
- Fruit sweeteners
- Honey
- Maple syrup
- Molasses
- Palm sugar
- Sorghum syrup
- Sucrose

[a] UW Health. 2015. Fructose-restricted diet [PDF file]. Retrieved from: https://www.uwhealth.org/healthfacts/nutrition/376.pdf.

RECOMMENDED DIETARY PATTERNS

The diet recommended most often to treat NAFLD is the Mediterranean diet. Following this diet has been shown to result in a reduction of liver fat, even if this reduction is not accompanied by weight loss. The DASH and Ketogenic diets have also been shown to be beneficial for those with NAFLD. More recently, a modified Mediterranean diet, which contains elements of both the Mediterranean and the Ketogenic diets, has been shown to have a lot of potential.

THE MEDITERRANEAN DIET

The Mediterranean diet has gained recognition for its ability to optimize cardiovascular and metabolic health, as it has been backed by more than 40 years of research (Sofi, Macchi, Abbate, Gensini, and Casini 2013). The data collected suggest that the cultural diet of the Mediterranean contributes to the low rates of chronic disease observed in that region of the world. The diet consists of foods such as fish, legumes, olives and olive oil, whole fruits and vegetables, nuts, seeds, and complex carbohydrates (Sofi and Casini 2014). The Mediterranean diet has also been proven to be effective for reducing the incidence of cardiovascular disease, metabolic syndrome, cognition, obesity, breast cancer, and type 2 diabetes (Guasch-Ferre et al. 2017). This diet is thought to prevent and treat such conditions, specifically NAFLD, due to it being a rich source of healthy fats and vitamins (Sofi and Casini 2014).

The Mediterranean diet includes increased consumption of the beneficial fats, monounsaturated (MUFA) and omega-3 polyunsaturated fatty acids (PUFA), and a reduced intake of carbohydrates, particularly refined carbohydrates and sugars. In a typical low-fat diet, fats constitute 30% of total calories and carbohydrates 50%–60%. However, with the Mediterranean diet, both fats and carbohydrates each make up 40% of total calories.

The Mediterranean diet is primarily plant-based and consists of a substantial intake of olive oil, an excellent source of monounsaturated fat. It also includes high intake of nuts, legumes, vegetables, fruit, whole grains, fish and seafood. In addition, it reduces intakes of both red and processed meats, as well as dairy products and sweets. The Mediterranean diet also recommends the consumption of wine, specifically red wine, in moderation.

Although fat intake contributes to much of the Mediterranean diet, it is the type of fat consumed which is crucial to its success. It is important to note that "the consumption of different types of fats have different effects on NAFLD and NASH; therefore, a reduction in total fat intake is not the simple solution" (Romero-Gómez, Zelber-Sagi, and Trenell 2017). Reducing the amount of fat eaten will not lead to reductions of fat in the liver alone. The two types of fats consumed on the Mediterranean diet (MUFA and Omega 3 PUFA) are particularly beneficial to NAFLD patients.

Omega-3 fatty acids are essential fatty acids and must be obtained through the diet as the human body cannot produce them. Fish can form omega-3 fatty acids by ingesting marine plants. The more fats fish can store in their flesh (versus their liver), the richer the fish will be in omega-3 fatty acids. Salmon and mackerel are examples of fish that do this. In fact, some consider that fish oil may offer a beneficial effect for NAFLD (Zelber-Sagi, Salomone, and Mlynarsky 2017). Research studies have shown that diets containing omega-3 PUFAs reduce triglycerides within the liver and increase insulin sensitivity. Both of these factors undoubtedly improve fat accumulation in the liver. Studies have also revealed that the omega-3 PUFAs, in fish oil, not only reduce fat accumulation but also liver enzyme levels and liver inflammation. A deficiency in these omega-3 PUFAs has been correlated with the development of steatosis of the liver and eventually NAFLD, NASH, and fibrosis.

Olive oil is comprised primarily of oleic acid (about 70%–80%), an omega 9 MUFA. Virgin and extra-virgin olive oil are higher grades that contain increased amounts of antioxidants, polyphenols, and phytochemicals – compounds found in plants that have been shown to benefit human health. Although MUFA is the major component of olive oil, the polyphenols it also contains have been demonstrated in randomized clinical trials to have both anti-inflammatory and metabolic advantages. In addition, these polyphenols have demonstrated antioxidant and antifibrotic effects on NAFLD. In essence, polyphenols inhibit the production of fat while stimulating the breakdown of fat in the liver. Polyphenols also suppress the activation of liver stellate cells and reduce cancer production.

The DASH (Dietary Approaches to Stop Hypertension) Diet

The DASH (Dietary Approaches to Stop Hypertension) diet is an eating plan developed to treat and prevent high blood pressure. It is a modified version of the USDA Diet Guidelines with considerations related to sodium consumption (Zivkovic, German, and Sanyal 2007). The DASH dietary pattern has similar components to the Mediterranean diet (i.e., high consumption of whole grains, vegetables, fruit, nuts and legumes and minimal intake of sweets and added sugars). However, it consists of different variations which differ in the level of sodium restriction (e.g., 2,300 or 1,500 mg/day) and the percentages of daily calories from fat and carbohydrates, respectively. In addition to reducing sodium, the DASH diet encourages the consumption of a variety of foods that are high in minerals which help to lower blood pressure (i.e., potassium, magnesium, and calcium).

The nutrient goal for a person consuming 2,100 calories/day on the DASH diet, with a 2,300 mg sodium *restriction*, is as follows:

Total fat: 28% of calories
Saturated fat: 6% of calories
Protein: 17% of calories
Carbohydrates: 55% of calories
Cholesterol: 114 mg
Potassium: 4,700 mg
Calcium: 1,370 mg
Magnesium: 535 mg
Fiber: 34 mg

Why Is the DASH Diet Effective for the Treatment of NAFLD?

NAFLD is associated with elevated blood pressure. The reduction of blood pressure can be of particular benefit to those with NAFLD not only in terms of cardiovascular disease prevention but also as it relates to the progression of liver disease. Due to its impact on lowering blood pressure, the DASH diet may be a viable and preferable eating plan for those with NAFLD. Rich in fruits, vegetables, whole grains and low in fat, a randomized control trial conducted by Razavi Zade et al. (2016) showed benefits of an 8-week DASH diet, in comparison to an isocaloric control diet, with weight, serum triglycerides, alanine aminotransferase, alkaline phosphatase, insulin and inflammatory and oxidative stress markers. Beneficial effects from the DASH diet may be especially true for African Americans, who appear to be especially sensitive to the blood pressure–lowering benefits of low-sodium diets (Zivkovic et al. 2007).

THE MODIFIED MEDITERRANEAN/KETOGENIC DIET

Two studies using a modified Mediterranean ketogenic diet had very profound results concerning its use therapeutically for NAFLD in clinical settings. A modified Mediterranean diet utilizes all the beneficial whole foods of the traditional Mediterranean diet while also including the metabolic benefits of a reduced-carbohydrate diet, such as ketogenic. In this case, 35% of calories come from complex carbohydrates, 45% of calories come from fats high in monounsaturated fat content, and 20% of calories come from protein (See Table 6.7).

Such a diet resulted in the significant reduction of the laboratory marker ALT associated with the progression of NAFLD among obese diabetic patients (Fraser, Abel, Lawlor, Fraser, and Elhayany 2008). Another related study conducted among obese men with metabolic syndrome and NAFLD found similar beneficial results using a Spanish ketogenic Mediterranean diet. To quote the authors, "complete fatty liver regression was observed in 21.4% of the patients, and an overall reduction was found in 92.86% of the patients [...] After the diet, all the subjects were free of MS according to the IDF definition, and 100% of them had normal triacylglycerols and HDL levels, in spite of the fact that 100% of them still had a BMI of > 30 kg = m2. We conclude that the SKMD could be an effective and safe way to treat patients suffering from MS and the associated NAFLD (Pérez-Guisado and Muñoz-Serrano 2011)."

While the modified Mediterranean ketogenic diet shows promising research, the typical ketogenic diet is still inconclusive. There are at least five variations of the ketogenic diet. The classic ketogenic diet is the strictest in terms of macronutrient ratios and is the one on which all other ketogenic diets are based. With the classic ketogenic diet, 90% of daily calories come from fat, 6% come from protein, and just 4% come from carbohydrates.

Studies have shown that low-carbohydrate diets promote weight loss, decrease the triglyceride content within the liver, and improve some metabolic factors in obese patients. However, there is not enough evidence to establish the role of very-low-carbohydrate ketogenic diets (VLCKD) in the long-term management of obesity (Bueno, Melo, Oliveira, and Ataide 2013).

TABLE 6.7
Modified Mediterranean Diet: Caloric Break Down[a]

Fat
- 45% of calories come from fats rich in monounsaturated and omega-3 fatty acids

Protein
- 20% of calories come from a mix of animal- and plant-based protein

Carbs
- 35% of calories come from predominantly non-starchy sources of carbohydrates

[a] Fraser, A. et al. 2008. A modified Mediterranean diet is associated with the greatest reduction in alanine aminotransferase levels in obese type 2 diabetes patients: results of a quasi-randomized controlled trial. *Diabetologia* 51 (9):1616–1622.

More significantly, laboratory studies of mice reported that long-term ketogenic diets can promote development of NAFLD and glucose intolerance (Schugar and Crawford 2012). This seems to occur for two reasons within mice. One, low intake of amino acids choline and methionine results in hepatic damage. Two, high fat intake induces hepatocyte cell injury in those hepatocytes that receive more fat than can be oxidized or exported by VLDL secretion (Schugar and Crawford 2012). Although ketogenic diets are recommended with increasing frequency for obesity, neurological diseases, and NAFLD, and despite having some beneficial attributes, their metabolic effects are not yet completely understood. The responses individuals have to these diets can vary (Schugar and Crawford 2012). So, if carbohydrate restriction is to be performed as therapy, types and amount of fat need be monitored without the restriction of protein intake (especially the amino acids, choline, and methionine).

Specific Nutrients, Food Sources, and Botanicals Beneficial for NAFLD

Currently, with the exception of vitamin E, there is limited evidence showing efficacy of the following compounds in human subjects (Barb, Portillo-Sanchez, and Cusi, 2016). However, the authors have seen efficacy in individuals within clinical settings. There is a need for additional randomized control trials for therapeutic micronutrients with regard to NAFLD.

Vitamins and Minerals

Vitamin C

Vitamin C is a very important antioxidant needed for biochemical, metabolic, and neurological health in the human body. It is also useful for the prevention of disease states such as cardiovascular disease, cancer, cataracts, gout, lead toxicity, and immune conditions. Vitamin C is also required in order for our cells to burn fat (Fry, 2017a). This may be an important consideration for the treatment of NAFLD considering the accumulation of fat surrounding the liver with this disease. Indeed, research suggests that vitamin C supplementation can reduce inflammatory markers and improve liver status in cases of NAFLD (Oliveira et al. 2003; Harrison, Torgerson, Hayashi, Ward, and Schenker 2003). Food sources of vitamin C by the highest concentration per cup include guavas, bell pepper, kiwifruit, strawberries, oranges, papaya, broccoli, tomato, kale, and snow peas (myfooddata.com).

Vitamin D

Vitamin D is needed for calcium metabolism in the body, blood pressure regulation, immune function, and insulin secretion. Low vitamin D status is linked with many chronic disease states and is useful for the prevention of high blood pressure, autoimmune conditions, osteoporosis, and cancer. Evidence from a systematic review of randomized controlled trials suggests that low serum vitamin D may cause NAFLD, in that hypovitaminosis D is associated with the severity and incidence of NAFLD (Hariri and Zohdi 2019). Low vitamin D levels may also increase the risk of developing NAFLD due to the lowered ability to counter inflammation when vitamin D deficiency is present (Barchetta et al. 2011).

Vitamin E

Vitamin E consists of four tocopherols (a-, b-, c-, and d-) and the corresponding tocotrienols (a-, b-, c-, and d-) which contain unsaturated side chains. Among the tocochromanol family, a-tocopherol is believed to present the most biological antioxidant activity, mainly attributed to inhibition of membrane lipid peroxidation (Bramley et al. 2000). It is at this location that vitamin E functions to protect cells from harmful substances. It is useful for the prevention of cardiovascular disease, cancer, and immune disorders while also being beneficial for the treatment of diabetes (Fry 2017b). Similar to vitamin C, vitamin E is beneficial for the treatment of NAFLD due to its ability to reduce the inflammatory status of the liver (Oliveria et al. 2003). However, please be aware that long-term vitamin E supplementation can increase the risk for the development of stroke and prostate cancer. A vitamin E dose of 800IU taken daily for 96 weeks showed significant improvement in the NAFLD Activity Score (a validated noninvasive tool used to assess changes in NAFLD status during therapeutic interventions; Brunt, Kleiner, Wilson, Belt, and Neuschwander-Tetri 2011) and no worsening fibrosis in adults with NASH (Barb, Portillo-Sanchez, and Cusi 2016).

Food sources of vitamin E by highest concentration per cup include sunflower seeds, almond, avocados, spinach, butternut squash, kiwifruit, broccoli, trout, olive oil, shrimp (myfooddata.com).

Fish Oils

Fish oils, mainly EPA and DHA-Omega 3 fatty acids, represent one of the most widely used supplements for many metabolic conditions as they can improve lipid homeostasis and inflammation. A 41 patient NASH study randomized patients to receive 3,000 mg/day of fish oil or placebo for 1 year and observed improved ALT in the treated patients. In another study, 52 obese NAFLD patients treated with 1000 mg fish oil reported improved AST, ALT, and steatosis (Perumpail et al. 2018).

Coenzyme Q-10

Like fish oil, coenzyme Q-10 (CoQ10) is used widely. CoQ10 has been known to improve inflammation and lipid homeostasis in the liver. A blinded RCT treated NAFLD patients with 100 mg of CoQ10 and noted reduced AST, ALT, and hepatic inflammation compared to placebo (Perumpail et al. 2018). Foods high in coenzyme Q10 include organ meat (heart, liver, and kidney), muscle meat of beef, chicken or pork, fatty fish such as trout, herring or sardines, and vegetables such as spinach, cauliflower, and broccoli (healthine.com/nutrition/coenzyme).

Spices

Ginger

Ginger, known as *Zingiber officinale*, is a root used as an ingredient and spice in many countries for centuries. This root contains many potent phytonutrients and has been used traditionally by many ancient cultures for the treatment of inflammatory diseases (Langner, Greifenberg, and Gruenwald 1998). Modern research has also provided evidence for its ability to be useful for the treatment of disease such as cancer, diabetes, and hyperlipidemia (Rahimlou, Yari, Hekmatdoost, Alavian, and Keshavarz 2016). In regard to NAFLD, research suggests that ginger may reduce inflammatory markers associated with the progression of NAFLD. In a double-blind randomized study of 44 patients with NAFLD, 2 g of ginger daily for 12 weeks along with a modified diet and physical activity program was found to have reduced NAFLD-related liver enzymes and inflammatory cytokines in comparison to placebo (Rahimlou et al. 2016).

Turmeric

Turmeric (*Curcuma longa*) is a root used traditionally in Indian food and herbal medicine. The active ingredient in turmeric is curcumin. There is abundant research indicating that curcumin is a powerful antioxidant and anti-inflammatory agent, with the ability to neutralize free radicals (Dinkova-Kostova and Talalay). Curcumin can decrease NAFLD risk factors (e.g., insulin resistance) via the reduction of lipids in the blood and decreasing the concentration of uric acid. In a study where 102 NAFLD patients were randomized to receive placebo or 1,000 mg/day of curcumin for 8 weeks, it was concluded that curcumin improved hepatic steatosis (determined via imaging and liver enzymes) in NAFLD patients without any issues of tolerance. A prospective cohort study involving 400 mg curcumin supplementation also noted statistically significantly improved liver ultrasound results (Perumpail et al. 2018). Research also indicates that the supplementation of 500 mg of curcumin per day is associated with a significant reduction of liver fat content and improvement in lipid, liver, and glucose markers when compared to a placebo group (Rahmani et al. 2016).

Flavonoids and Polyphenols

Flavonoids and polyphenols are classes of phytonutrients commonly stored in the pigmentation of various fruits, vegetables, and other plant material (Heneman and Zidenberg-Cherr 2008). These two classes of phytochemicals have been noted to be useful for the treatment and prevention of disease states such as cancer, cardiovascular disease, and other metabolic conditions such as NAFLD (Fry 2017c). Flavonoids, substances derived from citrus, have been observed to prevent hepatic steatosis, dyslipidemia, and insulin sensitivity by decreasing fat production in the liver while also decreasing inflammation of the liver (Assini, Mulvihill, and Huff 2013). Regulation of oxidative stress, inflammation, lipid metabolism, immune response, insulin resistance, and gut microbiota are fundamental characteristics of the effects of polyphenols on the body and contribute to the prevention and treatment of liver conditions (Li et al. 2018). Specifically, polyphenols inhibit lipogenesis, the metabolic formation of fat, reducing fat accumulation in the liver (Ben, Polimeni, Barrata, Pastori, and Angelico 2017).

Garlic and Onions

Garlic and onions contain a variety of chemical compounds that work as antioxidants, anti-inflammatory agents, and antimicrobials (Wilson and Demmig-Adams 2007). These two foods have been proven to be therapeutic for conditions such as cancer, coronary heart disease, obesity, hypercholesterolemia, type 2 diabetes, hypertension, and disturbances of the gastrointestinal tract. Garlic and onions have also been investigated as therapeutic foods for the treatment of NAFLD. Rodent studies have discovered that garlic and onions, particularly when utilized together, significantly reduce biochemical inflammatory markers associated with the progression of NAFLD (Lanzotti 2006; El-Din, Sabra, Hamman, Ebeid, and El-Lakkany 2014; Emamat et al. 2015).

Dark Chocolate and Cocoa Powder

Cocoa, the bean used to produce chocolate, contains antioxidant chemicals which include a variety of flavonoids and polyphenols (Emamat, Foroughi, Eini-Zinab, and Hekmatdoost 2018). Research investigating the therapeutic use of cocoa has concluded that it is beneficial for the treatment of cardiovascular conditions, reduces inflammation, and bolsters immune function (Lotito et al. 2000). As related to NAFLD, cocoa supplementation and the consumption of dark chocolate have led to the reduction of oxidative stress and inflammatory blood markers associated with the progression of NAFLD (Engler and Engler 2006; Rezazadeh, Mahmoodi, Mard, and Karimi Moghaddam 2015). Using nonalkalized sugar-free dark chocolate powder in smoothies or cooking may be a suitable way of incorporating this food into your diet.

Berries: Raspberries, Blueberries, and Strawberries

The Rosaceae and Ericaceae families of berries include strawberries, raspberries, and blueberries. These berries all contain compounds with antioxidant properties useful for the treatment and prevention of conditions such as inflammatory disorders, cardiovascular disease, and cancer (Skrovankova, Sumczynski, Mlcek, Jurikova, and Sochor 2015). The polyphenol anthocyanin in these berries have been used effectively to reduce inflammatory markers associated in *in vitro* models of NAFLD progression (Wang, Zhao, Wang, Huo, and Ji 2016). Be sure to contact a licensed health provider concerning optimal servings of berries considering the sugar content of berries.

Coffee

In many studies, coffee has been shown to have an inverse relationship with the progression of NAFLD. The benefits of coffee are due to polyphenols, which have a similar structure to milk thistle (silymarin), an herb beneficial to liver health. The polyphenols found in coffee can also increase the production of antioxidant proteins in the body. Antioxidants found within coffee include chlorogenic acids, melanoidin, and caffeine. Consumption of caffeinated coffee daily was shown to decrease liver transaminases (i.e., ALT and AST) and mitigate the progression to type 2 diabetes mellitus in those with NAFLD. This was not the case with the consumption of decaffeinated coffee (Dickson et al., 2015).

Green Tea

Green tea, like coffee, is well documented regarding having beneficial effects on those with NAFLD. It is made from the leaves of the *Camellia sinensis* plant and contains epigallocatechin-3-gallate (EGCG), the primary therapeutic agent in green tea. Both the polyphenols and EGCG in green tea result in its antioxidative effect. A double-blinded RCT with 80 NAFLD patients revealed improved ALT and AST levels in patients supplemented daily with 500 mg of green tea extract, compared to placebo. Another 12-week study, with 80 patients randomized to receive 500 mg of green tea extract or placebo daily, noted improvement in all parameters of NAFLD measured in the treatment group. The green tea group observed had improved inflammatory markers, aminotransferases, insulin resistance, adiponectin, and regression of fatty liver on ultrasound examination (Perumpail et al. 2018).

Resveratrol

Resveratrol is a phytochemical most notably found in the pigmentation of red grapes, black tea, green tea, and cocoa (Lee, Kim, Lee, and Lee 2003; Baur, 2006). This phytochemical is suspected to be a contributing factor to the reduced rates of metabolic conditions seen historically in the French populous due to the French incorporating red wine as a part of their diet. Much research has revealed resveratrol's ability to act as an antioxidant and its usefulness for the treatment of cancer, heart disease, hyperlipidemia, inflammatory conditions, and neurological conditions (Bauer and Sinclair 2006). Resveratrol has also shown to be beneficial for the treatment of NAFLD by slowing progression of fat accumulation in the liver and reducing inflammatory markers associated with NAFLD (Shang et al. 2008; Bujanda et al. 2008). In a double-blinded RCT, 50 NAFLD patients were divided to receive lifestyle modification and placebo or 500 mg of resveratrol, for 12 weeks. After the study period ended, the treatment group showed improved inflammatory cytokines, ALT, and hepatic steatosis compared to the placebo group. A similar RCT with 60 NAFLD patients randomized to either placebo or 600 mg of resveratrol, for 3 months, noted improved levels of ALT, AST, insulin resistance, and inflammatory factors (Perumpail et al. 2018).

Cocoa has the highest concentration of resveratrol compared to red wine and other sources (cocoa > red wine > green tea > black tea) (Lee et al. 2003). Adding two tablespoons of a nonalkalized sugar-free cocoa powder to smoothies, drinks, or cooking may therefore prove beneficial (Lee et al. 2003).

> All in all, there are many promising herbs and supplements that can be used as an alternative treatment for NAFLD…However, to say that they should be part of a treatment for NAFLD and/or NASH is to overstep, as there is no clinical data that support this notion. Milk thistle, turmeric, resveratrol, coffee, and green tea have been extensively researched in the NAFLD population and have not been shown to have toxic effects. We can only recommend that they be used with caution and that further research is necessary to confirm the therapeutic role of herbs in patients with NAFLD
>
> *Brandon J. Perumpail et al. (2018)*

COOKING AND FOOD PREPARATION METHODS FOR NAFLD

High-Fructose Corn Syrup

At least one study has indicated concerns regarding the heating of high-fructose corn syrup. In a study looking at the effect of feeding high-fructose corn syrup to bees as a honey replacement, it was noted that the heating of high-fructose corn syrup created a toxin called hydroxymethylfurfural, which is highly toxic to honey bees (LeBlanc et al., 2009). In a more recent article, the authors reviewed the effects of HMF from heating honey and other foods containing sugar molecules, including fruits and vegetables, and noted that there are both detrimental and health-promoting benefits when applying heat to certain foods (Shapla, Solayman, Alam, Khalil, and Gan 2018).

In this article, it is noted that HMF is not present naturally in food products. The compound is formed upon thermal treatment and in combination with other factors. As it is a product of the nonenzymatic Maillard reaction, there is no fixed concentration of HMF in different food items. The baking temperature, rate of saccharose degradation, concentration of reducing sugars, type of sugar (glucose, fructose, or others), water activity, the addition of other food additives such as HMF-containing sweeteners, coloring agents, caramelization, storage time and temperature, type of metallic storage, and processing container are all factors in the amount of HMFs a food contains, and thus, HMFs vary widely among different food items (Shapla et al. 2018). Storage temperature and storage duration in particular directly influence the development of HMF in stored honey. Unlike for honey, in the processing of other foodstuffs, comparatively higher temperatures (during baking, roasting), longer duration times, and different additives are required, which profoundly affect the HMF content in the foods. It is concluded that there are no heat-processed food products that are free of HMF (Shapla et al. 2018).

As the authors note, we consume several different food products, including bakery goods, milk, fruit juice, cereals, coffee, chocolate, soft drinks, vinegar, wine, nuts, and grilled meat in our daily lives. The majority of these products undergo thermal treatments prior to consumption, such as boiling, baking, extrusion cooking, roasting, pasteurization, and other processing. These processes are performed not only to make the products more edible but also (1) for preservation (by means of reducing microbial load and/or eliminating enzymatic activities) and (2) to generate more desirable sensory (color, aroma, and taste) and texture properties. With any of these techniques, there is a concern about not only HMFs but also other possible detrimental compounds being formed upon thermal treatment in combination with other factors. Extensive processing produces adverse effects both by introducing undesirable, harmful, and nonnutritive compounds and by reducing nutritive value, fresh appearance, and taste (Figure 6.2).

Vitamins E and C: discussed in the chapter on hyperlipidemia and hypertension.

Vitamin D

Cooking may cause detrimental loss of vitamin D, but it depends on the actual foodstuffs and the heating process. A study looking to evaluate retention of D2 and D3 from eggs, margarine, and bread found that for eggs and margarine, vitamin D during oven heating was retained at less than half, but frying resulted in higher retention. Boiled eggs were similar to frying retention amounts. For bread, retention of D3 and D2 occurred more for rye bread than for wheat bread. For mushrooms and trout fish, studies suggest higher retention of vitamin D2 and D3, respectively. With the exception of pan-frying for trout and oven baking for mushrooms, there was minimal changes to the percentage of vitamin D retained after cooking with boiling and steam and microwave cooking. Evaluating these foods are of particular importance as 100 g of trout fish and mushrooms in the raw state contain levels comparable to the recommended dietary allowance of 10–15 µg/day (400–600 IU).

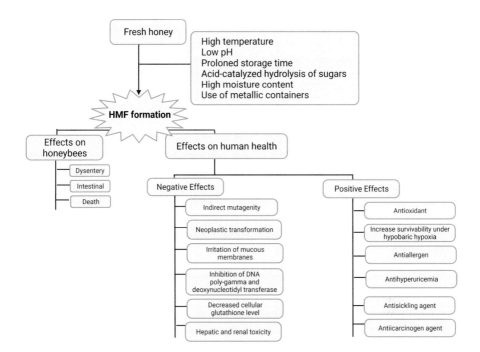

FIGURE 6.2   Causes of HMF formation from fresh honey and resultant effects on honeybees and human health. (Shapla, Ummay Mahfuza et al. 4 Apr. 2018. 5-Hydroxymethylfurfural (HMF) levels in honey and other food products: effects on bees and human health. *Chemistry Central Journal* 12(1):35.)

Additional culinary methods to maintain vitamin D levels are important to identify. Addition of lemon juice (2–5 drops) led to insignificant losses of vitamin D even when used with the cooking methods found to initially reduce levels in the aforementioned study.

Mixed results have occurred from studies evaluating the bioavailability of vitamin D, as measured by postprandial serum levels, from cooked foods. One study found that among prediabetics, there was no increase in serum levels after ingesting mushrooms cooked daily for 12 weeks; however, these mushrooms underwent not only cooking but freezing, thawing, and microwave reheating, while a randomized control study found that UV-enriched button mushrooms that were then cooked into a soup and consumed daily for 2 weeks led to increase in serum vitamin D levels among healthy adults.

Garlic and Onions: discussed in the chapter on hyperlipidemia and hypertension.

Coenzyme Q10

Coenzyme Q10 is a fat-soluble vitamin and is an important antioxidant. Levels in the body occur by endogenous synthesis or exogenously through food and supplement. Dietary sources of coenzyme Q10 are relatively understudied compared to supplements, despite the finding that low dose supplement and dietary source from organ meat can lead to similar serum levels (Weber, Bysted, and Hølmer 1997). With regard to cooking methods of animal products rich in coenzyme Q10, conflicting results exist if boiling versus frying can lead to retention. However, one study found no difference between the preparation methods and that coenzyme Q10 from organ meat had higher digestibility than that from muscle meat.

Resveratrol

Resveratrol is commonly consumed through berries, including consumption of wine. The relationship between polyphenols and culinary preparation can be complex. For example, wine production involves maceration of resveratrol-rich grape skins. Though the maceration, there is a diffusion-based increase in polyphenol concentration. In a study using berries as the source of resveratrol, baking of blueberries and bilberries for 18 minutes led to significant reduction in resveratrol concentrations. It is not known how the reduced levels for resveratrol with cooking affect its antioxidation function.

HEALTHY COOKING TECHNIQUES

For all of the recommended dietary protocols, food and herbal sources, proper preparation is key to retaining nutrients and enhancing digestibility of the foods. Moreover, there should always be a mixture of raw and cooked foods in every meal.

> The main rule of thumb for healthy cooking is to avoid methods that require excessive heat and fat. For that reason, I urge you not to fry food and especially to avoid deep-frying.
>
> *Dr. Andrew Weil, MD (2018a)*

Stir-frying: This method enables you to quickly cook foods over high heat, by combining and continually stirring vegetables and healthy sources of protein. Ideally, stir-frying can be done in a lightly oiled wok or in a stainless-steel frying pan. It is important to use a minimal amount of healthy oils (e.g., olive oil) and keep these oils below their respective smoking points.

Steam frying: This is another quick cooking technique in which you begin by sautéing food briefly in a pan, with a small amount of oil. You then add water or stock and cover the pan. When the food is almost done, simply uncover the pan and boil off any excess liquid (if applicable).

Sauté: Involves cooking food quickly, over direct heat, in a small amount of liquid or oil.

Steaming: Simply involves cooking food, over boiling water, in a pot or pan that is covered. This particular cooking technique does the least damage to nutrients and allows food to retain texture and shape.

Broiling, baking, and roasting are also healthy methods of food preparation, as long as you don't add unnecessary or unhealthy fat.

Broiling: Cooking food at a high temperature, directly under the heat source.

Baking: Cooking food in an oven.

Roasting: Cooking food uncovered in an oven.

COOKWARE RECOMMENDATIONS

It is advised to not cook food in aluminum cookware as the ingestion of aluminum can be harmful to the kidneys. In addition, it can deplete the body of phosphorus and calcium, weakening the bones.

However, if you simply love the look of aluminum pots, be sure the aluminum is only used on the exterior surface of the cookware. The interior should ideally be constructed of stainless steel or another material that does not pose health risks such as ceramic.

As Dr. Weil has pointed out, "There is no need for aluminum in human nutrition, and because it is so chemically reactive, it is probably not good for us" (Weil 2018b). He suggests using stainless-steel cookware as it is completely nontoxic, highly durable, and provides excellent cooking results.

He also recommends ceramic-coated (eco) pans. Dr. Weil states that "I think they're a great advance over earlier nonstick pans and bakeware and are safer because they're made without perfluorooctanoic acid, known as PFOA, the potentially toxic chemical used in the manufacture of coatings for nonstick pans such as Teflon. The nonstick surface of the new green pans uses ceramic-based nanotechnology that is said – unlike older nonstick coatings – to be stable on exposure to high heat."

NAFLD KEY POINTS

- Fructose also plays a key role in the development of NAFLD, specifically in its processed form as high-fructose corn syrup.
- Dietary patterns such as the Dash and Mediterranean diet can be helpful in reducing RISK factors and for improving NAFLD.
- Mediterranean ketogenic diet shows favorable results in NAFLD patients.
- Nutrients shown to protect against NAFLD include vitamin E, vitamin D, and omega-3.
- Relevant cooking methods helps to maintain NAFLD protective nutrients:
  - High-fructose corn syrup – eating and especially the heating of foods with HFCS should be avoided.
  - Vitamin D – mushrooms may be a good source to provide protective levels even when cooked.
  - Use of lemon juice may maintain vitamin D levels in some cooked dishes.

REFERENCES

Assini, J. M., E. E. Mulvihill, and M. W. Huff. 2013. Citrus flavonoids and lipid metabolism. *Current Opinion in Lipidology* 24 (1):34–40.

Barb, D., P. Portillo-Sanchez, and K. Cusi. 2016. Pharmacological management of nonalcoholic fatty liver disease. *Metabolism* 65 (8):1183–1195. doi:10.1016/j.metabol.2016.04.004.

Barchetta, I., F. Angelico, M. Del Ben, et al. 2011. Strong association between non alcoholic fatty liver disease (NAFLD) and low 25 (OH) vitamin D levels in an adult population with normal serum liver enzymes. *BMC Medicine* 9 (1):85.

Baur, J. A., and D. A. Sinclair. 2006. Therapeutic potential of resveratrol: The in vivo evidence. *Nature Reviews Drug Discovery* 5 (6):493.

Ben M. D., L. Polimeni, F. Baratta, D. Pastori, F. Angelico. 2017. The role of nutraceuticals for the treatment of non-alcoholic fatty liver disease. *British Journal of Clinical Pharmacology* 83(1):88–95. doi: 10.1111/bcp.12899.

Bramley, P. M., A. Kafatos, F. J. Kelly, Y. Manios, H. E. Roxborough, W. Schuch, P. J. A. Sheehy, and K. H. Wagner. 2000. Review vitamin E. *Journal of the Science of Food and Agriculture* 80:913–938.

Brunt, E. M., D. E. Kleiner, L. A. Wilson, P. Belt, and B. A. Neuschwander-Tetri. 2011. Nonalcoholic fatty liver disease (NAFLD) activity score and the histopathologic diagnosis in NAFLD: Distinct clinicopathologic meanings. *Hepatology* 53 (3):810–820. doi:10.1002/hep.24127.

Bueno, N. B., I. S. Melo, S. L. Oliveira, and T. D. Ataide. 2013. Very-low-carbohydrate ketogenic diet v. low-fat diet for long-term weight loss: A meta-analysis of randomised controlled trials. *British Journal of Nutrition* 110 (07):1178–1187. doi:10.1017/s0007114513000548.

Bujanda, L., E. Hijona, M. Larzabal, et al. 2008. Resveratrol inhibits nonalcoholic fatty liver disease in rats. *BMC Gastroenterology* 8 (1):40.

Dickson, J. C., A. D. Liese, C. Lorenzo, et al. 2015. Associations of coffee consumption with of liver injury in the insulin resistance atherosclerosis study. *BMC Gastroenterology* 15 (1):88. doi:10.1186/s12876-015-0321-3.

Dinkova-Kostova, A. T., and P. Talalay. 1999. Relation of structure of curcumin analogs to their potencies as inducers of Phase 2 detoxification enzymes. *Carcinogenesis* 20 (5):911–914.

Drewnowski, A. and N. Darmon. 2005. Food choices and diet costs: An economic analysis. *The Journal of Nutrition* 135(4):900–904.

El-Din, S. H., A. N. Sabra, O. A. Hammam, F. A. Ebeid, and N. M. El-Lakkany. 2014. Pharmacological and antioxidant actions of garlic and. or onion in non-alcoholic fatty liver disease (NAFLD) in rats. *Journal of the Egyptian Society of Parasitology* 44 (2):295–308.

Emamat, H., F. Foroughi, H. Eini-Zinab, and A. Hekmatdoost. 2018. The effects of onion consumption on prevention of nonalcoholic fatty liver disease. *Indian Journal of Clinical Biochemistry* 33 (1):75–80.

Emamat, H., F. Foroughi, H. Eini–Zinab, M. Taghizadeh, M. Rismanchi, and A. Hekmatdoost. 2015. The effects of onion consumption on treatment of metabolic, histologic, and inflammatory features of nonalcoholic fatty liver disease. *Journal of Diabetes & Metabolic Disorders* 15 (1):25.

Engler, M. B. and M. M. Engler. 2006. The emerging role of flavonoid-rich cocoa and chocolate in cardiovascular health and disease. *Nutrition Reviews* 64 (3):109–118.

Fan, J. G., and H. X. Cao. 2013. Role of diet and nutritional management in non-alcoholic fatty liver disease. *Journal of Gastroenterology and Hepatology* 28 (S4):81–87.

Fraser, A., R. Abel, D. A. Lawlor, D. Fraser, and A. Elhayany. 2008. A modified Mediterranean diet is associated with the greatest reduction in alanine aminotransferase levels in obese type 2 diabetes patients: Results of a quasi-randomised controlled trial. *Diabetologia* 51 (9):1616–1622.

Fry, M. 2017a. Module 11: Vitamin C [PDF file]. Retrieved from Maryland University of Integrative Health, NUTR612 Human Nutrition II: Micronutrients. Canvas: https://learn.muih.edu.

Fry, M. 2017b. Module 8: Vitamin D [PDF file]. Retrieved from Maryland University of Integrative Health, NUTR612 Human Nutrition II: Micronutrients. Canvas: https://learn.muih.edu.

Fry, M. 2017c. Module 13: Flavonoids & polyphenols [PDF file]. Retrieved from Maryland University of Integrative Health, NUTR612 Human Nutrition II: Micronutrients. Canvas: https://learn.muih.edu.

Guasch-Ferré M., J. Merino, Q. Sun, M. Fitó, J. Salas-Salvadó. 2017. Dietary polyphenols, mediterranean diet, prediabetes, and type 2 diabetes: A narrative review of the evidence. *Oxidative Medicine Cellular Longevity* 2017:6723931. doi: 10.1155/2017/6723931.

Harrison, S. A., S. Torgerson, P. Hayashi, J. Ward, and S. Schenker. 2003. Vitamin E and vitamin C treatment improves fibrosis in patients with nonalcoholic steatohepatitis. *The American Journal of Gastroenterology* 98 (11):2485–2490.

Hariri, M., and S. Zohdi. 2019. Effect of vitamin D on non-alcoholic fatty liver disease: A systematic review of randomized controlled clinical trials. *International Journal of Preventive Medicine* 10:14. Published 2019 Jan 15. doi:10.4103/ijpvm. IJPVM_499_17.

Heneman, K., and S. Zidenberg-Cherr. 2008. *Nutrition and health info sheet: Phytochemicals*. Oakland, CA: University of California, Division of Agriculture and Natural Resources.

Iser, D., and M. Ryan. 2013. Fatty liver disease: A practical guide for GPs. *Australian Family Physician* 42 (7):444–447. http://www.racgp.org.au/afp/2013/july/fatty-liver-disease/.

Jakobsen, J., and P. Knuthsen. 2014. Stability of vitamin D in foodstuffs during cooking. *Food Chemistry* 148:170–175.

Jensen, T., M. F. Abdelmalek, S. Sullivan, et al. 2018. Fructose and sugar: A major mediator of nonalcoholic fatty liver disease. *Journal of Hepatology* 68 (5):1063–1075.

Jin, R., J. A. Welsh, N. A. Le, et al. 2014. Dietary fructose reduction improves markers of cardiovascular disease risk in Hispanic-American adolescents with NAFLD. *Nutrients* 6 (8):3187–3201.

Kanerva, N., S. Sandboge, N. E. Kaartinen, S. Männistö, and J. G. Eriksson. 2014. Higher fructose intake is inversely associated with risk of nonalcoholic fatty liver disease in older Finnish adults. *American Journal of Clinical Nutrition* 100 (4):1133–1138.

Kawasaki, T., K. Igarashi, and T. Koeda, et al. 2009. Rats fed fructose-enriched diets have characteristics of nonalcoholic hepatic steatosis. *The Journal of Nutrition* 139 (11):2067–2071.

LaBrecque, D., A. Zaigham, A. Frank, et al. 2014. Nonalcoholic fatty liver disease and non-alcoholic steatohepatitis. World Gastroenterology Organization Global Guidelines. *Journal of Clinical Gastroenterology* 48 (6):467–473 Retrieved from http://www. worldgastroenterology.org/assets/export/userfiles/2012_NASH%20and%20NAFLD_ Final_lo ng.pdf.

Lanaspa, M. A., L. G. Sanchez-Lozada, Y. Choi, et al. 2012. Uric acid induces hepatic steatosis by generation of mitochondrial oxidative stress. *Journal of Biological Chemistry* 287 (48):40732–40744. doi:10.1074/jbc.m112.399899.

Langner, E., S. Greifenberg, and J. Gruenwald. 1998. Ginger: History and use. *Advances in Therapy* 15 (1):25–44.

Lanzotti, V. 2006. The analysis of onion and garlic. *Journal of Chromatography A* 1112 (1–2):3–22.

LeBlanc, B. W., G. Eggleston, D. Sammataro, C. Cornett, R. Dufault, T. Deeby, E. St Cyr. 2009. Formation of hydroxymethylfurfural in domestic high-fructose corn syrup and its toxicity to the honey bee (Apis mellifera). *Journal of Agricultural and Food Chemistry* 26;57(16):7369–76.

Lee, K. W., Y. J. Kim, H. J. Lee, and C. Y. Lee. 2003. Cocoa has more phenolic phytochemicals and a higher antioxidant capacity than teas and red wine. *Journal of Agricultural and Food Chemistry* 51 (25):7292–7295.

Li, S., H. Y. Tan, N. Wang, F. Cheung, M. Hong, and Y. Feng. 2018. The potential and action mechanism of polyphenols in the treatment of liver diseases. *Oxidative Medicine and Cellular Longevity* 2018 (5):1–25. doi:10.1155/2018/8394818.

Lim, J. S., M. Mietus-Snyder, A. Valente, J. M. Schwarz, and R. H. Lustig. 2010. The role of fructose in the pathogenesis of NAFLD and the metabolic syndrome. *Nature Reviews Gastroenterology and Hepatology* 7 (5):251.

Lotito, S. B., L. Actis-Goretta, M. L. Renart, et al. 2000. Influence of oligomer chain length on the antioxidant activity of procyanidins. *Biochemical and Biophysical Research Communications* 276 (3):945–951.

Mahan, L. K., and J. L. Raymond. 2012. *Krause's food & the nutrition care process* (13th ed.). St. Louis, MO: Elsevier Saunders.

Martínez Steele, E., L. G. Baraldi, M. L. Louzada, J. C. Moubarac, D. Mozaffarian, and C. A. Monteiro. 2016. Ultra-processed foods and added sugars in the US diet: Evidence from a nationally representative cross-sectional study. *BMJ Open* 6(3):e009892.

Mirmiran, P., Z. Amirhamidi, H. S. Ejtahed, Z. Bahadoran, and F. Azizi. 2017. Relationship between diet and non-alcoholic fatty liver disease: A review article. *Iranian Journal of Public Health* 46(8):1007–1017.

Oliveira, C. P., L. C. da Costa Gayotto, C. Tatai, et al. 2003. Vitamin C and vitamin E in prevention of nonalcoholic fatty liver disease (NAFLD) in choline deficient diet fed rats. *Nutrition Journal* 2 (1):9.

Pérez-Guisado, J., and A. Muñoz-Serrano. 2011. The effect of the Spanish Ketogenic Mediterranean Diet on nonalcoholic fatty liver disease: A pilot study. *Journal of Medicinal Food* 14 (7–8):677–680.

Perumpail, B., A. Li, U. Iqbal, et al. 2018. Potential therapeutic benefits of herbs and supplements in patients with NAFLD. *Diseases* 6 (3):80. doi:10.3390/diseases6030080.

Popkin, B. M., and C. Hawkes. 2016. Sweetening of the global diet, particularly beverages: Patterns, trends, and policy responses. *The Lancet Diabetes & Endocrinology* 4 (2):174–186.

Rahimlou, M., Z. Yari, A. Hekmatdoost, S. M. Alavian, and S. A. Keshavarz. 2016. Ginger supplementation in nonalcoholic fatty liver disease: A randomized, double-blind, placebo-controlled pilot study. *Hepatitis Monthly* 16 (1).

Rahmani, S., S. Asgary, G. Askari, et al. 2016. Treatment of non-alcoholic fatty liver disease with curcumin: A randomized placebo-controlled trial. *Phytotherapy Research* 30 (9):1540–1548.

Razavi Zade, M., M. H. Telkabadi, F. Bahmani, B. Salehi, S. Farshbaf, and Z. Asemi. 2016. The effects of DASH diet on weight loss and metabolic status in adults with non-alcoholic fatty liver disease: A randomized clinical trial. *Liver International* 36 (4):563–571.

Rezazadeh, A., M. Mahmoodi, S. A. Mard, and E. Karimi Moghaddam. 2015. The effects of dark chocolate consumption on lipid profile, fasting blood sugar, liver enzymes, inflammation, and antioxidant status in patients with non-alcoholic fatty liver disease: A randomized, placebo-controlled, pilot study. *Journal of Gastroenterology and Hepatology Research* 4 (12):1858–1864.

Romero-Gómez, M., S. Zelber-Sagi, and M. Trenell. 2017. Treatment of NAFLD with diet, physical activity and exercise. *Journal of Hepatology* 67 (4):829–846. doi:10.1016/j.jhep.2017.05.016.

Schugar, R. C., and P. A. Crawford. 2012. Low-carbohydrate ketogenic diets, glucose homeostasis, and nonalcoholic fatty liver disease. *Current Opinion in Clinical Nutrition and Metabolic Care* 15 (4):374–380. doi:10.1097/mco.0b013e3283547157.

Shang, J., L. L. Chen, F. X. Xiao, H. Sun, H. C. Ding, and H. Xiao. 2008. Resveratrol improves non- alcoholic fatty liver disease by activating AMP-activated protein kinase. *Acta Pharmacologica Sinica* 29 (6):698.

Shapla, U. M., M. Solayman, N. Alam, M. I. Khalil, and S. H. Gan. 2018. 5-Hydroxymethylfurfural (HMF) levels in honey and other food products: Effects on bees and human health. *Chemistry Central Journal* 12 (1):35.

Skrovankova, S., D. Sumczynski, J. Mlcek, T. Jurikova, and J. Sochor. 2015. Bioactive compounds and antioxidant activity in different types of berries. *International Journal of Molecular Sciences* 16 (10):24673–24706.

Sofi, F., and A. Casini. 2014. Mediterranean diet and non-alcoholic fatty liver disease: New therapeutic option around the corner? *World Journal of Gastroenterology* 20 (23):7339.

Sofi, F., C. Macchi, R. Abbate, G. F. Gensini, and A. Casini. 2013. Mediterranean diet and health. *Biofactors* 39 (4):335–342.

Tetri, L. H., M. Basaranoglu, E. M. Brunt, L. M. Yerian, and B. A. Neuschwander-Tetri. 2008. Severe NAFLD with hepatic necroinflammatory changes in mice fed trans fats and a high-fructose corn syrup equivalent. *American Journal of Physiology-Gastrointestinal and Liver Physiology* 295 (5):G987–G995.

Urbain, P., F. Singler, G. Ihorst, H. K. Biesalski, and H. Bertz. 2011. Bioavailability of vitamin D_2 from UV-B-irradiated button mushrooms in healthy adults deficient in serum 25-hydroxyvitamin D: A randomized controlled trial. *European Journal of Clinical Nutrition* 65 (8):965–971.

UW Health. 2015. Fructose-restricted diet [PDF file]. Retrieved from: https://www.uwhealth.org/healthfacts/nutrition/376.pdf.

Vasdev, S., V. Gill, S. Parai, L. Longerich, and V. Gadag. 2002. Dietary vitamin E and C supplementation prevents fructose induced hypertension in rats. *Molecular and Cellular Biochemistry* 241 (1–2):107–114.

Wang, Y., L. Zhao, D. Wang, Y. Huo, and B. Ji. 2016. Anthocyanin-rich extracts from blackberry, wild blueberry, strawberry, and chokeberry: Antioxidant activity and inhibitory effect on oleic acid-induced hepatic steatosis in vitro. *Journal of the Science of Food and Agriculture* 96 (7):2494–2503.

Weber, C., A. Bysted, and G. Hølmer. 1997. Intestinal absorption of coenzyme Q 10 administered in a meal or as capsules to healthy subjects. *Nutrition Research* 17:941–945.

Weil, A. 2018a. Healthy cooking techniques? *Dr. Weil*, (July 2, 2017). http://www.drweil.com/diet-nutrition/cooking-cookware/healthy-cooking-techniques/.

Weil, A. 2018b. Anxious about anodized aluminum? *Dr. Weil*, (October 23, 2008). http://www.drweil.com/diet-nutrition/cooking-cookware/anxious-about-anodized-aluminum/.

Wilson, E. A., and B. Demmig-Adams. 2007. Antioxidant, anti-inflammatory, and antimicrobial properties of garlic and onions. *Nutrition & Food Science* 37 (3):178–183.

Yasutake, K., M. Kohjima, K. Kotoh, M. Nakashima, M. Nakamuta, and M. Enjoji. 2014. Dietary habits and behaviors associated with nonalcoholic fatty liver disease. *World Journal of Gastroenterology* 20 (7):1756–1767.

Zelber-Sagi, S., F. Salomone, and L. Mlynarsky. 2017. The Mediterranean dietary pattern as the diet of choice for non-alcoholic fatty liver disease: Evidence and plausible mechanisms. *Liver International* 37 (7):936–949. doi:10.1111/liv.13435.

Zivkovic, A. M., J. B. German, and A. J. Sanyal. 2007. Comparative review of diets for the metabolic syndrome: Implications for nonalcoholic fatty liver disease. *The American Journal of Clinical Nutrition* 86 (2):285–300. doi:10.1093/ajcn/86.2.285.

GRAPHIC/FOOTNOTE:

Lanaspa, M. A., Sanchez-Lozada, L. G., Choi, Y., Cicerchi, C., Kanbay, M., Roncal-Jimenez, C. A., . . . Johnson, R. J. 2012. Uric acid induces hepatic steatosis by generation of mitochondrial oxidative stress. *Journal of Biological Chemistry* 287 (48):40732–40744. doi:10.1074/jbc.m112.399899.

ADDITIONAL REFERENCES

Anstee, Q. M., G. Targher, and C. P. Day. 2013. Progression of NAFLD to diabetes mellitus, cardiovascular disease or cirrhosis. *Nature Reviews Gastroenterology & Hepatology* 10 (6):330–344. doi: 10.1038/nrgastro.2013.41.

Byrne, C. D., and G. Targher. 2015. NAFLD: A multisystem disease. *Journal of Hepatology* 62 (1). doi:10.1016/j.jhep.2014.12.012.

Charlie Foundation for Ketogenic Therapies. 2018. 5 variations of the ketogenic diet. https://charliefoundation.org/diet-plans/.

Ekstedt, M., L. E. Franzén, U. L. Mathiesen, et al. 2006. Long-term follow-up of patients with NAFLD and elevated liver enzymes. *Hepatology* 44 (4):865–873. doi:10.1002/hep.21327.

Gaggini, M., M. Morelli, E. Buzzigoli, R. Defronzo, E. Bugianesi, and A. Gastaldelli. 2013. Non-alcoholic fatty liver disease (NAFLD) and its connection with insulin resistance, dyslipidemia, atherosclerosis and coronary heart disease. *Nutrients* 5 (5):1544–1560. doi:10.3390/nu5051544.

National Heart, Lung and Blood Institute. August 2015. In brief: Your guide to lowering your blood pressure with DASH. http://www.nhlbi.nih.gov/files/docs/public/heart/dash_brief.pdf.

Ratziu, V., S. Bellentani, H. Cortez-Pinto Day, and G. Marchesini. 2010. A position statement on NAFLD/NASH based on the EASL 2009 special conference. *Journal of Hepatology* 53 (2):372–384. doi:10.1016/j.jhep.2010.04.008.

Zelber-Sagi, S., D. Nitzan-Kaluski, R. Goldsmith, M. Webb, L. Blendis, Z. Halpern, et al. 2007. Long term nutritional intake and the risk for non-alcoholic fatty liver disease (NAFLD): A population based study. *Journal of Hepatology* 47 (5):711–717. doi:10.1016/j.jhep.2007.06.020.

7 Irritable Bowel Syndrome

Joshua Z. Goldenberg
The Goldenberg GI Center, LLC
Helfgott Research Institute

CONTENTS

DOI: 10.1201/b22377-7

INTRODUCTION

Irritable bowel syndrome (IBS) is a functional bowel disorder characterized by pain and bowel movement changes (Drossman and Hasler 2016). It affects a large percentage of humanity. Estimates put the global prevalence of IBS at anywhere between 10% and 25% of the world's population. From a demographics perspective, more women report an IBS diagnosis than men, with prevalence rates one and a half to three times higher. IBS is not more frequently reported by age as people report IBS similarly across the age spectrum. Evidence is mixed on whether higher or lower socioeconomic status has an increased prevalence of IBS (Canavan, West, and Card 2014).

QUALITY OF LIFE

IBS can have a large impact on quality of life. The SF-36 is a commonly utilized health-related quality of life survey developed by the Rand Corporation. It is a scale-based assessment that measures domains involving limitations in physical, social, and usual role activities because of physical or emotional problems, bodily pain, general mental health, vitality, and general health perceptions (Ware and Sherbourne 1992). In a study of 877 IBS patients, people with IBS scored lower on every one of the domain subscores of the SF-36 when compared to the general population (Gralnek et al. 2000). Most pronounced were lower scores in energy/fatigue, role limitations caused by physical health problems, bodily pain, and general health perceptions.

Qualitative research studies can help us understand the impact on the daily life of patients through their own words (Chapman, Hadfield, and Chapman 2015). Dr. Cecilia Håkanson reviewed numerous qualitative studies of the life-limiting impacts of IBS to look for common themes among patients' descriptions. What she found was that first, IBS patients inevitably think of their body and symptoms as shameful and unpredictable. Second, they commonly speak of the syndrome's impact on limiting their activities of daily living such as their ability to "move about freely, fulfill ambitions or commitments at work, maintain social activities, uphold or develop close and/or sexual relationships and parenting, and live a life with spontaneity" (Håkanson 2014). Third, they feel "as if life was controlled by the bowels" (McCormick et al. 2012), which leads to a forth common theme that many IBS patients tend to avoid activities in anticipation that they may run into bowel issues (Dancey and Backhouse 1993).

Sadly, because of the feelings of shame many experience, very few patients discuss the full extent of how IBS has affected their lives with their physicians (Casiday et al. 2008; Rønnevig, Vandvik, and Bergbom 2009). And those that do often struggle with healthcare providers "who trivialized or dismissed their symptoms" (Bertram et al. 2001) or even worse, made them feel like they were "exaggerating or even imagining their illness" (Dancey and Backhouse 1993).

COSTS

The effects of this incredibly common and often debilitating syndrome play out in out-of-pocket expenses for patients and in the overall cost to the health care system. For example, in the United States, people with constipation predominant IBS

(IBS-C) will spend on average almost $4,000 more a year on health care related to gastrointestinal disorders compared to people without IBS or constipation symptoms (Doshi et al. 2014). This perhaps isn't too surprising when we consider that the same study found that IBS-C patients saw the doctor more and were hospitalized more. Of course, for many who choose to see a natural medicine provider, there are also the costs of supplements (usually not covered by insurance) as well as other noncovered diagnostic testing. Use of complementary and alternative medicine (CAM) is very common with IBS patients. In fact, large surveys estimate that about 1/3 of IBS sufferers will use one form of CAM or another. The median cost per year for that was found to be $240 a person but ranged up to $2,200 (van Tilburg et al. 2008).

DIAGNOSIS

The diagnosis of IBS is a complex process because there is no stellar test that exists to diagnose IBS. Unlike with inflammatory bowel disease (IBD), colonoscopy cannot serve as a diagnostic tool. Thus, doctors are left with the symptoms that patients report which include diarrhea or constipation, abdominal pain, and perhaps bloating. Because these symptoms are common to many diseases, doctors will often order tests to rule out other causes for which good tests are available, such as celiac disease, ulcerative colitis, Crohn's disease, microscopic colitis, etc. Once those have been ruled out, the physician will often default to an IBS diagnosis. In this way, IBS is sometimes diagnosed through "exclusion."

Many studies now have suggested that simply using the criteria set out by the Rome Foundation in the absence of red flag or alarm symptoms (like new onset after age 50 or blood per rectum for example) can adequately diagnose IBS in most cases (Whitehead and Drossman 2010). To be diagnosed with IBS, one must meet the Rome Foundation criteria. The Rome Foundation is a not-for-profit that seeks to "improve the lives of people with functional GI disorders (FGIDs)." It has two stated goals: "To promote clinical recognition and legitimization of the FGIDs and to develop a scientific understanding of their pathophysiological mechanisms to achieve optimal treatment" (Drossman 2007).

There are even indications now that certain tests can make colonoscopies unnecessary in many cases – although this is still being worked out (van Rheenen, Van de Vijver, and Fidler 2010). Two exciting examples of this are the fecal calprotectin test (to rule out Crohn's and ulcerative colitis) and the blood tests anti-CDTB and anti-vinculin to make a positive diagnosis of IBS-D which follows food poisoning (post-infectious IBS) (van Rheenen, Van de Vijver, and Fidler 2010; Pimentel et al. 2015).

In 2016, the Rome Foundation published its latest version of the Rome criteria for IBS:

Recurrent abdominal pain on average at least 1 day/week in the last 3 months, associated with **two or more** of the following criteria:

1. Related to defecation
2. Associated with a change in frequency of stool
3. Associated with a change in form (appearance) of stool

The Rome Foundation recognizes the following subtypes of IBS: IBS with predominate constipation (IBS-C), IBS with predominate diarrhea (IBS-D), IBS with mixed bowel habits (IBS-M), and IBS unclassified (IBS-U) (Drossman and Hasler 2016).

PATHOPHYSIOLOGY

The current understanding of IBS is that it is a fluid disorder with a spectrum of presentations. In fact, the latest iteration of the Rome Foundation's approach is that functional bowel disorders themselves are on a spectrum. For example, we now view functional constipation and constipation predominate IBS as distinct but different ends of a shared spectrum. People can absolutely transition from one to another if, for example, pain was not present initially but developed later (Drossman and Hasler 2016).

Many still consider IBS idiopathic. That being said, research accumulating over many decades now points to a few potential pathophysiologic mechanisms. These include altered GI motility, infection, visceral hypersensitivity, increased intestinal permeability, immune activation, altered microbiota, and bile acid malabsorption. A brief description of these follows below.

ALTERED GI MOTILITY

The normal gut motility essential to a healthy digestion may, at least in a subset of individuals with IBS, be altered (Gasbarrini et al. 2008). However, it is still unclear to what extent this may be driving IBS symptoms. In other words, just because we see this association in some people with IBS, that doesn't mean that it is the motility issues themselves causing the IBS.

INFECTION

Interestingly, around 10% or so of people with IBS recall a precipitating enteric infection. What is particularly interesting is that these people are developing IBS *after* the infection clears. The body's reaction to the infection, not the infection itself, is causing lasting physiologic responses which cause symptoms that meet criteria for IBS (Beatty, Bhargava, and Buret 2014). One particularly interesting hypothesis, driven primarily by researchers at Cedar Sinai Hospital, argues that there are a handful of infective organisms that share a particular toxin (cytolethal distending toxin B), and an exposed person may develop antibodies to this toxin. As normally occurs when the body creates antibodies, the body retains a "memory" of the infection in the form of antibodies that circulate "looking" for this invader again, in order to have a faster response next time. Unfortunately, as the hypothesis argues, the body's antibodies may attack elements of the motility system of the gut particularly the protein vinculin which is involved in gut motility (Pimentel et al. 2015).

VISCERAL HYPERSENSITIVITY

Visceral hypersensitivity is a fascinating area of research in IBS. In short, a subset of people (about 1/3 of people with IBS) will have an increased pain, bloating, or discomfort response to a given distention of the colon compared to healthy controls (Zhou and Verne 2011). The unfortunate test for this (not clinical, only used in research settings) is to insert a balloon into the rectum and fill it with a gas to exert a very specific pressure on the rectal walls. IBS patients with visceral hypersensitivity will report discomfort and pain while healthy controls receiving identical pressure will not. The exact mechanism for how this happens is still being worked out but many believe that this altered and overly sensitive response may cause some of the symptoms that IBS patients have such as sensations of bloating, discomfort, and pain (Keszthelyi, Troost, and Masclee 2012).

INTESTINAL HYPERPERMEABILITY AND FOOD SENSITIVITY

One of the more fascinating areas of research in terms of potential causes of IBS is intestinal hyperpermeability, more commonly referred to in the lay media as "leaky gut." Different lines of evidence regarding this phenomenon are now pointing toward an alteration in the functionality of the mucosal barrier in the digestive tract, caused, for example, by bacterial toxins and allergic/immune responses. This may cause an increase in permeability that, in turn, may lead to an increase in antigens passing from the gastrointestinal tract into the "sacred space" of the body where immune cells may be activated (Camilleri and Gorman 2007). This is one of the thoughts behind the food sensitivity and IBS hypothesis, namely, that increased permeability of the gut wall allows inappropriate food antigens to pass through to the immune system which then reacts causing inflammation, worsening the permeability further and presumably leading to symptoms. While the details are still being investigated, the overall picture of the evidence suggests that a certain subset of IBS patients may indeed have leaky gut (Camilleri and Gorman 2007).

Elimination diets followed by rechallenge testing administered by qualified medical personnel may help IBS patients identify food sensitivities. Removing these inflammatory triggers, together with other gut healing approaches, may lead to restoration of normal mucosal permeability. Elimination diets are generally considered the gold standard but they are certainly not for everybody. There is some early clinical trial evidence suggesting that using IgG or ALCAT blood tests may help guide an elimination diet in IBS patients leading to improvement in symptoms (Atkinson et al. 2004; Ali et al. 2017).

IMMUNE ACTIVATION

This is one of the more interesting areas in irritable bowel syndrome research. IBS can present clinically like many other conditions. Specifically, one that often looks similar from a clinical perspective is inflammatory bowel disease. The difference in this terminology, 'inflammatory' versus 'irritable,' underlines what was considered a fundamental difference between IBS and IBD for years, that of inflammation. Gastroenterologists typically perform a colonoscopy when a patient presents with symptoms consistent with IBD because the inflammation of IBD is very obvious visually (or at least microscopically when biopsies are examined by a pathologist later). IBS, it was traditionally thought, it not characterized by inflammation. Fascinatingly, new research is showing that IBS involves an inflammatory process as well. Inflammatory cell types are seen in increased number in the mucosa of IBS patients compared to healthy controls (Bhattarai, Muniz Pedrogo, and Kashyap 2017). This has shifted researchers' and doctors' focus toward inflammatory mechanisms as causes of IBS.

ALTERED MICROBIOTA

Small Intestine

Small intestinal bacterial overgrowth (SIBO) is one of the exciting but still somewhat controversial areas of IBS research. In general, it is thought that the bacteria of the gut microbiome belong, primarily, in the colon (large intestine) with a transition zone in the terminal ileum. For the most part, there shouldn't be a large population of bacteria in the small intestine. This is because the high acidity of the stomach as well as the effects of digestive enzymes and bile retard the colonization of bacteria introduced to the small intestine via our food and, whatever does make it past these defenses, are swept down to the colon via the migrating motor complex (peristalsis). Finally, an intact ileocecal valve prevents bacteria from moving upwards from the colon to the small intestine. However, when these defenses break down, colonic bacteria can proliferate in the small intestine, and this can often cause problems. This is known as SIBO.

It is thought that when we eat foods that contain elements that these bacteria (and sometimes archaea) can ferment, the resultant gases (methane, hydrogen, hydrogen sulfide, and others) can directly or indirectly cause symptoms. For example, these may include diarrhea, constipation, bloating, distension, cramping, and pain. Of course, these are similar to symptoms described by people with IBS. This has led to the hypothesis that, at least in some people with IBS, IBS may be caused by SIBO (Lin 2004). Indeed, some studies of people with IBS have shown that over 80% test positive for SIBO (e.g., Pimentel, Chow, and Lin 2003). However, studies by other groups have not been able to replicate this and indeed find that a similar number of people test positive for SIBO whether they have IBS or not (Posserud et al. 2007). While fascinating, this is still an area of controversy (Quigley 2014).

Large Intestine

There have been some interesting findings in terms of the microbiota of the large intestine and IBS. Indeed, shifts in the gut microbiota population have been found in patients with IBS, and there are even suggestions that the severity of a patient's IBS symptoms is associated with a lack of microbial complexity in the microbiome. Unfortunately, despite these fascinating early findings, the conclusion of these studies is not consistent. This may be related to the heterogeneity in IBS patients, in study design, or it may simply just be too early for a clear signal from this early research (Bhattarai, Muniz Pedrogo, and Kashyap 2017).

BILE ACID MALABSORPTION

It has been reported that up to 1/3 of people with IBS-D have bile acid malabsorption. Bile is made by the liver, stored in the gall bladder, and used to emulsify fats to help with absorption along the small intestine. Normally, the bile should be reabsorbed in the last section of the small intestine, the terminal ileum. In fact, in a healthy working digestive tract, it is estimated that 95% of the bile is reabsorbed. When this doesn't happen, the bile acids make their way into the large intestine where they can cause diarrhea by various mechanisms. Removal of, or disease activity in, the terminal ileum can of course cause issues here, but this is less likely a cause of bile acid malabsorption in people with functional bowel disease like IBS. While there are tests for this, usually physicians will prescribe a therapeutic trial of bile acid sequestrants like colestipol to see if this improves the patient's diarrhea (Camilleri 2015).

PREVENTION

IBS is not a condition that most researchers and clinicians speak of in terms of prevention. This is likely because, as discussed above, most consider IBS to be idiopathic. However, some of the proposed mechanisms of pathology suggest that some risk factors for IBS could be preventable including infection, increased intestinal permeability, and altered microbiota. We may be able to hypothesize that limiting one's exposure/risk of food poisoning, avoiding triggers of intestinal permeability, and eating a diversity of foods in pursuit of a diverse microbiome may prevent the incidence of IBS, although at this point, this is speculative.

TREATMENT

Nondietary Treatment

There are many nondietary approaches to IBS that have varying levels of evidence to support their use. From a mind–body perspective, there are a small number of randomized controlled trials showing cognitive behavioral therapy to be effective in IBS, and fascinatingly, people with a specific genetic variant (a single nucleotide polymorphism, or SNP) find CBT for IBS particularly effective (Han et al. 2017). Hypnosis has also been shown to be effective in well-conducted randomized controlled trials (Dobbin et al. 2013). This author has recently published a large systematic review and meta-analysis of randomized controlled trials using various forms of biofeedback to help manage IBS symptoms (Goldenberg et al., 2019). Biofeedback is a therapy where participants use technology to track a process that is not normally under conscious control (e.g., heart rate, the tension of the anal sphincter) intending to see how relaxed states of the mind affect these measures (Goldenberg, 2019). Our research has shown that the evidence base investigating the effects of biofeedback on IBS is small, and the results of RCTs to date are mixed. Additionally, exercise, yoga, and acupuncture have also been shown to be effective (Hajizadeh et al. 2018; Schumann et al. 2016; Manheimer et al. 2012).

Various medications have been shown to be effective in managing IBS symptoms with varying degrees of success such as loperamide, lubiprostone, linaclotide, amitriptyline, dicyclomine, rifaximin, and others (Trinkley and Nahata 2014).

Many IBS patients will pursue complementary and alternative approaches for their IBS in one form or another, including nutraceuticals (Hussain and Quigley 2006). Commercially available IBS nutraceutical options are myriad, and there is some well-conducted trial evidence for a limited selection of them (Currò et al. 2017).

Dietary Approaches to IBS

Traditionally, the role of diet in IBS has been overlooked (Eswaran, Tack, and Chey 2011). Despite this, 2/3 of IBS sufferers report that they believe food to have an important role in their symptoms (Simrén et al. 2001), and now new research is beginning to support what patients have known all along that there certainly is a food and diet connection with IBS (Singh et al. 2018).

In the following sections, we review what is known about food, diet, and IBS.

Alcohol

Alcohol has been known to affect intestinal hyperpermeability (leaky gut), and many patients report that consumption of alcohol seems to worsen their IBS symptoms. While data on this question is limited, one observational study of women with IBS found that whereas binge drinking (greater than four drinks) was associated with worsening symptoms, moderate or mild drinking was either weakly associated or not associated with gastrointestinal symptoms at all (Reding et al. 2013). Guidelines for the dietary management of IBS have noted that alcohol can induce or worsen IBS symptoms, and recommend limiting alcohol intake and insuring such intake is "within safe national levels" (McKenzie et al. 2016; Dalrymple and Bullock 2008).

Caffeine

There have been no randomized controlled studies looking at whether reducing coffee or caffeine intake would lead to better IBS outcomes. The other types of evidence available are a bit mixed but many IBS patients do self-report that coffee worsens symptoms for them (Cozma-Petruţ et al. 2017).

Fiber

Surprisingly, using fiber with IBS patients is still debated. Fiber can help with constipation in some people, but many patients report that it can make their constipation worse. It seems to be person-specific and likely dose- and possibly fiber type/form-specific as well. But because of the low side effect profile, many doctors may discuss trying it out with patients, at least initially (Ford and Talley 2012). Furthermore, a systematic review of 12 studies found that even the use of psyllium husk, the most recommended initial fiber supplement for IBS symptoms, has limited and conflicting evidence to support its recommendation (Chouinard, 2011).

FODMAP (Fermentable Oligosaccharide, Disaccharide, Monosaccharides, and Polyols)

The past few years have seen an explosion of research on the low FODMAP diet in particular for patients with IBS. While initial studies were limited by study design, later follow-up studies were much more rigorous and continue to be promising (Marsh, Eslick, and Eslick 2016).

Some examples of high FODMAP foods can be seen in Table 7.1. High FODMAP foods have high concentrations of poorly absorbed carbohydrates. To date, we have two mechanisms to explain how these foods might cause problems. The first is via water retention in the small intestine. These foods get poorly absorbed and will draw

TABLE 7.1

Examples of High FODMAP Foods Organized by Types of FODMAPs

Excess

Fructose	Lactose	Fructans	Mannitol[a]	Sorbitol[a]	Galactans
Fruit: Apple, boysenberry, mango, Nashi fruit, pear, tamarillo, watermelon	**Cow's/goat's/ sheep:** Milk, custard, dairy desserts, evaporated milk, ice cream, milk powder, sweetened condensed milk	**Fruit:** Custard apples, white peaches, tamarillo, nectarines, persimmon, watermelon	**Fruit:** Clingstone, peach, watermelon	**Fruit:** Apples, apricots, blackberries, Nashi fruit, nectarines, peaches, pears, plums	**Legumes:** Chickpeas, legumes, lentils
Vegetables: Asparagus, artichokes, sugar snap peas		**Vegetables**: Artichokes, garlic, leek, onion, spring onion (white part only), shallot	**Vegetables:** Cauliflower, mushrooms, snow peas	**Other:** Sorbitol	
Other: agave, high-fructose corn syrup, honey		**Grains/cereals:** Barley-, rye-, and wheat-based bread; crackers; pasta; cereal couscous; gnocchi; noodles; croissants; muffins; crumpets			
		Nuts and legumes: Cashews, pistachios, chickpeas, legumes (e.g., red kidney beans, soy beans), lentils			
		Other: Fructooligosaccharides, inulin			

Source: From Mullin, et al. (2014).

[a] Used as sweeteners in "diet," "sugar-free," or "low-carb" foods.

water into the small intestine and possibly the colon. In people who are susceptible, this swelling is experienced as pain, bloating, and cramping and can lead to diarrhea. We now actually have a fascinating MRI study which shows that lactulose (a nonabsorbed fermentable carbohydrate) when delivered to patients with IBS, versus healthy control subjects, causes more symptoms in the IBS patients and causes more water absorption in the small bowel than in healthy controls (Undseth et al. 2014).

Another proposed mechanism for the effect of FODMAPs has to do with bacterial fermentation and SIBO (Sachdeva et al., 2011). The theory goes that these poorly absorbed carbohydrates are excellent sources of food for an overgrowth of bacteria in the small intestine. These bacteria and sometimes archaea (single-celled nonbacterial organisms) ferment the carbohydrates and release different gases such as hydrogen and methane (recent evidence points to hydrogen sulfide, as well) (Banik et al. 2016). The gases released can cause the symptoms of bloating and also lead to cramping, pain, and changes in the motility of the small intestine.

Dairy

Dairy is often mentioned by patients when asked what foods trigger their IBS symptoms (Böhn et al. 2013). This isn't too surprising as there are numerous potential mechanisms for dairy to worsen IBS. For example, many people may have undiagnosed lactose malabsorption/lactose intolerance. In people with lactose intolerance, exposure to lactose such as in milk and other dairy products can cause symptoms similar to IBS (Zar, Kumar, and Benson 2001). In other words, IBS could be misdiagnosed, and a patient could actually have lactose intolerance instead. Also, an IBS patient may have lactose intolerance AND IBS. Consumption of dairy could cause increased symptom severity due to the overlapping nature of the symptoms of these two disorders. A trial removal of dairy (specifically lactose containing foods in this case) could lower their overall symptom burden. Oddly, apparently in a very small number of people, removing diary and then reintroducing it may cause a dangerous anaphylactic reaction (Flinterman et al. 2006), and therefore, patients must be sure to review any diet changes with their doctor ahead of time.

In addition to lactose intolerance issues, milk itself is a high FODMAP food because of the lactose content (Tuck et al. 2018). FODMAP foods have high concentrations of poorly absorbed carbohydrates which can cause gastrointestinal symptoms. Lactose products could cause IBS symptoms in people even without lactose intolerance due to the osmatic effects of FODMAP foods as well as the potential for SIBO.

More so than the sugar content in dairy (lactose), the milk proteins themselves may cause food allergies and/or sensitivity reactions. Food sensitivity testing in IBS patients often show reactivity to dairy proteins (Ali et al. 2017; Atkinson et al. 2004).

For these reasons, many physicians will consider a trial off of dairy to see if it impacts a patient's IBS symptoms. For example, the guidelines from the British Dietetics Association state "In individuals with IBS where sensitivity to milk is suspected and a lactose hydrogen breath test is not available or dairy products appropriate, a trial period of a low lactose diet is recommended. This is particularly useful in individuals with an ethnic background with a high prevalence of primary lactase deficiency" (McKenzie et al. 2016). Additionally, this author has conducted a Delphi study of North American Naturopathic experts in IBS. There was consensus among these experts that the exclusion of dairy in elimination/rechallenge diets for IBS was reasonable (Goldenberg et al. 2018). For more on elimination diets, see below.

Elemental Diet

The elemental diet is not really a "food" diet at all but rather powdered predigested nutrients which one mixes with water, and drinks, in many cases exclusively, for 2 weeks or more. The idea behind it is that all of the nutrients are absorbed high up in the small intestine not leaving any left over for subsequent fermentation lower down in the intestine. Elemental diets have been used for a while now with Crohn's disease (Ohara et al. 2017), but more recently, people are looking at using it for IBS/SIBO. One study by a very prominent SIBO researcher, Dr. Mark Pimentel, MD, conducted on IBS patients with an abnormal breath test reading for SIBO, found that 85% of patients had an improvement in their breath test results following a 2-week elemental diet (Pimentel et al. 2004).

Elimination Diets

Elimination rechallenge testing diets either conducted on common trigger foods or guided by IgG or ALCAT-based food sensitivity testing are often used for IBS (Ali et al. 2017; Atkinson et al. 2004). This author has conducted a Delphi study of North American Naturopathic experts in IBS which resulted in consensus on detailed elimination diet guidance from a naturopathic perspective (Goldenberg et al. 2018).

Gluten

The role of gluten in IBS continues to be somewhat controversial. Many people who have an IBS diagnosis and avoid gluten do better. However, the reason it is controversial is as follows. It is thought that some people with an IBS diagnosis may actually have celiac disease that was just falsely negative on blood testing. So, while the patients may have an existing IBS diagnosis because their doctor felt they ruled out celiac disease with a negative blood test, in reality, they be "seronegative celiac" meaning they have it, but their blood test is negative. It follows that the IBS diagnosis is false since the patient's symptoms are coming from the hidden celiac disease not the IBS. Therefore, the improvement off of gluten may be due to the fact that celiac patients do better off of gluten (Tack et al. 2010).

Another argument making avoiding gluten controversial in IBS is that removal of gluten-containing foods also leads to the reduction or elimination of other foods such as those high in FODMAPs and others that are thought to cause IBS-like symptoms (Aziz, Hadjivassiliou, and Sanders 2015). While it is difficult to determine if gluten is the causative element, its elimination is associated with symptom amelioration in many IBS patients. Thus, a significant percentage of patients with an IBS diagnosis (whether a false diagnosis or not) may benefit from a trial of avoiding gluten-containing foods. Whether that benefit is because their IBS diagnosis is false (and in reality, they have hidden celiac disease) or because in avoiding gluten-containing foods the person avoids other troublesome components as well, the fact remains that these patients benefit.

One additional note on avoiding gluten: just because a product is "gluten-free" doesn't mean it is healthy. In fact, many processed gluten-free foods are still full of simple carbohydrates which are not generally considered part of a healthy diet (Dehghan et al. 2017). It is likely prudent to discuss dietary choices with a registered dietician or nutritionist to ensure one's diet is still a healthy one. Additionally, by avoiding all gluten for an extended period of time, one may make it less likely to get a firm celiac disease diagnosis in the future, as biopsies may lead to false negatives in such cases. If a firm celiac diagnosis is important to one's medical care, it may make more sense to get that answer first and then try a gluten elimination afterwards (Kowalski et al. 2017).

Histamine

Many IBS sufferers identify histamine-releasing foods as triggers of their IBS symptoms. In one survey of 197 IBS sufferers, two thirds of the studied population claimed that foods thought to be histamine releasing triggered their IBS symptoms. Identified histamine-rich food triggers included milk, wine/beer, pork, chocolate, orange, shellfish, strawberries, tomato, and fish (Böhn et al. 2013).

Specific Carbohydrate Diet

Another dietary approach to IBS, although with limited formal research support, is the specific carbohydrate diet (SCD). This diet was first described in 1924 but became more popular after the publication of "Breaking the Vicious Cycle" by Elaine Gottschall who was a biochemist and described using it to help her daughter with ulcerative colitis (Gottschall 1994). The premise of the SCD is based on the theory that disaccharides and polysaccharides are malabsorbed and can result in bacterial and yeast overgrowth and intestinal injury. This diet severely limits intake of simple carbohydrates (Knight-Sepulveda et al. 2015). You can see examples of foods not permitted on the SCD in Table 7.2. Research on this diet is preliminary, and most of it was not done on IBS patients but rather on patients with IBD. In one study comparing the SCD diet to the low FODMAP diet in patients with IBS, IBS patients ($n = 60$) were randomized to either the SCD or the low FODMAP diet for 3 months. While the IBS patients showed a statistically significant improvement after 3 months when randomized to the low FODMAP diet, the patients randomized to the SCD diet did not (Vincenzi et al. 2017).

Spicy Food

Patients with IBS may report association with spicy foods. In a 2016 review of the literature on diet and IBS, seven studies were identified looking at this association, two of which were randomized controlled trials. Ironically, one study found that high dose chili powder improved abdominal pain thresholds (Bortolotti and Porta 2011),

---

TABLE 7.2
Examples of Foods to Include and to Avoid When Following the SCD

	Include	Avoid
Grains	None	All cereal grains
Fruits	All but canned or frozen fruits	None
Vegetables	All but canned or frozen vegetable	Potato, yam, corn
Proteins	All others	Processed, canned, or smoked meats
Nuts, seeds, legumes	Lentil and split pea	Most legumes (e.g., chickpea and soybean)
Dairy	Lactose-free	All others
Beverages	Wine	Milk, instant tea, instant coffee, soybean, milk, beer
Other	Saccharin, honey, butter	Chocolate, margarine, corn syrup

Source: From Knight-Sepulveda et al. (2015).

but all the other studies suggested that spicy foods worsened IBS symptoms. After a review of the evidence, The British Dietetics Association guidelines suggest that spicy foods may exacerbate symptoms in IBS patients particularly men and those with IBS-D (McKenzie et al. 2016).

Eating Hygiene

Finally, eating habits may have an impact on IBS symptoms. Rushing through meals, mindless eating, irregular meals, and missing meals may adversely affect IBS symptoms in some people. Therefore, eating hygiene (chewing food thoroughly, eating mindfully, etc.) and a regular meal pattern (frequency and timing of food consumption) have been adopted by some guidelines including this author's research on expert naturopathic approaches to IBS (Goldenberg et al. 2018).

COOKING AND FOOD PREPARATION METHODS

Cooking and food preparation methods can have an impact on some food constituents relevant in IBS. For example, as discussed above, food sensitivities (such as nonceliac gluten sensitivity) are thought to potentially be contributory to IBS (Ali et al. 2017). One proposed mechanism is thought to be low-level immunological reactions to triggering proteins (Cuomo et al. 2014). Studies suggest that baking can alter the immunologic properties of gluten and other cereal proteins (Smith et al. 2015). And, it isn't just proteins affected, fiber quantity and form (soluble and insoluble) are impacted by cooking techniques as well. In one study, the steaming of vegetables caused a shift from insoluble to soluble fiber – in some cases by three-fold (Kalala et al. 2018). For IBS patients sensitive to food-derived histamine, selection of cooking methods may be important. Histamine formed in food is heat-stable and thus remains intact in cooked food. A study evaluating the effect of different cooking methods on histamine from namely seafood, processed meats, and fermented foods found that frying and grilling significantly increased measured histamine levels, whereas boiling, likely due to dilution, produced lower levels (Chun et al., 2017).

Short-chain carbohydrates, such as FODMAPs, are modified by food preparation techniques as well. This was well documented in one study (Tuck et al. 2018), where sprouted grains and legumes were shown to have a lower FODMAP content than those which were unsprouted. Most impressively, pickling caused 87%–97% reductions in the FODMAP content of artichokes, onions, beets, and garlic. It is hypothesized that because of the water solubility of FODMAPs, there is leaching into the pickling liquid and thus reduction in the consumed food. Additionally, canned kidney beans were shown to be lower in FODMAPs than the equivalent uncanned versions (Tuck et al. 2018). Other researchers have shown that soaking or cooking legumes (e.g., chickpeas, kidney beans, and lentils) and then draining the water can have favorable decreases in the fermentable sugar content. For example, fructose and sucrose levels dropped 38% and 50%, respectively, once legumes were cooked and drained (Vidal-Valverde, Frías, and Valverde 1993). In terms of optimal cooking times before straining of cooked legumes, Tuck et al. (2018) found that for red lentils, 5 minutes of simmering reduced fermentable sugar content by 43% and for red kidney beans 30 minutes of simmering led to the most reduction in fermentable sugars.

SUMMARY

IBS is a condition that leads to a tremendous amount of frustration and suffering in a surprisingly large percentage of people throughout the world. Researchers are still elucidating the mechanisms of why and how this happens and attempting to support patients with dietary and nondietary approaches which may alleviate their symptoms. Much of the difficulty in finding a "cure" for IBS surely rests on the fact that one person's IBS is unlikely to be the same (from a causal perspective) as another's, despite a similar symptom picture. It is the opinion of this author, and many others, that IBS is caused by a constellation of varying issues. The cause of IBS is not alike in all IBS patients, and therefore, all IBS patients should not be treated alike. There should be work done with caring and understanding medical providers to help identify the likely cause or mechanisms behind each individual's IBS symptoms and subsequently a personalized plan crafted to help that specific person based on the presumed specific causes of their IBS.

Certainly, the good news is that recently, there has been an explosion of interest and recognition that diet plays a role in IBS – mostly due to a recent flurry of research into the relationship between high FODMAP foods and IBS. With any luck, this trend will continue, and the value of dietary approaches for IBS will be accepted within the larger medical community and established as part of standards of care.

REFERENCES

Ali, A., T. R. Weiss, D. McKee, A. Scherban, S. Khan, M. R. Fields, D. Apollo, and W. Z. Mehal. 2017. "Efficacy of Individualised Diets in Patients with Irritable Bowel Syndrome: A Randomised Controlled Trial." *BMJ Open Gastroenterology* 4 (1): e000164. doi:10.1136/bmjgast-2017-000164.

Atkinson, W, T. A. Sheldon, N. Shaath, and P. J. Whorwell. 2004. "Food Elimination Based on IgG Antibodies in Irritable Bowel Syndrome: A Randomised Controlled Trial." *Gut* 53 (10): 1459–64. doi:10.1136/gut.2003.037697.

Aziz, I., M. Hadjivassiliou, and D. S. Sanders. 2015. "The Spectrum of Noncoeliac Gluten Sensitivity." *Nature Reviews Gastroenterology & Hepatology* 12 (9): 516–26. doi:10.1038/nrgastro.2015.107.

Banik, G. D., A. De, S. Som, S. Jana, S. B. Daschakraborty, S. Chaudhuri, and M. Pradhan. 2016. "Hydrogen Sulphide in Exhaled Breath: A Potential Biomarker for Small Intestinal Bacterial Overgrowth in IBS." *Journal of Breath Research* 10 (2): 026010. doi:10.1088/1752-7155/10/2/026010.

Beatty, J. K, A. Bhargava, and A. G Buret. 2014. "Post-Infectious Irritable Bowel Syndrome: Mechanistic Insights into Chronic Disturbances Following Enteric Infection." *World Journal of Gastroenterology* 20 (14): 3976. doi:10.3748/wjg.v20.i14.3976.

Bertram, S., M. Kurland, E. Lydick, G. R. Locke, and B. P. Yawn. 2001. "The Patient's Perspective of Irritable Bowel Syndrome." *The Journal of Family Practice* 50 (6): 521–25.

Bhattarai, Y., D. A. Muniz Pedrogo, and P. C. Kashyap. 2017. "Irritable Bowel Syndrome: A Gut Microbiota-Related Disorder?" *American Journal of Physiology-Gastrointestinal and Liver Physiology* 312 (1): G52–62. doi:10.1152/ajpgi.00338.2016.

Böhn, L., S. Störsrud, H. Törnblom, U. Bengtsson, and M. Simrén. 2013. "Self-Reported Food-Related Gastrointestinal Symptoms in IBS Are Common and Associated with More Severe Symptoms and Reduced Quality of Life." *American Journal of Gastroenterology* 108 (5): 634–41. doi:10.1038/ajg.2013.105.

Bortolotti, M., and S. Porta. 2011. "Effect of Red Pepper on Symptoms of Irritable Bowel Syndrome: Preliminary Study." *Digestive Diseases and Sciences* 56 (11): 3288–95. doi:10.1007/s10620-011-1740-9.

Camilleri, M. 2015. "Bile Acid Diarrhea: Prevalence, Pathogenesis, and Therapy." *Gut and Liver* 9 (3): 332–39. doi:10.5009/gnl14397.

Camilleri, M., and H. Gorman. 2007. "Intestinal Permeability and Irritable Bowel Syndrome." *Neurogastroenterology & Motility* 19 (7): 545–52. doi:10.1111/j.1365-2982.2007.00925.x.

Canavan, C., J. West, and T. Card. 2014. "The Epidemiology of Irritable Bowel Syndrome." *Clinical Epidemiology* 6. Dove Press: 71–80. doi:10.2147/CLEP.S40245.

Casiday, R. E, A. P. S. Hungin, C. S. Cornford, N. J de Wit, and M. T Blell. 2008. "Patients' Explanatory Models for Irritable Bowel Syndrome: Symptoms and Treatment More Important than Explaining Aetiology." *Family Practice* 26 (1): 40–47. doi:10.1093/fampra/cmn087.

Chapman, A. L., M. Hadfield, and C. J. Chapman. 2015. "Qualitative Research in Healthcare: An Introduction to Grounded Theory Using Thematic Analysis." *Journal of the Royal College of Physicians of Edinburgh* 45 (3): 201–5. doi:10.4997/JRCPE.2015.305.

Chouinard, L. E. 2011 Spring. The role of Psyllium Fibre Supplementation in Treating Irritable Bowel Syndrome. *Canadian Journal of Dietetic Practice and Research* 72(1): e107–14.

Chun, B. Y., et al. Dec 2017. Effect of Different Cooking Methods on Histamine Levels in Selected Foods. *Annals of Dermatology* 29(6): 706–714.

Cozma-Petruţ, A., F. Loghin, D. Miere, and D. L. Dumitraşcu. 2017. "Diet in Irritable Bowel Syndrome: What to Recommend, Not What to Forbid to Patients!" *World Journal of Gastroenterology* 23 (21): 3771. doi:10.3748/wjg.v23.i21.3771.

Cuomo, R., P. Andreozzi, F. P. Zito, V. Passananti, G. De Carlo, and G. Sarnelli. 2014. "Irritable Bowel Syndrome and Food Interaction." *World Journal of Gastroenterology* 20 (27): 8837–45. doi:10.3748/wjg.v20.i27.8837.

Currò, D, G. Ianiro, S. Pecere, S. Bibbò, and G. Cammarota. 2017. "Probiotics, Fibre and Herbal Medicinal Products for Functional and Inflammatory Bowel Disorders." *British Journal of Pharmacology* 174 (11): 1426–49. doi:10.1111/bph.13632.

Dalrymple, J., and I. Bullock. 2008. "Diagnosis and Management of Irritable Bowel Syndrome in Adults in Primary Care: Summary of NICE Guidance." *BMJ* 336 (7643): 556–58. doi:10.1136/bmj.39484.712616.AD.

Dancey, C. P., and S. Backhouse. 1993. "Towards a Better Understanding of Patients with Irritable Bowel Syndrome." *Journal of Advanced Nursing* 18 (9): 1443–50.

Dehghan, M., A. Mente, X. Zhang, S. Swaminathan, W. Li, V. Mohan, R. Iqbal, et al. 2017. "Associations of Fats and Carbohydrate Intake with Cardiovascular Disease and Mortality in 18 Countries from Five Continents (PURE): A Prospective Cohort Study." *The Lancet* 390 (10107): 2050–62. doi:10.1016/S0140-6736(17)32252-3.

Dobbin, A., J. Dobbin, S. C. Ross, C. Graham, and M. J. Ford. 2013. "Randomised Controlled Trial of Brief Intervention with Biofeedback and Hypnotherapy in Patients with Refractory Irritable Bowel Syndrome." *The Journal of the Royal College of Physicians of Edinburgh* 43 (1): 15–23. doi:10.4997/JRCPE.2013.104.

Doshi, J. A., Q. Cai, J. L. Buono, W. M. Spalding, P. Sarocco, H. Tan, J. J. Stephenson, and R. T. Carson. 2014. "Economic Burden of Irritable Bowel Syndrome with Constipation: A Retrospective Analysis of Health Care Costs in a Commercially Insured Population." *Journal of Managed Care Pharmacy* 20 (4): 382–90. doi:10.18553/jmcp.2014.20.4.382.

Drossman, D. A. 2007. "Introduction. The Rome Foundation and Rome III." *Neurogastroenterology & Motility* 19 (10): 783–86. doi:10.1111/j.1365-2982.2007.01001.x.

Drossman, D. A., and W. L. Hasler. 2016. "Rome IV—Functional GI Disorders: Disorders of Gut-Brain Interaction." *Gastroenterology* 150 (6): 1257–61. doi:10.1053/j.gastro.2016.03.035.

Eswaran, S., J. Tack, and W. D. Chey. 2011. "Food: The Forgotten Factor in the Irritable Bowel Syndrome." *Gastroenterology Clinics of North America* 40 (1): 141–62. doi:10.1016/j.gtc.2010.12.012.

Flinterman, A. E., A. C. Knulst, Y. Meijer, C. A. F. M. Bruijnzeel-Koomen, and S. G. M. A. Pasmans. 2006. "Acute Allergic Reactions in Children with AEDS after Prolonged Cow's Milk Elimination Diets." *Allergy* 61 (3): 370–74. doi:10.1111/j.1398-9995.2006.01018.x.

Ford, A. C., and N. J. Talley. 2012. "Irritable Bowel Syndrome." *BMJ* 345 (sep04 1): e5836–e5836. doi:10.1136/bmj.e5836.

Gasbarrini, A., E. C. Lauritano, M. Garcovich, L. Sparano, and G. Gasbarrini. 2008. "New Insights into the Pathophysiology of IBS: Intestinal Microflora, Gas Production and Gut Motility." *European Review for Medical and Pharmacological Sciences* 12 Suppl 1 (August): 111–17.

Goldenberg, J. Z., L. Ward, A. Day, and K. Cooley. 2018. "Naturopathic Approaches to Irritable Bowel Syndrome—A Delphi Study." *The Journal of Alternative and Complementary Medicine*, September, acm.2018.0255. doi:10.1089/acm.2018.0255.

Goldenberg, J. Z., M. Brignall, M. Hamilton, et al. 2019. "Biofeedback for Treatment of Irritable Bowel Syndrome." *Cochrane Database of Systematic Reviews* 2019 (11). doi:10.1002/14651858.CD012530.pub2

Gottschall, E. G. 1994. *Breaking the Vicious Cycle : Intestinal Health through Diet.* Baltimore, ON: Kirkton Press.

Gralnek, I. M., R. D. Hays, A. Kilbourne, B. Naliboff, and E. A. Mayer. 2000. "The Impact of Irritable Bowel Syndrome on Health-Related Quality of Life." *Gastroenterology* 119 (3): 654–60.

Hajizadeh, M., B. Bakhtyar Tartibian, F. C. Mooren, L. Z. FitzGerald, K. Krüger, M. Chehrazi, and A. Malandish. 2018. "Low-to-Moderate Intensity Aerobic Exercise Training Modulates Irritable Bowel Syndrome through Antioxidative and Inflammatory Mechanisms in Women: Results of a Randomized Controlled Trial." *Cytokine* 102 (February): 18–25. doi:10.1016/j.cyto.2017.12.016.

Håkanson, C. 2014. "Everyday Life, Healthcare, and Self-Care Management Among People With Irritable Bowel Syndrome." *Gastroenterology Nursing* 37 (3): 217–25. doi:10.1097/SGA.0000000000000048.

Han, C. J., R. Kohen, S. Jun, M. E. Jarrett, K. C. Cain, R. Burr, and M. M. Heitkemper. 2017. "COMT Val158Met Polymorphism and Symptom Improvement Following a Cognitively Focused Intervention for Irritable Bowel Syndrome." *Nursing Research* 66 (2): 75–84. doi:10.1097/NNR.0000000000000199.

Hussain, Z., and E. M. M. Quigley. 2006. "Systematic Review: Complementary and Alternative Medicine in the Irritable Bowel Syndrome." *Alimentary Pharmacology and Therapeutics* 23 (4): 465–71. doi:10.1111/j.1365-2036.2006.02776.x.

Kalala, G., B. Kambashi, N. Everaert, Y. Beckers, A. Richel, B. Pachikian, A. M. Neyrinck, N. M. Delzenne, and J. Bindelle. 2018. "Characterization of Fructans and Dietary Fibre Profiles in Raw and Steamed Vegetables." *International Journal of Food Sciences and Nutrition* 69 (6): 682–89. doi:10.1080/09637486.2017.1412404.

Keszthelyi, D., F. J. Troost, and A. A. Masclee. 2012. "Irritable Bowel Syndrome: Methods, Mechanisms, and Pathophysiology. Methods to Assess Visceral Hypersensitivity in Irritable Bowel Syndrome." *American Journal of Physiology-Gastrointestinal and Liver Physiology* 303 (2): G141–54. doi:10.1152/ajpgi.00060.2012.

Knight-Sepulveda, K., S. Kais, R. Santaolalla, and M. T. Abreu. 2015. "Diet and Inflammatory Bowel Disease." *Gastroenterology & Hepatology* 11 (8): 511–20.

Kowalski, K., A. Mulak, M. Jasińska, and L. Paradowski. 2017. "Diagnostic Challenges in Celiac Disease." *Advances in Clinical and Experimental Medicine* 26 (4): 729–37. doi:10.17219/acem/62452.

Lin, H. C. 2004. "Small Intestinal Bacterial Overgrowth: A Framework for Understanding Irritable Bowel Syndrome." *JAMA* 292 (7): 852–58. doi:10.1001/jama.292.7.852.

Manheimer, E., L. Susan Wieland, Ke Cheng, S. M. Li, X. Shen, B. M. Berman, and L. Lao. 2012. "Acupuncture for Irritable Bowel Syndrome: Systematic Review and Meta-Analysis." *The American Journal of Gastroenterology* 107 (6): 835–47. doi:10.1038/ajg.2012.66.

Marsh, A., E. M. Eslick, and G. D. Eslick. 2016. "Does a Diet Low in FODMAPs Reduce Symptoms Associated with Functional Gastrointestinal Disorders? A Comprehensive Systematic Review and Meta-Analysis." *European Journal of Nutrition* 55 (3): 897–906. doi:10.1007/s00394-015-0922-1.

McCormick, J. B., R. R. Hammer, R. M. Farrell, G. Geller, K. M. James, E. V. Loftus, M. Mercer, J. C. Tilburt, and R. R. Sharp. 2012. "Experiences of Patients with Chronic Gastrointestinal Conditions: In Their Own Words." *Health and Quality of Life Outcomes* 10 (1): 25. doi:10.1186/1477-7525-10-25.

McKenzie, Y. A., R. K. Bowyer, H. Leach, P. Gulia, J. Horobin, N. A. O'Sullivan, C. Pettitt, et al. 2016. "British Dietetic Association Systematic Review and Evidence-Based Practice Guidelines for the Dietary Management of Irritable Bowel Syndrome in Adults (2016 Update)." *Journal of Human Nutrition and Dietetics* 29 (5): 549–75. doi:10.1111/jhn.12385.

Mullin, G., S. J. Shepherd, B. Roland, C. Ireton-Jones, and L. Matarese. 2014. "Irritable Bowel Syndrome." *JPEN. Journal of Parenteral and Enteral Nutrition* 38. doi:10.1177/0148607114545329.

Ohara, N., T. Mizushima, H. Iijima, H. Takahashi, S. Hiyama, N. Haraguchi, T. Inoue, et al. 2017. "Adherence to an Elemental Diet for Preventing Postoperative Recurrence of Crohn's Disease." *Surgery Today* 47 (12): 1519–25. doi:10.1007/s00595-017-1543-5.

Pimentel, M., E. J. Chow, and H. C. Lin. 2003. "Normalization of Lactulose Breath Testing Correlates with Symptom Improvement in Irritable Bowel Syndrome. a Double-Blind, Randomized, Placebo-Controlled Study." *The American Journal of Gastroenterology* 98 (2): 412–19. doi:10.1111/j.1572-0241.2003.07234.x.

Pimentel, M., T. Constantino, Y. Kong, M. Bajwa, A. Rezaei, and S. Park. 2004. "A 14-Day Elemental Diet Is Highly Effective in Normalizing the Lactulose Breath Test." *Digestive Diseases and Sciences* 49 (1): 73–77.

Pimentel, M., W. Morales, A. Rezaie, E. Marsh, A. Lembo, J. Mirocha, D. A. Leffler, et al. 2015. "Development and Validation of a Biomarker for Diarrhea-Predominant Irritable Bowel Syndrome in Human Subjects." Edited by Seungil Ro. *PLoS One* 10 (5): e0126438. doi:10.1371/journal.pone.0126438.

Posserud, I., P.-O. Stotzer, E. S Bjornsson, H. Abrahamsson, and M. Simren. 2007. "Small Intestinal Bacterial Overgrowth in Patients with Irritable Bowel Syndrome." *Gut* 56 (6): 802–8. doi:10.1136/gut.2006.108712.

Quigley, E. M. M. 2014. "Small Intestinal Bacterial Overgrowth." *Current Opinion in Gastroenterology* 30 (2): 141–46. doi:10.1097/MOG.0000000000000040.

Reding, K. W., K. C. Cain, M. E. Jarrett, M. D. Eugenio, and M. M. Heitkemper. 2013. "Relationship Between Patterns of Alcohol Consumption and Gastrointestinal Symptoms Among Patients With Irritable Bowel Syndrome." *The American Journal of Gastroenterology* 108 (2): 270–76. doi:10.1038/ajg.2012.414.

van Rheenen, P. F., E. Van de Vijver, and V. Fidler. 2010. "Faecal Calprotectin for Screening of Patients with Suspected Inflammatory Bowel Disease: Diagnostic Meta-Analysis." *BMJ (Clinical Research Ed.)* 341 (July): c3369.

Rønnevig, M., P. O. Vandvik, and I. Bergbom. 2009. "Patients' Experiences of Living with Irritable Bowel Syndrome." *Journal of Advanced Nursing* 65 (8): 1676–85. doi:10.1111/j.1365-2648.2009.05030.x.

Sachdeva, S, et al. 2011 Apr. "SIBO in Irritable Bowel Syndrome: Frequency and Predictors. *Journal of Gastroenterology and Hepatology* 26 (Suppl 3): 135–8.

Schumann, D., D. Anheyer, R. Lauche, G. Dobos, J. Langhorst, and H. Cramer. 2016. "Effect of Yoga in the Therapy of Irritable Bowel Syndrome: A Systematic Review." *Clinical Gastroenterology and Hepatology* 14 (12): 1720–31. doi:10.1016/j.cgh.2016.04.026.

Simrén, M., A. Månsson, A. M. Langkilde, J. Svedlund, H. Abrahamsson, U. Bengtsson, and E. S. Björnsson. 2001. "Food-Related Gastrointestinal Symptoms in the Irritable Bowel Syndrome." *Digestion* 63 (2): 108–15. doi:10.1159/000051878.

Singh, R., A. Salem, J. Nanavati, and G. E. Mullin. 2018. "The Role of Diet in the Treatment of Irritable Bowel Syndrome." *Gastroenterology Clinics of North America* 47 (1): 107–37. doi:10.1016/j.gtc.2017.10.003.

Smith, F., X. Pan, V. Bellido, G. A. Toole, F. K. Gates, M. S. J. Wickham, P. R. Shewry, S. Bakalis, P. Padfield, and E. N. Clare Mills. 2015. "Digestibility of Gluten Proteins Is Reduced by Baking and Enhanced by Starch Digestion." *Molecular Nutrition & Food Research* 59 (10). Wiley-Blackwell: 2034–43. doi:10.1002/mnfr.201500262.

Tack, G. J., W. H. Verbeek, M. W. Schreurs, and C. J. Mulder. 2010. "The Spectrum of Celiac Disease: Epidemiology, Clinical Aspects and Treatment." *Nature Reviews Gastroenterology & Hepatology* 7 (4): 204–13. doi:10.1038/nrgastro.2010.23.

van Tilburg, M. A. L., O. S. Palsson, R. L. Levy, A. D. Feld, M. J. Turner, D. A. Drossman, and W. E. Whitehead. 2008. "Complementary and Alternative Medicine Use and Cost in Functional Bowel Disorders: A Six Month Prospective Study in a Large HMO." *BMC Complementary and Alternative Medicine* 8 (1). BioMed Central: 46. doi:10.1186/1472-6882-8-46.

Trinkley, K. E., and M. C. Nahata. 2014. "Medication Management of Irritable Bowel Syndrome." *Digestion* 89 (4): 253–67. doi:10.1159/000362405.

Tuck, C., E. Ly, A. Bogatyrev, I. Costetsou, P. Gibson, J. Barrett, and J. Muir. 2018. "Fermentable Short Chain Carbohydrate (FODMAP) Content of Common Plant-Based Foods and Processed Foods Suitable for Vegetarian- and Vegan-Based Eating Patterns." *Journal of Human Nutrition and Dietetics* 31 (3): 422–35. doi:10.1111/jhn.12546.

Undseth, R., A. Berstad, N.-E. Kløw, K. Arnljot, K. S. Moi, and J. Valeur. 2014. "Abnormal Accumulation of Intestinal Fluid Following Ingestion of an Unabsorbable Carbohydrate in Patients with Irritable Bowel Syndrome: An MRI Study." *Neurogastroenterology & Motility* 26 (12): 1686–93. doi:10.1111/nmo.12449.

Vidal-Valverde, C., J. Frías, and S. Valverde. 1993. "Changes in the Carbohydrate Composition of Legumes after Soaking and Cooking." *Journal of the American Dietetic Association* 93 (5): 547–50.

Vincenzi, M., I. Del Ciondolo, E. Pasquini, K. Gennai, and B. Paolini. 2017. "Effects of a Low FODMAP Diet and Specific Carbohydrate Diet on Symptoms and Nutritional Adequacy of Patients with Irritable Bowel Syndrome: Preliminary Results of a Single-Blinded Randomized Trial." *Journal of Translational Internal Medicine* 5 (2): 120–26. doi:10.1515/jtim-2017-0004.

Ware, J. E., and C. D. Sherbourne. 1992. "The MOS 36-Item Short-Form Health Survey (SF-36) I. Conceptual Framework and Item Selection." *Medical Care* 30 (6): 473–83.

Whitehead, W. E., and D. A Drossman. 2010. "Validation of Symptom-Based Diagnostic Criteria for Irritable Bowel Syndrome: A Critical Review." *The American Journal of Gastroenterology* 105 (4): 814–20; quiz 813, 821. doi:10.1038/ajg.2010.56.

Zar, S., D. Kumar, and M. J. Benson. 2001. "Food Hypersensitivity and Irritable Bowel Syndrome." *Alimentary Pharmacology & Therapeutics* 15 (4): 439–49.

Zhou, Q. Q., and G. N. Verne. 2011. "New Insights into Visceral Hypersensitivity—Clinical Implications in IBS." *Nature Reviews Gastroenterology & Hepatology* 8 (6): 349–55. doi:10.1038/nrgastro.2011.83.

8 Osteoarthritis

Nicole M. Farmer
National Institutes of Health, Clinical Center

CONTENTS

OSTEOARTHRITIS OVERVIEW

Osteoarthritis (OA) is one of the most common chronic health conditions in the world and a leading cause of pain and disability among adults (Allen, 2015). OA is caused by injury, loss of cartilage, structure, and function, and dysregulation of pro-inflammatory pathways (Goldring, 2011). It was not until the early 21st century (2001) that the pro-inflammatory pathways became recognized as a significant

DOI: 10.1201/b22377-8

contributor to the disease process for OA (Sokolove, 2013). With this inflammatory characterization came the realization that approaches to preventing both, the onset of OA and further joint destruction, may extend beyond strategies for weight management and mitigation of repetitive motion. Thus, decreasing inflammation and oxidative stress may be advantageous in reducing symptoms and result in improved management of OA progression. To date, no drug has been approved to improve structural protection of the joint or to prolong joint life in OA despite the high prevalence, individual impact of disability, and high societal cost of OA (Ma, 2017). This chapter will provide an overview of epidemiology and pathophysiology of OA and a review of nutrition-related factors that may aid in the prevention or slowing of disease progression through prevention of inflammation. This chapter will also include food science-based knowledge in relation to cooking methods that can help to maintain nutrition factors relevant for OA.

EPIDEMIOLOGY

The epidemiology of OA is related to an array of person-level and disease-level factors. Person-level factors related to OA are age, obesity status, and race/ethnicity, and systemic risk factors such as hyperlipidemia or metabolic syndrome. In contrast, disease-level factors are related to disease phenotype, as well as joint or localized risk factors such as prior injury or leg muscle weakness. Overall, in the U.S., it is estimated that about 14 million Americans have symptomatic OA, with about half having advanced disease. More than half of these cases present in individuals who are less than 65 years of age (Deshpande et al., 2016). Thus, many of these patients with symptomatic OA will foreseeably deal with decades of treatment and management requirements. The rising prevalence of obesity plays a significant role in the prevalence of OA, especially with respect to certain disease phenotypes (Deveza et al., 2017). Worldwide estimates for prevalence of OA vary by country and region. For instance, prevalence among adults in India is 28.7% (Prakash et al., 2016), 16.9% in Iran (Davatchi et al., 2016), and 64.9% in South Korea (Lee and Kim, 2017).

Determining the severity of OA involves multiple assessments including quality of life questionnaires related to pain, physical examination, and radiographic findings. The most commonly used quality of life measure is the Western Ontario McMaster Index (WOMAC). The WOMAC questionnaire contains several parts and contains questions related to severity and frequency of symptoms such as swelling of the joint, grinding and clicking noises, knee catching or hanging up, and the ability to straighten or bend knees, pain in the knees in different positions, knee functions, and ability to perform daily functions (McConnell et al., 2001). Higher scores indicate greater severity.

Traditionally, OA is diagnosed with X-ray radiographs from different angles to look for joint space width and asymmetry and for the presence of osteophytes. More recent methods such as magnetic resonance imaging (MRI), ultrasound, and optical coherence tomography have enhanced the OA diagnosis (Hunter et al., 2011). Most trials, however, utilize the assessment of pain and function as access to advanced imaging may be limited and not cost-effective.

Knee OA remains the most prevalent type of OA followed by hip and then hand OA. Within knee OA, there are six described clinical phenotypes: (1) chronic pain (with prominent central mechanism), (2) inflammation, (3) metabolic syndrome, (4) bone and cartilage metabolism, (5) mechanical overload, and (6) minimal joint disease (Dell'Isola et al., 2016). All of these phenotypes present with distinct clinical symptoms. In fact, Dell'Isola et al. found that of the clinical phenotypes, pain sensitization, psychological distress, radiographic severity, body mass index (BMI), muscle strength, inflammation, and comorbidities (especially metabolic syndrome) play significant parts in distinguishing clinically distinct phenotypes. A better definition of OA is expected by delineating different phenotypes of the disease and developing treatment targeted more specifically at these phenotypes which might lead to improved outcomes. Most of the treatment focus for OA is related to pharmacological, nonpharmacological including surgical and rehabilitation therapies, whereas preventive focus has remained focused on obesity prevention. However, current dietary recommendations for OA do not deviate greatly from general weight-management guidelines. While effective for obesity-related prevention, these guidelines treat obesity as a required factor for OA. However, analysis of adults in the general U.S. population shows that obesity classification was not a contributor to the association between metabolic syndrome and OA (Puenpatom and Victor, 2009). A diet-intensive intervention of overweight or obese adults greater than 55 years of age found that despite weight loss, there were no significant changes in structural progression of OA by X-ray or MRI after 18 months (Hunter, 2015). Suggesting, the issue regarding the obese, type 2 diabetes (DM) and metabolic syndrome phenotype for OA may have a more nuanced relationship and that it may be best to base dietary guidelines for OA on current understanding of the role of inflammation in the pathophysiology of OA.

Despite disease-level, person-level, and possibly, genetic distinctions, OA ultimately has a unifying mechanism: the disruption in the tribology of the joint that is initiated through an inflammatory process. Tribology refers to the study of the coordinated movement and load bearing of the joint's synovium and cartilage for protection. Through exploring the components of the tribology and how each component may be influenced by inflammation, a potential for role of nutrition and diet-related factors may arise.

There is evidence in the literature for overlap of the primary risk factors for OA with the clinical phenotypes (Deveza et al., 2017). Systemic risk factors include obesity, hyperlipidemia, and sociodemographic factors, of which sex is important. Due to their association with inflammation, a triad of obesity, diabetes, and metabolic syndrome is reported to directly influence the development of OA (Yoshimura, 2012). In fact, the prevalence of metabolic syndrome in patients with OA is 59% compared to 23% in the general U.S. population (Puenpatom and Victor, 2009). In terms of biological sex, compared to men women are more likely to develop hand, foot, and knee OA but are less likely to develop cervical spine OA (Johnson, 2014). In comparing cases and controls, hyperlipidemia was an independent risk factor for hand OA in a U.K. study, whereas other studies show that higher levels of HDL can be protective against incidence of OA (Vinna, 2018). Local risk factors which should be considered and which overlap with clinical phenotypes include ACL injury, muscle weakness, and various gait abnormalities.

The advancement of genome wide assessment studies has led to the identification of specific genomic alleles (genes) as other systemic risk factors, which may increase predisposition to OA. Although the conventional alleles linked to major histocompatibility complex (MHC) 1 are involved, other genetic pathways related to cytokine production and hormone receptors are considered candidate genes for knee OA. In fact, polymorphisms in the estrogen receptor may play a role in the higher prevalence of knee OA among postmenopausal women, while single nucleotide polymorphisms in the GDF5 gene responsible for the production of the inflammatory cytokine, transdermal growth factor (TGFβ), are thought to contribute to the increased prevalence of knee OA among Caucasians and Asian populations due to the higher frequency of the polymorphisms in these populations (Reynard and Loughlin, 2013).

PATHOPHYSIOLOGY

Cartilage is a strong and spongy tissue that forms round the end of the ball and socket of a joint. It allows for the hinge and pivot action to protect the end of a bone. When we move, cartilage acts to reduce friction. Thus, when cartilage wears down, the protection to the bone and nerve endings along the bone are lost. Maintenance of tribology-related protection within a joint involves a balance between cartilage breakdown (catabolism) and synthesis (anabolism). As illustrated in Figure 8.1, inflammatory cytokines, interleukin (IL)-beta and tumor necrosis factor (TNF)-alpha drive catabolic pathways and perpetuate loss of this protection (Thomas et al., 2018) (Figure 8.1).

The pathology of OA also involves degeneration of a synovial joint and involves the remodeling of subchondral bone, synovial inflammation, and loss of articular cartilage OA, affecting the entire diarthrodial (moveable) joint, where layers of cartilage lining two opposing joint surfaces and a layer of synovium containing synovial fluid for lubrication allow for easy joint movement. Within the diarthrodial joint, the cartilage is damaged, the underlying subchondral bone structure is remodeled, and a chronic

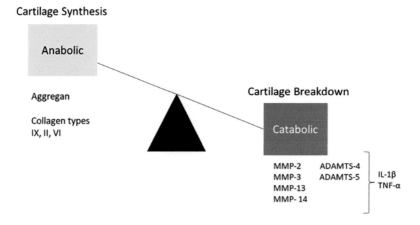

FIGURE 8.1 The pathology of OA results from an imbalance in cartilage synthesis and breakdown within a joint. Inflammatory factors IL-1β and TNF-α are principally involved in the cartilage breakdown.

inflammation of the synovium develops (Grover, 2016). Chondrocytes then produce and maintain the cartilaginous matrix, which is a large amount of extracellular matrix (ECM) composed of type II collagen fibers and substance rich in proteoglycan (PG) and elastin. The ECM helps allow for joint stability. PGs, such as aggrecan, in the ECM protect the joint from greater mechanical stress. In fact, glucosamine – an effective supplement for preventing OA – is a precursor for the PG, glycosaminoglycan. Chondroitin, another effective supplement for OA, is itself a PG. Healthy cartilage contains type II collagen. In the early stages of OA, collagen synthesis increases, but the composition type changes from type II to type I. This composition change ultimately affects the mechanical stability of the ECM network of the joint as type II collagen contains fibrils which allow for entrapping of PGs which lend stability to the joint. A morphological feature of early OA is that chondrocytes form clusters; this occurs because the normally quiescent cells start to proliferation (Grover, 2016) (Figure 8.2).

When damage, such as an injury, occurs to the joint, immune cells produce an inflammatory process generated from T cells, B cells, and macrophages occurring in the synovial space. The immune cells in turn lead to cytokine and chemokine activation which also leads to increased activity of matrix metalloproteinases (MMPs). MMPs are responsible for the degradation of the articular cartilage, such as type II collagen and ECM proteins, like PG. There are several principle MMPs in the pathology of OA: MMP-1, MMP-3, MMP-2, MMP-9, and MMP-13. A special type of MMP is one that also functions as a disintegrin, ADAM, as it inhibits platelet aggregation started from integrin. Within the ADAM class, ADAMTS has a special adhesive glycoprotein that can mediate cell to cell and cell to matrix interactions. ADAMTS-4 and ADAMTS-5 appear to be the most critical of the ADAMTS family for initiating the degradation of the aggrecan in early OA (Verma P, Dalal K, J Cell

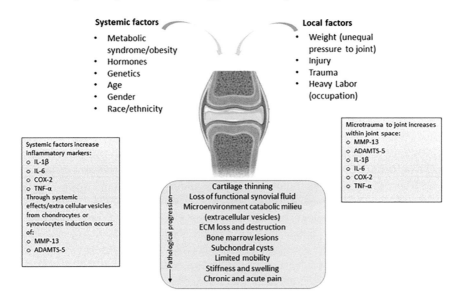

FIGURE 8.2 Risk factors for OA and pathophysiology including systematic and joint inflammatory mediators.

Biochem 2011). Inflammatory factors which promote inflammation can stimulate transcription of MMPs and ADAMTs genes in normal and OA human chondrocyte cells. These same inflammatory factors lead to COX-2 expression in the joints, which then promotes production of prostaglandins thought to be involved in the creation of pain from the joint. Pro-inflammatory cytokines are also found at increased levels within synovial fluid of patients with OA (Malemud, 2015). Inflammatory cytokines may also lead to the progression of OA by leading to programmed cell death (apoptosis) of chondrocytes. Apoptosis is mediated by the cell adhesion molecules, integrins, which help to maintain connection of chondrocytes with the ECM. After signaling from inflammatory cytokines, like IL-1β, integrins turn on intracellular signals that ultimately lead to apoptosis through the expression of the protein, caspase-3.

IL-1β stimulates the production of ROS such as peroxides and hydroxylated radicals and the production of NO and a deficiency in SOD. The deficiency in SOD leads to higher levels of superoxide. NO and superoxide react to form peroxynitrite which can lead to a decrease in the synthesis of collagen type II. ROS created from IL-1β may also damage the joint through creation of lipid peroxidation products which then induce cleavage of type II collagen. Additionally, expression of Nrf2 (nuclear factor erythroid 2-related factor 2), the anti-inflammatory transcription factor, may suppress the IL-1β induced ROS in chondrocytes (Khan et al., 2017). Hence, there may be a role for antioxidants in preserving the integrity of type II collagen in OA.

As mentioned earlier, the role of the synovium is to provide lubrication for the joint. It comprises the synovial membrane and the encompassed fluids. The membrane lines the joint cavity and acts as a semipermeable membrane that regulates transfer of molecules into and out of the joint. The membrane allows the essential synovial fluid components into the synovium: hyaluronic acid and lubricin and plasma like proteins such as globulin and albumin. All of the components have an influence on film thickness, friction coefficient, and wear rate within the joint. Lubricin in fact serves as a critical lubricant between opposing cartilage surfaces. In fact, when a joint injury occurs, there is an initial release of cytokines, which leads to decreased lubricin expression (Musumeci et al., 2013). This reduced expression predisposes to cartilage denegation and places the joint at risk for OA. Inflammation of the synovium, synovitis, is recognized as a key factor associated with the signs and symptoms of OA, particularly joint swelling, stiffness, and pain. Synovitis involves the infiltration of immune cells into the synovial membrane and the production of pro-inflammatory cytokines, IL-1, IL-6, and TNF-α, as well as increased expression of MMPs in synovial tissue (Sofat, 2014). One hypothesis that may explain how the synovium becomes inflamed is through advanced glycation end products that contact the synovium and are recognized as foreign prompting synovial cells to produce inflammatory mediators (Sofat, 2014). Advanced glycation products not only have a role in the synovium but are also linked to chondrocyte function. Hyperglycemia prompts accumulation of advanced glycation end products (Zhuo, 2012), and the receptor for advanced glycation end products is increased in OA articular chondrocytes. Taking into consideration the role of inflammation and advanced glycation end products in OA, the potential for identifying dietary changes that may be protective against OA becomes evident.

In addition to advanced glycation products, another dietary factor that may be involved in OA is the intake of high uric acid-containing foods. Association studies have long found a relationship between the diagnosis of gout and OA. Although a linked inflammatory mechanism was long suspected, it was not until *in vitro* studies on the cellular effects of uric acid became known that a plausible pathway existed. Uric acid, either systemically or within a joint, can activate IL-1β and TNF-α pathways responsible for OA development. Uric acid can form into monosodium uric acid crystals, which can activate the Il-1β stimulating inflammasome (NALP-3) or can activate complement of T cells which directly promote MMP activity (Ma, 2017). Clinical studies offer evidence of this potential pathway. The Prediction of Osteoarthritis Progression study found that subjects with knee OA but without prior gout history had uric acid within the fluid that was strongly associated with IL-1β and radiographic severity of knee OA (Denoble et al., 2011).

As evidenced through the pathophysiological steps in OA, the joint is a system in which the cartilage, the bone, and the synovium engage in crosstalk between all the tissues (Grover, 2016). This system crosstalk can be detrimental when uncontrolled inflammation is present but may be beneficial in the setting of exposure to anti-inflammatory or antioxidant-based foods that can leverage the system to return the joint to its protective functional state.

DIETARY PATTERNS AND OA

For rheumatoid arthritis and gout arthritis, recommendations for dietary patterns, such as low uric acid or vegan diet, are established in the literature (Badsha, 2018; Chiu, 2020). For OA, beneficial dietary patterns are focused mostly on the Mediterranean diet. The Mediterranean diet consists of regular daily consumption of fruit, vegetables, legumes, nuts, seeds, and cereals in high amounts, regular weekly intake of seafood, and moderate consumption of dairy products, poultry, and eggs. The diet also promotes olive oil, a source of monounsaturated fatty acid (MUFA), as the main type of dietary lipids (Trichopoulou et al., 2014). The diet has consistently shown association with lowered risk for metabolic syndrome and protective effect against inflammation. Therefore, it is logical to assess for a role for the Mediterranean diet in OA.

In theory, the Mediterranean diet may help OA through its anti-inflammatory actions and by increasing antioxidant capacity, which may enhance collagen type II and aggrecan expression and inhibit apoptosis-related protein expression (Veronese et al., 2016). Cross-sectional analysis of participants with symptomatic knee OA or who were at high risk for developing knee OA showed that higher Mediterranean diet scores were associated with lower prevalence of knee OA (Veronese et al., 2016), lower symptoms of OA as assessed by WOMAC scores (Veronese et al., 2017), and better cartilage thickness and volume as assessed by MR images of the knee (Veronese et al., 2019). However, these studies are limited by being cross-sectional in nature and thus cannot show any causal role of the Mediterranean diet. Intervention studies may provide additional evidence. In fact, one study of a 16- week dietary intervention comparing Mediterranean diet vs. Western diet found a decrease in the OA-related cytokine, IL-1, decrease in cartilage degradation markers, and increase in knee flexion and rotation after 4 months with the Mediterranean diet (Dyer et al., 2017). Further intervention-based evidence of the role of Mediterranean diet on OA is provided by the following study. Rats given a surgically induced knee injury subsequently had reduced lubricin (PG 4) levels as expected. The rats were then given an extra virgin olive oil-supplemented diet along with daily treadmill activity. Following the supplemented diet and activity, the rats with the intervention had a return of lubricin levels back to normal in comparison to the control rats (Musumeci et al., 2013).

A whole food, plant-based dietary pattern is also reported as helping to alleviate OA symptoms. A 6-week randomized study using a nutrition education curriculum from the Physician's Committee for Responsible Medicine (PCRM) as the dietary intervention found that for the intervention group, there was greater improvement in pain scale compared to the control group occurring after 2 weeks on the whole food plant-based diet (Clinton et al., 2015). Of note, the intervention group was asked to restrict animal protein to 10% of their total calorie intake. The study authors attributed the positive outcomes for the study to a presumed increase in consumption of phytonutrients, minerals, and essential fatty acids in the intervention group as a result of the PCRM diet.

Dietary patterns to be aware of for OA symptom management may also relate to development, not just prevention, of OA. Based on the pathophysiology evidence presented earlier, adverse dietary patterns may include high glycemic diets and diets that promote production of uric acid. Dietary factors related to uric acid exposure actually overlap with dietary patterns related to hyperglycemia. Added sugars that provide fructose either from sugar sweetened or naturally occurring fructose from fruit juices are linked to higher risk of uric acid formation and gout. Additionally, consumption of purine-rich animal foods, but not purine-rich vegetables, is linked to increased risk for gout. This suggests an adverse role for foods that contain stearic acid such as lard and tallow when present in a diet or meal that may lead to uric acid synthesis.

NUTRIENTS RELATED TO OA

The traditional use of herbs such as frankincense for OA has long been published in the literature and supports the notion that plant molecules of phytonutrients may play a protective role in the condition (Dragos et al., 2017). Two popular natural supplements for OA, glucosamine chondroitin and SAM (S-adenyl methionine), have long been touted for pain relief from OA. Exact mechanisms for their function are not known, but suspected mechanisms include reduction of MMP through anti-inflammatory processes and protection of the PG, aggrecan, and network within the cartilage (Vasilladis, 2017). While developments in genotyping and proteomic expression have led to novel potential pharmacologics for OA, it has also brought the ability to identify nutrients likely to favorably impact inflammatory pathways in OA. For example, luteolin, apigenin, sulforaphane, and isoliquiritigenin (nutrient bioactives to be described in later sections) were found to significantly suppress IL-1β production in chondrocytes (Davidson et al., 2018). Identification of these nutrient bioactives highlights the role of specific food based nutrients in the pathophysiology of OA, and the thus the necessity to explore each nutrient and its response to food preparation techniques.

MINERALS

Magnesium

Epidemiological studies show that approximately half of the US population consumes less than the daily requirement of magnesium from foods (Hafsi et al., 2019). Magnesium is a mineral necessary for smooth muscle relaxation throughout the body. Its connection to OA may lie within its secondary role in promoting an anti-inflammatory effect within cells. A recent cross-sectional analysis of the Osteoarthritis Initiative (OAI) database study, which enrolled adults with knee OA living in four different U.S. cities, found that magnesium intake levels of 100 mg/day were associated with more cartilage volume on MRI imaging (Veronese et al., 2019). The finding was consistent with other studies that show a relationship between magnesium intake (Qin et al., 2012) and serum levels (Zeng et al., 2015) with radiographic evidence of OA. Within the Veronese et al. study, the association persisted after adjusting for BMI, socioeconomic indicators, physical activity, and Mediterranean diet score. In terms of food equivalents, 100 mg/day is found readily in one cooked cup of black beans, edamame, whole grains, or quinoa. And animal models show that magnesium deficiency is associated with a decrease in the knee chondrocytes and consequent decrease cartilage (Vormann et al., 1997). However, intervention studies are needed to determine if magnesium has a direct role in protection from OA or if factors such as most magnesium consumption coming from vegetables are actually responsible for the association.

Zinc

Similar to calcium, higher urine zinc levels are associated with knee OA. Specific accumulation of Zn^{2+} is reported in cartilage regions exposed to either loading or stretching in aged populations (Roschger et al., 2013). Zinc, like calcium, also has an important role with MMPs, which degrade cartilage, for MMPs are not only calcium-dependent but also zinc-dependent. Recent molecular investigations suggest a role of zinc through activation of the zinc transporter, ZIP8, with catabolic cascade of cartilage breakdown prior to the initiation of MMP activity (Kim et al., 2014). Although the evidence appears divergent on zinc and OA, taken together, the evidence may suggest that overall zinc homeostasis is important in OA.

Vitamin D

There is evidence for a role of Vitamin D in OA. Expression of the vitamin D receptor (VDR) is increased in areas of erosion in OA (Orfanidou et al., 2012). It's also been shown that patients with OA have decreased serum vitamin D levels (Bassiouni et al., 2017). When at deficient levels, vitamin D is associated in both prospective and cross-sectional studies with increased risk for OA and increased radiographic arthritic changes, respectively (Goula et al., 2015). It's also been shown that patients with OA have decreased serum vitamin D levels (Bassiouni et al., 2017). However, imaging studies looking at increased vitamin D serum levels as a way to decrease the risk for OA have been inconclusive (Garfinkel et al., 2017). VDRs present in immune cells are activated upon vitamin D binding. This activation then leads to activation of VDR response elements that can block transcription of inflammatory cytokines such as NF-κB and allows for upregulation of the anti-inflammatory cytokines, IL-10

(Garfinkel et al., 2017). Therefore, the association of vitamin D deficiency with OA may be based in its modulation if inflammation. Vitamin D may also work in synergy with other nutrients related to OA, such as magnesium or calcium. Magnesium is able to potentiate the effects of vitamin D on the skeletal system, further reinforcing a possible positive effect of for both magnesium and vitamin D with knee OA. Calcium is required for muscle contraction and nerve signaling; the serum concentration of calcium has obvious significance for the musculoskeletal system. Calcium is mostly located in the skeleton. Only a fraction of the stored calcium is present in extracellular fluid and available for use in the form of ionized calcium. Levels in the extracellular fluid represent the action of two hormones, parathyroid (PTH) and vitamin D. Thus, studies which find an inverse association with serum calcium levels (Hui et al., 2016) and OA are likely indicative of regulation of these hormones. However, some studies focused on the role of calcium within the skeleton, as an important element for the MMP enzymes, suggest that calcium availability within the joint may contribute to knee OA for some patients (Corr et al., 2017). However, how this reflects or is related to dietary intake of calcium, independent of vitamin D, is unknown.

Vitamin C

Given the role of inflammation in breaking down the ECM of joints effected by OA, identifying nutrients in foods which may help to combat the inflammatory process may be beneficial. For example, vitamin C is involved in the synthesis of collagen type II needed to help trap PGs in the ECM to form a stable supportive matrix. Thus, its presence in a diet maybe protective of the downward effects of inflammation. Vitamin C is also an antioxidant, and these properties may protect a joint against inflammatory-related oxidation. In a prospective analysis from the Framingham study, knee OA progression and development of knee pain were reduced in people with high intakes of vitamin C (McAlindon et al., 1996). The effective intakes of vitamin C ranged from 2.5 times to 7.1 times the recommended daily intake of 60 mg a day. Vitamin C may have a particular advantage over other antioxidants, especially those that are fat-soluble, as it is water-soluble and thus can exist in the aqueous ECM joint. Interestingly in this same study, vitamin E, a fat-soluble vitamin, only had a protective association with OA when not controlling for vitamin C levels in the same individuals.

In relation to the role of uric acid to stimulate OA progression, use of vitamin C-rich foods may have another protective role for OA. Cherries are a source of several types of antioxidants, especially vitamin C. Consumption of approximately 1–2 cups of cherries a day (280 g) led to decrease in uric acid levels and inflammatory markers, including the OA cytokine IL-1β (Torralba et al., 2012).

Despite these beneficial findings, there may be a need for precaution with vitamin C supplementation and OA. Vitamin C may increase production of TGF-β on chondrocytes, and animal model studies have shown an association between vitamin C supplementation of 200 mg/day and development of OA. Another consideration is that there may be a differential effect of vitamin C from foods versus vitamin C supplements on OA. For example, vitamin C-rich foods may also provide flavonoids (discussed in further sections) that could counter effects of vitamin C's ability to increase TGF-β. And this synergistic effect may be what was ultimately measured in the population-based studies such as the Framingham study.

Essential Fatty Acids: Omega-6 (LA, AA), Omega-3s (ALA, EPA, and DHA)

Linoleic acid (LA; 18:2n26) and ALA (18:3n23) and their long-chain derivatives arachidonic acid (AA; 20:4), eicosapentaenoic acid (EPA; 20:5n23), and docosahexaenoic (DHA; 22:6n23) are polyunsaturated fatty acids (PUFAs) that are important components of animal and plant cell membranes and contribute to human growth and development. These fatty acids were identified as essential to get from dietary intake when it was demonstrated in 1963 that humans do not have the enzymes to synthesize LA and ALA *de novo* (Candela, 2011). The difference between LA and ALA is in the presence of the first double bond (3 versus 6 location), counting from the methyl end of the fatty acid structure. Epidemiological studies, both cross-sectional and prospective, show that consumption of both LA and ALA has favorable effects on blood lipids. And LA, when consumed as 15% of daily calories, has anti-inflammatory and insulin-sensitizing effects (Mozzaffarian, 2016).

ALA and LA are found in plant food sources. ALA can be found in green leafy vegetables, inside of plant chloroplasts, and in seeds, such as flax and chia. LA is found in abundant amounts in most plant seeds and oils, except for most saturated fat plant oils such as coconut or palm oils. Upon ingestion from plant food sources, ALA and LA are elongated to EPA, DHA, and AA, respectively, by desaturase enzymes. However, this elongation process is not very efficient. For example, for conversion of ALA, only 5%–10% is converted to EPA and 2%–5% to DHA (Arterburn, 2006). Food sources for the long forms of the essential fatty acids are also recommended. AA can be found in animal-based food sources, while EPA and DHA are found in mostly fish fatty acids or in algae.

A key enzyme shared by both ALA and LA is delta-6 desaturase. It starts the elongation cascade and has a higher affinity for ALA versus LA. This preference for ALA leads to a 10-fold greater proportion of LA that is needed versus ALA to inhibit the formation of the ALA long chains, EPA and DHA. Experimental evidence based on this factor differential leads to the recommendation for an optimal ratio of LA to ALA of 4-5:1 (Candela, 2011). It is important to note that omega-6 and omega-3 fatty acids are not interconvertible (Simopoulos, 2016). In other words, humans cannot convert omega-6 to omega -3 fatty acids. This means that dietary choices lead to a fixed exposure to a particular essential fatty acid, thus having dietary balance become ever more important.

In assessing the value of omega 6 and omega 3 to inflammation, it is important to highlight that both omega 6 and omega 3 are metabolically and functionally distinct and often have important opposing physiological effects. For instance, ingestion of EPA and DHA leads to displacement of AA from cellular membranes (Simopoulos, 2016). It also leads to (1) decreased production of prostaglandin E2 metabolites; (2) decreased concentrations of thromboxane A2, a potent platelet aggregator and vasoconstrictor; (3) decreased formation of leukotriene B4, an inducer of inflammation and a powerful inducer of leukocyte chemotaxis and adherence; (4) increased concentrations of thromboxane A3, a weak platelet aggregator and vasoconstrictor; (5) increased concentrations of prostacyclin PGI3, leading to an overall increase in total prostacyclin by increasing PGI3 without decreasing PGI2 (both PGI2 and PGI3 are active vasodilators and inhibitors of platelet aggregation); and (6) increased concentrations of leukotriene B5, a weak inducer of inflammation and chemotactic agent (Simopoulos, 2016). With regard to OA, the omega 3 essential fatty acids may therefore be involved in altering inflammatory response in chondrocytes through inhibiting IL-1-induced MMP3, MMP13, ADAMTS4, and ADAMTS5.

In terms of OA, studies to date in the literature have utilized long-chain omega-3 fatty acids when determining the association with OA. A large prospective study in OA patients found that higher intakes of total and saturated fat were associated with increased joint space-width loss. Interestingly in this study, higher intakes MUFA and PUFAs were associated with reduced radiographic OA progression (Lu et al., 2017). Other studies support these findings. An inverse relationship was found between the total plasma omega-3, DHA with patellofemoral cartilage loss, as measured by MRI, in the MOST (Multicenter Osteoarthritis Study) cohort study (Baker et al., 2012). Human clinical studies focused on fish oil supplementation and OA are limited but offer intriguing and promising results. One efficacy study of 1,000 mg and 2,000 mg fish oil with EPA (400 mg) and DHA (200 mg) given to 75 participants with knee OA showed an improvement in walking velocity, knee pain, and function after 8 weeks of use. It is interesting that the results also showed that post intervention, there was a significant difference up to 12 weeks after stopping the intervention (Peanpadungrat, 2015). In terms of effective dose, results from a randomized double-blind study in Australia suggest that a low-dose of 0.45 g resulted in the same reduction in pain symptom as 4.5 g of fish oil after 24 months of supplementation (Hill, 2015).

OA joints and OA-affected synovium tend to accumulate high levels of omega-6 fatty acids which are precursors of potentially pro-inflammatory eicosanoids (Plumb and Aspden, 2004). Omega-6 levels have a positive association with synovitis, inflammation in the synovium, but association with serum levels and omega-6 remain unclear. Omega-6 levels and omega-3 levels depend on the same enzyme-based desaturation system in order to form from the longer-chain essential fatty acids. Therefore, evaluating their interrelationship may be important. A cross-sectional study evaluating the role of omega 6: omega 3 serum levels in patients with OA-related pain found that a lower ratio of 5.08 was associated with less clinical pain. The sources of omega-3 included both supplement and diet. Although causality could not be established, this study further suggests the important role of omega-3 in OA symptoms. The importance of omega-3 may lie in the fact that omega-3-fatty acids have anti-inflammatory effects via suppression of IL-1Beta, TNF-alpha, and IL-6, but omega-6 levels do not (Simopoulos, 2016). Recommendations regarding omega-6 and OA may also be harder to determine given the null or protective role identified for omega-6 in conditions with similar risk factors as OA, such as type 2 diabetes and CVD (Hooper et al., 2018).

CURCUMIN

Curcumin is the main bioactive anti-inflammatory polyphenol in the plant rhizome turmeric. In cell studies, curcumin has the ability to block several inflammatory mediators. *In vitro* curcumin can inhibit NF-κB and COX-2, and chondrocyte studies show an ability to block the expression of MMP. There have been several clinical studies published showing some effectiveness for use of curcumin in OA. In one study, over a period of 4 weeks, patients with OA received a daily dose of 2 g of curcumin in comparison to patients given the NSAID, ibuprofen. After 4 weeks, there was no difference in pain score or function score between the two groups, leading to the conclusion that turmeric is as effective as ibuprofen for OA (Kuptniratsaikul et al., 2014). Other studies also show reduction in patient reports of pain as well as reduction of inflammatory markers with lower doses of curcumin, 200 mg, for 3 months or 8 months (Belcaro et al., 2010a; Belcaro et al., 2010b).

Overall, curcumin has poor bioavailability in supplement form. Since only 3% of turmeric's weight comes from curcumin, equivalent doses of OA effective doses translate to extremely large intakes of turmeric, possibly more than the average diet allows. Nevertheless, to increase bioavailability of curcumin, turmeric needs fatty acid, such as phosphatidylcholine, or piperine, an active ingredient in black pepper. Interestingly, there may be a synergy with use of resveratrol and curcumin together in inhibiting NF-κB in chondrocytes and preventing chondrocyte apoptosis (Shakibaei et al., 2011). In terms of food preparation, this would suggest that there is a benefit to serving foods high in resveratrol, such as red wine, grapes, red onions, and peanuts with foods incorporating turmeric to see a possible effect on OA without unrealistically increasing turmeric consumption (Figure 8.3).

Cruciferous Foods and Glucosinolates

The cruciferous vegetables, kale, Brussels sprouts, and particularly broccoli, contain glucosinolates, which are sulfur-containing molecules derived from the amino acids methionine or tryptophan. Glucosinolates are precursors to isothiocyanates, which become activated by the enzyme myrosinase upon shear pressures such as chewing or chopping. The cruciferous vegetable broccoli contains the glucosinolate glucoraphanin, which becomes sulforaphane (SFN) through activation by the enzyme myosinase. SFN is actually a chondroprotective substance found *in vivo* and *in vitro* to repress expression of MMPs, regulates NF-κB, and inhibits the production of prostaglandin E2 and NO in chondrocytes. As well, SFN is effective in inhibiting expression of ADAMTS4 and TS5 in mouse models through direct inhibition of NF-κB (Davidson et al., 2013). And through its epigenetic action, SFN is involved in the disinhibition of Nrf2 through removing an epigenetically silenced status of Nrf2 (Zhang et al., 2013). To test the potential usefulness of dietary glucosinolates as a protective bioactive for OA, a clinical study of patients with OA about to undergo total knee replacement (TKR) found that after a 14-day high-glucoraphanin diet from broccoli, the presence of sulforaphane was higher in synovial joints than in patients who stayed on a low glucoraphanin diet. Those patients on the high-glucoraphanin diet also had lower inflammation markers in the synovium. However, clinical outcomes of these patients in relation to lower inflammation markers were not measured in this study.

Flavonoids

Diets rich in fruits and vegetables are thought to be beneficial to health due to the presence of flavonoids, polyphenols widely distributed in the fruits and vegetables. The range of foods containing flavonoids includes tea, citrus foods, herbs,

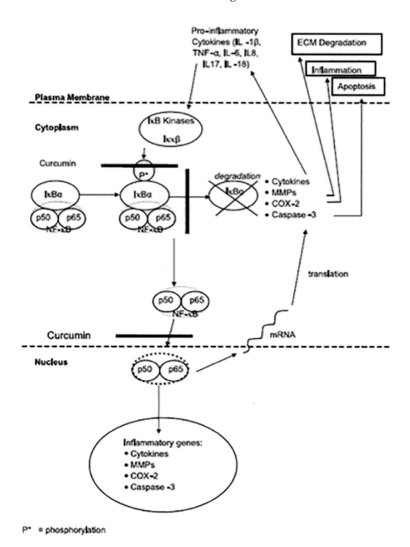

FIGURE 8.3 Inflammatory cell signaling responses in joint cells with schematic illustrations of potential sites of action for curcumin (C) in a typical joint cell. (From Henrotin et al. 2010. Biological actions of curcumin on articular chondrocytes. *Osteoarthr Cartil.* 18: 141–149.)

and some commonly consumed vegetables such as celery. With regard to OA, there are particular categories of flavonoids that are protective of chondrocytes and joint damage. Flavones, a category of flavonoids located predominately in the leaves and in the outer parts of plants (Ewald et al., 1999) contain apigenin and luteolin. Often, apigenin and luteolin are found together in the same plant foods, such a parsley and celery. In a study of human chondrocytes, micromolar (μM) amounts of apigenin and lutein were found to prevent expression of joint destroying MMPs (Davidson et al., 2018). Pharmacokinetic studies in humans show that absorption of apigenin and luteolin from parsley or celery leads to serum levels in the µM range (Hostetler et al., 2017). Thus, it is logical to preclude that consumption of foods such as parsley, spinach, and celery which contain both apigenin and luteolin may be helpful for OA.

Nobiletin, a polymethoxy flavone found in citrus skin, may be particularly protective for OA. *In vitro* studies show that synovial cells and cartilage chondrocytes when exposed to nobiletin (16–64 µM) inhibited cartilage degradation by interfering with ADAMTS-4 and 5 activity as well as activating an MMP inhibitor (Xie et al., 2019). Other *in vitro* studies report the mechanism of nobiletin's ability to reduce the expression of inflammatory mediators maybe from the inhibition of the phosphorylation of the pro-inflammatory factor, NF-κB (Lin et al., 2019).

Wogonin is a unique aglycone flavone that may offer protection from OA. The flavone is primarily found in Chinese herbal teas. Unlike other flavonoids that originate from the flower parts of a plant, wogonin originates from the root of the herb *Scutellaria baicalensis* (Zhao et al., 2016). *In vitro* studies show that the flavone exerts direct anti-inflammatory and chondroprotective effects through suppressing the expression and production of inflammatory mediators including IL-6, COX-2, PGE_2, iNOS, and NO in IL-1β-stimulated OA chondrocytes (Khan et al., 2017). Wogonin also exhibited chondroprotective potential through inhibiting the expression, production, and activities of matrix-degrading proteases including MMP-13, MMP-3, MMP-9, and ADAMTS-4 in OA chondrocytes (Khan et al., 2017).

GINGER

Ginger is a member of the cardamom and turmeric plant family. The edible portion of the ginger plant is the rhizome, the horizontal stem from which the roots grow, containing chemical components with antioxidative and anti-inflammatory properties. These properties provide an explanation for ginger's positive effects on arthritis, specifically OA. Several studies have shown lowered inflammatory markers, such as C-reactive protein after ginger supplementation (Vaishya et al., 2018), and randomized studies have found that ginger and the anti-inflammatory medicine diclofenac both improved pain-related symptoms better than the each alone (Paramdeep, 2013).

Ginger contains certain chemical components which are responsible for its inflammatory actions; 6-gingerol, shogaols, and pungent constituents (gingerdione). Both gingerol and shogaol *in vitro* have the ability to decrease COX-2 activity, and the pungent components *in vitro* show the ability to also attenuate COX-2 but also Il-β, IL-6, and TNF-α. Both also have the ability to target the potentially chondroprotective pathway, Nrf2 (Schadich et al., 2016); however, the role in chondrocytes has yet to be reported.

SESAME OIL

Sesame oil has been used in traditional medicine to alleviate pain from inflammatory conditions. The oil is extracted from *Sesamum indicum*, and animal OA models show an ability for sesame oil to alleviate joint pain by inhibiting oxidative progression and serum inflammatory markers (Dragos et al., 2017). Human studies show that five tablespoons of sesame seeds in conjunction with standard drug therapy for OA led to improvement in pain and mobility after 2 months compared to control

(Sadat et al., 2013). And in another study, the same amount of sesame seed was associated with a statistically significant drop in serum levels of IL-6 and C-reactive protein after 2 months of treatment (Haghighian et al., 2015).

SOLANACEAE (NIGHTSHADES)

For long, the consumption of nightshades has been linked to occurrence of arthritic symptoms in patient-based anecdotes. Some common fruits and vegetables belong to the biological family of nightshades: tomatoes, potatoes, eggplant (aubergine), and peppers. Consumption of these foods in various forms is included within these anecdotes. Characteristically, nightshades contain plant alkaloids such as nicotine, solanine, and anatabine. Published studies directly evaluating the role of these chemicals have not found a relationship with increased arthritic inflammatory markers. In fact, a survey study on the use of anatabine as a dietary supplement found that most users reported improvement in musculoskeletal aches, pains, and stiffness (Lanier et al., 2013). Similar studies linking nicotine or solanine with musculoskeletal symptoms have not been reported as of yet. As with all foods, the nightshade alkaloids do not exist alone. For example, nightshades also characteristically contain lectins, a class of chemicals linked to molecular mimicry and T-cell activation. However, it is the alkaloids in nightshades which have been linked to arthritis and led to the cautionary advice of limiting nightshade consumption. However, nightshades, especially tomatoes and pigmented potatoes, may contain anti-inflammatory chemicals, such as lycopene or carotenoids that can be protective for OA (Kaspar et al., 2010).

COOKING METHODS FOR NUTRIENTS AND FOODS RELATED TO OA

OMEGA-3 FATTY ACIDS: FISH

The current evidence in relation to OA suggests an advantage of omega-3s in the diet as protective. Long-chain omega-3s, DHA and EPA, are mostly consumed from fish sources. However, the availability of omega 3 fatty acids in fish is sensitive to preparation methods including cooking method, cooking time, and oils utilized. Therefore, exploring how long-chain omega-3s in fish may be affected by cooking processes is important.

Current recommendations from the WHO (World Health Organization) are for adults to consume at least 500 mg of EPA and DHA daily (Bastias et al., 2017). Fish is commonly prepared for consumption by steaming, boiling, pan-frying, baking, or roasting. Theoretically, the high temperature could degrade EPA and DHA. Given the current recommendations for consumption of omega-3-rich fish within the Mediterranean diet, the following section will focus on omega-3-rich species commonly recommended with this dietary pattern but also offer information on lean fish species.

In a study using deskinned salmon cooked either by boiling (99°C), pan-frying for 10 minutes without oil (200°C ±10°C), or oven-baking (200°C) compared to non-cooked salmon, Leung et al (2018) found that EPA and DHA levels were unchanged. In contrast, a prior study on pan-fried salmon found that when cooked for 15–20 minutes in sunflower oil, there was a loss of EPA and DHA (Gladyshev et al., 2006), suggesting that length of time of pan-frying and the presence of cooking oil, are important factors. The role for cooking oil is based on the hypothesis that EPA and DHA levels reduce after cooking because the lipid component of the cooked fish represents the lipid component of the oil. Similar to salmon, use of cooking oil (sunflower oil) with pan-frying of trout can decrease EPA and DHA, but less so for cod and herring (Gladyshev et al., 2006). The difference between trout, cod and herring may be explained by location of omega3s within fish. With leaner fish, the omega-3s are present within phospholipids (Liisberg et al., 2016) which are more bioavailable than the omega-3s in fatty fish that are present within triglycerides.

The selection of the cooking oil for omega3 retention in fish can be further illustrated through studies that use the same type of fish with different cooking oils. Flaskerud et al. (2017) found that pan-frying trout in corn oil or canola led to no effect on EPA and DHA levels. But peanut oil reduced EPA levels, and sunflower oil reduced both EPA and DHA, as in aforementioned studies. Similar results have been reported for scallops, a fish with high concentration of omega-3 and relatively low amount of omega-6. In comparison to raw, steaming for 2.3 minutes, and pan-frying for 2.4 minutes, deep frying scallops for 1.4 minutes (in a batter of flour, salt, and water) using vegetable oil led to significant lowering of omega3/omega6 ratio (Su and Babb, 2007) in the deep fried and pan fried scallops. There was higher maintenance of omega-3 with steaming compared to the other methods, as well as an increase in amount of DHA compared to EPA in the steamed scallops (Su and Babb, 2007).

To further support the effect of cooking methods on EPA and DHA, Bastias et al. (2017) found that EPA and DHA amounts significantly increased , from raw, when salmon was steamed for 25 minutes to a center temperature of $83.5°C \pm 2°C$, but not when oven-cooked for 25 minutes at $250°C$ to a center temperature of $76.2°C \pm 0.5°C$. Similar findings occurred for the omega-3-rich fish, mackerel, but the EPA and DHA levels increased with microwaving for 12 minutes to center temp of $86.3°C \pm 1°C$. Placing their findings in the context of the WHO recommendations for EPA and DHA, for an individual to meet the guidelines the authors recommended 25 g of steamed salmon and larger portion for oven-cooked salmon, of 41 g of oven-cooked salmon (about 1.5 ounces or approximately half adult palm size). For mackerel, 77 g steamed or microwaved was recommended by the authors.

Omega-3 availability is also impacted by oxidation during the cooking process, for which the type of oil used with cooking and the cooking method is important. Fish are highly susceptible to oxidation due to their higher content of PUFAs. Thermal treatment of omega-3s is known to increase their susceptibility toward lipid oxidation. Al-Saghir et al. (2004) found that among farmed salmon, pan-frying for 6 minutes did not increase lipid peroxidation, but did increase cholesterol oxidation products. The highest level of cholesterol oxidation products occurred from the steaming of the farmed fish, suggesting that the fish oils present in the farmed fish themselves can be a significant source of oxidation when oil is not present. But not all oxidation leads to harmful free radicals. Some oxidation creates oxidized fatty acids that actually may offer health benefits. For example, the long-chain omega-3 fatty acid DHA when oxidized can become 4-HHE. This oxidized fatty acid is actually helpful in decreasing inflammation through activation of the Nrf2 pathway (Ishikado et al., 2013). In the same study assessing EPA and DHA levels in salmon, Leung et al. found that pan-frying salmon for 10 minutes leads to elevation of 4-HHE.

The proposed mechanism for this is that the high heat used in pan-frying promotes secondary lipid peroxidation that generates the 4HHE, which are aldehydes, that can cross-link with the fish protein (Leung et al., 2018). In total, the current evidence regarding lipid oxidation with cooking of fish is limited especially when taking into context the important role of certain cooking methods, such as steaming, in retaining overall EPA and DHA levels.

CRUCIFEROUS FOODS AND GLUCOSINOLATES: BROCCOLI

As stated in the prior section, the presence of a glucosinolate-rich diet through broccoli led to the presence of the chondroprotective isothiocyanate SFN in synovial joints. Interestingly, the instructed preparation of broccoli for patients on the high-glucoraphanin diet was to steam the broccoli. Steaming of broccoli is reported to lower myrosinase activity, the enzyme needed to change glucosinolates to the protective isothiocyanates, unless light steaming occurs (Yuan et al., 2009). Myrosinase is activated in precooking through chopping but is heat-sensitive to cooking methods. During cooking, inactivation of plant myrosinase, loss of enzymatic cofactors, thermal breakdown and/or leaching of glucosinolates and their metabolites, or volatilization of metabolites may occur (Rungapamestry et al., 2007). Thus, common home-cooking methods such as boiling, microwaving, stir-frying, and stir-frying with boiling lead to lower levels when comparing cooked to uncooked freshly harvested broccoli heads (Rungapamestry et al., 2007). However, one study found that myrosinase activity can be maintained under quick high heat during stir-frying if chopped broccoli is allowed to sit first for at least 30 minutes before cooking (Wu et al., 2018). Addition of exogenous sources of myrosinase to cooked broccoli, such as half a teaspoon (1 g) of powdered brown mustard seed while cooking, can increase bioavailability of SFN by four times that of broccoli cooked without mustard seed (Okunade et al., 2018). Of note, studies show that brown mustard has higher myrosinase activity than black or yellow mustard (Okunade et al., 2015).

For cruciferous vegetables, particularly broccoli, there may be mechanisms that protect against OA despite loss of SFN. For example, broccoli not only contains high amounts of glucoraphanin but also contains high amounts of the antioxidant, vitamin C. Both of these nutrients are maintained with light steaming (Yuan et al., 2009). Thus, use of lightly steamed broccoli as a therapeutic food for OA could represent synergistic benefits of these two classes of molecules.

GINGER

The traditional use of ginger includes processing and heating. When ginger is dried, gingerol undergoes a dehydration reaction to form shogaols. And heating of the chemical components related to ginger's inflammatory actions is relatively preserved during processing and heating. During heating, gingerol is transformed into the component zingerone which is less pungent and provides a spicy sweet aroma. This transformation may account for the reduced amount of gingerol with heating. One study of preparation temperatures for ginger found that gingerol reduced with a 3-hour exposure to 125°C but shogaols increased (Ho and Su, 2016).

FLAVONES

Nobiletin

Dried citrus fruit peels are used as remedies for respiratory symptoms, notably because heat treatment is applied to the citrus peels during the drying process. *In vitro* studies show that the effect of water heat treatment actually increases both antioxidant and anti-inflammatory action of citrus peels (Xu et al., 2008). One study found that the anti-inflammatory activity of citrus peel was elevated significantly after 100°C for period up to 120 minutes. And the anti-inflammatory activity of the citrus peel was highly associated with the content of the hydrophobic flavone, nobiletin.

Curcumin

The role of cooking methods for maintaining curcumin activity within turmeric is covered in Chapter 5 Cardiovascular Risk Factors: Hypertension and Hyperlipidemia.

Minerals

The role of cooking methods for maintaining minerals within foods was covered in Chapter 2.

OA KEY POINTS

- OA has several different phenotypes including inflammatory and metabolic syndrome.
- Dietary patterns such as the Mediterranean diet can be helpful particularly with use of EVOO and regular physical activity. Avoiding dietary patterns that increase uric acid may also be helpful.
- Most nutrients that are protective for OA work by decreasing inflammation. Some such as the flavone nobiletin (skin of citrus fruits) may reduce cartilage breakdown.
- Foods shown to protect against OA include broccoli, ginger, curcumin, skin of citrus foods, and omega-3-rich foods.
- Relevant cooking methods to maintain OA protective nutrients:
  - Broccoli – consume raw, lightly steamed, or allow the chopped vegetable to sit for at least 30 minutes before heating or CONSIDER adding sweet mustard sauce to cooked broccoli
  - Citrus foods – add small amounts of raw or heated citrus skin to dishes as garnishes (gremolata) or flavor addition to baked goods (zesting)
  - Omega-3-rich foods – when eating omega-rich seafood, limit the amount of cooking oil in order to maintain omega-3 levels; consider adding olive oil after fish is cooked

REFERENCES

Allen K.D. and Y.M. Golightly. 2015. State of the evidence. *Curr Opin Rheum.* 27: 276–283.

Al-Saghir S., K. Thurner, K.H. Wagner, et al. 2004. Effects of different cooking procedures on lipid quality and cholesterol oxidation of farmed salmon fish. *J Agric Food Chem.* 52: 5290–5296.

Arterburn L. 2006. Distribution and dose response of omega-3 fatty acids in humans. *Am J Clin Nutr.* 83: 1467S–1476S.

Badsha H. 2018. Role of diet in influencing rheumatoid arthritis disease activity. *Open Rheumatol J.* 12: 19–28.

Baker K.R., N.R. Matthan, L.H. Lichtenstein, et al. 2012. Association of plasma omega-6 and omega-3 polyunsaturated fatty acids with synovitis in the knee: the MOST study. *Osteoarthr Cartil.* 5: 382–387.

Bassiouni H., H. Aly, K. Zaky, et al. 2017. Probing the relation between Vitamin D deficiency and progression of medial femoro-tibial osteoarthritis of the knee. *Curr Rheumatol Rev.* 13: 65–71.

Bastias J.M, P. Balladares, and S. Acuna. 2017. Determining the effect of different cooking methods on the nutritional composition of salmon and Chilean jack mackerel. *PLoS One.* 12(7): e0180993.

Belcaro, G., et al. 2010a. Product evaluation registry of Meriva. *Panminerva Med.* 52: 55–62.

Belcaro, G., et al. 2010b. Efficacy and safety of Meriva®, a curcumin-phosphatidylcholine complex, during extended administration in osteoarthritis patients. *Altern Med Rev.* 15(4): 337–344.

Candela C.G., L.M. Bermejo López, and V. Loria Kohen. 2011. Importance of a balanced omega 6/3 ratio for the maintenance of health. *Nutr Hosp.* 26(2): 323–329. doi: 10.1590/S0212-16112011000200013

Chiu T.H.T., C.H. Liu, C.C. Chang, M.N. Lin, and C.L. Lin. 2020. Vegetarian diet and risk of gout in two separate prospective cohort studies. *Clin Nutr.* 39(3): 837–844. doi: 10.1016/j.clnu.2019.03.016.

Clinton M.C., S. O'Brien, J. Law, C.M. Renier, and M.R. Wendt. 2015. Whole-foods, plant-based diet alleviates the symptoms of Osteoarthritis. *Arthritis* 2015: 708152. doi:10.1155/2015/708152.

Corr E.M., C. Cunningham, and L. Helbert. 2017. Osteoarthritis-associated basic calcium phosphate crystals activate membrane proximal kinases in human innate immune cells. *Arthritis Res Ther.* 19: 23.

Davatchi F., M. Sandoughi, N. Moghimi, et al. 2016. Epidemiology of rheumatic diseases in Iran from analysis of four COPCORD studies. *Int J Rheum Dis.* 19: 1056–1062.

Davidson R.K., et al. 2013. Sulforaphane repressed matrix-degrading proteases and protects cartilage from destruction in invitro and in vivo. *Arthritis and Rhematism.* 65: 3130–3140.

Davidson R.K., J. Green, S. Gardner, et al. 2018. Identifying chondroprotective diet-derived bioactives and investigating their synergism. *Sci Rep.* 8: 17173. doi: 10.1038/s41598-018-35455-8

Dell'Isola A., R. Allan, S.L. Smith, et al. 2016. Identification of clinical phenotypes in knee osteoarthritis: a systematic review of the literature. *BMC Musculoskelet Disord.* 17: 425. [PubMed: 27733199].

Denoble A.E., K.M. Huffman, T.V. Stabler, and et al. 2011. Uric acid is a danger signal of increasing risk for osteoarthritis through inflammasome activation. *Proc Nat Acad Sci.* 108: 2088–2093.

Deshpande B.R., et al. 2016 December. The number of persons with symptomatic knee osteoarthritis in the United States: impact of race/ethnicity, age, sex, and obesity. *Arthritis Care Res (Hoboken).* 68(12): 1743–1750.

Deveza L.A., L. Melo, and T.P. Yamato, et al. 2017. Knee osteoarthritis phenotypes and their relevance for outcomes: a systematic review. *Osteoarthr. Cartil.* 25: 1926–1941.

Dragos D., G. Marilena, L. Gaman, et al. 2017. Phytomedicine in Joint Disorders. *Nutrients.* 9: 70.

Dyer J., G. Davison, S.M. Marcora, and A.R. Mauger. 2017. Effect of a Mediterranean type diet on inflammatory and cartilage degradation biomarkers in patients with osteoarthritis. *J Nutr Health Aging.* 21: 562–566.

Ewald K., S. Fjelkner-Modig, K. Johansson, L. Sjoholm, and B. Akesson. 1999. Effect of processing on major flavonoids in processed onions, green beans, and peas. *Food Chem.* 64: 231–235.

Flaskerud K., M. Bkowski, M. Golovko, et al. 2017. Effects of cooking techniques on fatty acid and oxylipin content of farmed rainbow trout. *Food Sci Nutr.* 5: 1195–1204.

Garfinkel R.J., M.F. Dilisio, and D.K. Agrawal. 2017. Vitamin D and its effects on articular cartilage and *Orthop J Sports Med..* 5(6): 2325967117711376

Gladyshev M.I., N.N. Sushchik, G.A. Gubanenko, et al. 2006. Effect of way of cooking on content of essential polyunsaturated fatty acids in muscle tissue of humpback salmon. *Food Chem.* 96: 446–451.

Goldring, M.B. and M. Otero. 2011. Inflammation in osteoarthritis. *Curr Opin Rheumatol.* 23: 471–482.

Goula T., A. Kouskoukis, G. Drosos, et al. 2015. Vitamin D status in patients with knee or hip osteoarthritis in a Mediterranean country. *J Orthop Traumatol.* 16: 35–39.

Grover A.K. and S.E. Samson. 2016. Benefits of antioxidant supplements for knee osteoarthritis: rational and reality. *Nutr J.* 15: 1.

Hafsi K., J. McKay, J. Li, et al. 2019. Nutritional, metabolic and genetic considerations to optimize regenerative medicine outcome for knee osteoarthritis. *J Clin Orthop Trauma.* 10: 2–8.

Haghighian M.K., Alipoor B., A.M. Mahdavi, et al. 2015. Effects of sesame seed supplementation on inflammatory factors and oxidative stress biomarkers in patients with knee osteoarthritis. *Acta medica Iranica.* 53: 207–213.

Henrotin Y. et al. 2010. Biological actions of curcumin on articular chondrocytes. *Osteoarthr Cartil.* 18: 141–149.

Hill C.L., L.M. March, D. Aitken, S.E. Lester, R. Battersby, K. Hynes, T. Fedorova, S.M. Proudman, M. James, L.G. Cleland, and G. Jones. 2016. Fish oil in knee osteoarthritis: a randomised clinical trial of low dose versus high dose. *Ann Rheum Dis.* 75(1): 23–29. doi: 10.1136/annrheumdis-2014-207169.

Ho S.C. and M.S. Su. 2016. Optimized heat treatment enhances the anti-inflammatory capacity of ginger. *Int J Food Properties.* 19(8): 1884–1898.

Hooper J.M., Deshmukh, A.J., and Schwarzkopf, R. 2018. The role of bariatric surgery in the obese total joint arthroplasty patient. *Orthop Clin North Am.* 49: 297–306.

Hostetler G.L., et al. 2017. Flavones: food sources, bioavilability, metabolism, and bioactivity. *Adv Nutr.* 8: 423–435.

Hui L., C. Zeng, J. Wei, et al. 2016. Serum calcium concentration is inversely associated with radiographic knee osteoarthritis: a cross-sectional study. *Medicine.* 95: e2838.

Hunter D.J., D.P. Beavers, F. Eckstein, A. Guermazi, R.F. Loeser, B.J. Nicklas, S.L. Mihalko, G.D. Miller, M. Lyles, P. DeVita, C. Legault, J.J. Carr, J.D. Williamson, and S.P.Messier. 2015. The Intensive Diet and Exercise for Arthritis (IDEA) trial: 18-month radiographic and MRI outcomes. *Osteoarthritis Cartilage.* 23(7):1090–1098. doi: 10.1016/j.joca.2015.03.034.

Hunter D.J., W. Zhang, W. Conaghan, et al. 2011. Systematic review of the concurrent, and predictive validity of MRI biomarkers in OA. *Osteoarthr Cartil.* 19: 557–588

Ishikado A., K. Morino, Y. Nishio, F. Nakagawa, et al. 2013. 4-Hydroxy hexenel derived from docosahexaenoic acid protects endothelial cells via Nrf2 activation. *PLoS One.* 8: e69415.

Johnson V.L. and D.J. Hunter. 2014. The epidemiology of osteoarthritis. *Best Pract Res Clin Rheumatol*. 28: 5–15.

Kaspar K.L., et al. 2010. Pigmented potato consumption alters oxidative stress and inflammatory damage in men. *J Nutr*. 141(1): 108–111.

Khan N.M., A. Haseeb, M.Y. Ansari, P. Devarapalli, et al. 2017. Wogonin, a plant derived small molecule, exerts potent anti-inflammatory and chrondroprotective effects through the activation of ROS/ERK/Nrf2 signaling pathways in human osteoarthritis chondrocytes. *Free Rad Bio Med*. 106: 288–301.

Kim J.H., et al. 2014. Regulation of the catabolic cascade in osteoarthritis by the Zinc-ZIP8-MTF1 Axis. *Cell*. 156: 730–743.

Kuptniratsaikul, V., P. Dajpratham, W. Taechaapornkul, et al. 2014. Efficacy and safety of Curcuma domestica extracts compared with ibuprofen in patients with knee osteoarthritis: a multicenter study. *Clin Inter Aging*. 9: 451–458.

Lanier R.K., et al. 2013. Effects of dietary supplementation with the solanaceae plant alkaloid anatabine on joint pain and stiffness: results from an internet-based survey study. *Clin Med Insights Arthritis MSK Disord*. 6: 73–84.

Lee S. and S.J. Kim. 2017. Prevalence of knee osteoarthritis, risk factors, and quality of life: the Fifth Korean National Health and Nutrition Examination Survey. *Int J Rheum Dis*. 20: 809–817.

Leung K.S., J.M. Galeno, T. Durand, and J.C.Y. Lee. 2018. Profiling of Omega-Polyunsaturated fatty acids and their oxidized products in salmon after different cooking methods. *Antioxidants*. 7: 96.

Liisberg U., K.R. Fauske, O. Kuda, E. Fjaere, et al. 2016. Intake of a Western diet containing cod instead of pork alters fatty acid composition in tissue phospholipids and attenuates obesity and hepatic lipid accumulation in mice. *J Nutr Biochem*. 33: 119–127.

Lin Z, D. Wu, L. Huang, et al. 2019. Nobiletin inhibits IL-1B induced inflammation in chondrocytes via suppression of NF-κB signaling and attenuates osteoarthritis in mice. *Front Pharmacol*. 10: 570.

Lu B., J.B. Driban, C. Xu, et al. 2017. Dietary fat intake and radiographic progression of knee osteoarthritis: data from the osteoarthritis initiative. *Arthritis Care Res*. 69: 368–375.

Ma C.A. and Y.Y. Leung. 2017. Exploring the link between Uric Acid and OA. *Front Med*. 4: 225.

Malemud C.J. 2015. Biologic basis of osteoarthritis: state of the evidence. *Curr Opin Rheumatol*. 27(3): 289–294. doi:10.1097/BOR.0000000000000162

McAlindon T.E., P. Jacques, Y. Zhang, et al. 1996. Do antioxidant micronutrients protect against the development and progression of knee osteoarthritis? *Arthritis Rheum*. 39: 648–656.

McConnell S., P. Kolopack, and A.M. Davis. 2001. The Western Ontario and McMaster Universities Osteoarthritis Index (WOMAC): a review of its utility and measurement properties. *Arthritis Rheum*. 45: 453–461.

Mozzaffarian D. 2016. Dietary and policy priorities for cardiovascular disease, diabetes, and obesity: a comprehensive review. *Circulation*. 133: 187–225.

Musumeci G., et al. 2013 Dec. Extra-virgin olive oil diet and mild physical activity prevent cartilage degeneration in an osteoarthritis model: an in vivo and in vitro study on lubricin expression. *J Nutr Biochem*. 24(12): 2064–2075.

Okunade O.A., S.K. Ghawi, L. Methven, and K. Nirnajan. 2015. Thermal and pressure stability of myrosinase enzymes from black mustard and yellow mustard seeds. *Food Chem*. 187: 485–490.

Okunade O., K. Niranjan, S.K. Ghawi, et al. 2018. Supplementation of the diet by exogenous myrosinase via mustard seeds to increase the bioavailability of sulforaphane in healthy human subjects after the consumption of cooked broccoli. *Mol Nutr Food*. 62: e1700980.

Orfanidou T., K.N. Malizos, S. Varitimidis, and A. Tseuzou. 2012. 1,25-Dihydroxyvitamin D(3) and extracellular inorganic phosphate activate mitogen-activated protein kinase pathway through fibroblast growth factor 23 contributing to hypertrophy and mineralization in osteoarthritic chondrocytes. *Exp Biol Med.* 3: 241–253.

Paramdeep G. 2013. Efficacy and tolerability of ginger in patients with osteoarthritis of knee. *Ind J Physiol Pharmacol.* 57: 177–83.

Peanpadungrat P. 2015. Efficacy and safety of fish oil in treatment of knee osteoarthritis. *J Med Assoc Thai.* 3: S110–S114.

Plumb M.S. and R.M. Aspden. 2004. High levels of fat and (omega-6) fatty acids in cancellous bone in osteoarthritis. *Lipids Health Dis.* 3: 12.

Prakash C.P., P. Singh, S. Chaturvedi, et al. 2016. Epidemiology of knee osteoarthritis in India and related factors. *Ind J Orthop.* 50: 518.

Puenpatom R.A. and T.W. Victor. 2009. Increased prevalence of metabolic syndrome in individuals with osteoarthritis: an analysis of NHANES III data. *Postgrad Med.* 121: 9–20.

Qin B., X. Shi, P.S. Samai, et al. 2012. Association of dietary magnesium intake with radiographic knee osteoarthritis: results from a population-based study. *Arthritis Care Res.* 9: 1306–1311.

Reynard L.N. and J. Loughlin. 2013. The genetics and functional analysis of primary OA susceptibility. *Expert Rev Mol Med.* 15: e2.

Roschger A., J.G. Hofsaetter, B. Pemmer, et al. 2013. Differential accumulation of lead and zinc in double tidemarks of articular cartilage. *Osteoarthr Cartil.* 21: 1707–1715.

Rungapamestry V., et al. 2007. Effect of cooking brassica vegetables on the subsequent hydrolysis and metabolic fate of glucosinolates. *Proc Nutr Soc.* 66: 69–81.

Sadat B.E., M.K. Haghighian, B. Alipoor, A.M. Mahdavi, et al. 2013. Effects of sesame seed supplementation on clinical signs and symptoms in patients with knee osteoarthritis. *Int J Rheum Dis.* 5: 578–582.

Sant'ana L.S. and J.M. Filho. 2000. Influence of the addition of antioxidants in vivo on the fatty acid composition of fish fillets. *Food Chem.* 68: 175–178.

Schadich E., J. Hlavac, T. Volna, et al. 2016. Effects of ginger phenylpropanoids and quercetin on Nrf2-ARE pathway in human BJ fibroblasts and HaCaT keratinocytes. *Biomed Res Int.* 2016: 2173275.

Shakibaei M., A. Mobasheri, and C. Buhrmann. 2011. Curcumin synergizes with resveratrol to stimulate the MAPK signaling pathway in human articular chondrocytes in vitro. *Genes Nutr.* 6: 171–179.

Simopoulos P. 2016. An increase in the omega-6/omega-3 fatty acid ratio increases the risk for obesity. *Nutrients.* 8: 128.

Sofat N., and A. Kuttapitiya. 2014. Future directions for the management of pain in osteoarthritis. *Int J Clin Rheumtol.* 9(2): 197–276. doi: 10.2217/ijr.14.10.

Sokolove J. and C.M. Lepus. 2013. Role of Inflammation in the pathogenesis of osteoarthritis: latest findings and interpretations. *Ther Adv Musculoskeletal Dis.* 5: 77–94.

Su X.Q. and J.R. Babb. 2007. The effect of cooking process on the total lipid and omega PUFA contents of Bass Strait scallops. *Asia Pac J Clin Nutr.* 16: 407–411.

Thomas S., H. Browne, A. Mobasheri, and M.P. Rayman. 2018. What is the evidence for a role for diet and nutrition in osteoarthritis? *Rheumatology.* 57: iv61–iv74.

Torralba K.D., E. DeJesus, and S. Rachabattula. 2012. The interplay between diet, urate transporters and the risk for gout and hyperuricemia: current and future directions. *Int J Rheum Dis.* 15: 499–506.

Trichopoulou A., M.A. Martinez-Gonzalez, T.Y.N. Tong, et al. 2014. Definitions and potential health benefits of the Mediterranean diet: views from experts around the world. *BMC Med.* 12: 112.

Vaishya R., A.K. Agarwal, A. Shah, et al. 2018. Current status of top 10 nutraceuticals used for Knee Osteoarthritis in India. *J Clin Orthop Trauma.* 9: 338–348.

Vasilladis H.S. and K. Tsikopoulos. 2017. Glucosamine and chondroitin for the treatment of osteoarthritis. *World J Orthop.* 8: 1–11.

Verma P., and K. Dalal. 2011. ADAMTS-4 and ADAMTS-5: key enzymes in osteoarthritis. *J Cell Biochem.* 112(12): 3507–3514. doi: 10.1002/jcb.23298.

Veronese N., B. Stubbs, M. Noale, et al. 2016. Adherence to the Mediterranean diet is associated with better diet quality of life: data from the Osteoarthritis Initiative. *Am J Clin Nutr.* 104: 1403–1409.

Veronese N., B. Stubbs, M. Noale et al. 2017. Adherence to a Mediterranean diet is associated with lower prevalence of osteoarthritis: data from the Osteoarthritis Initiative. *Clin Nutr* 36: 1609–1614.

Veronese N., et al. 2019. The association between dietary magnesium intake and magnetic resonance parameters for knee osteoarthritis. *Nutrients.* 11: 1387.

Vinna E.R. and K. Kwoh. 2018. Epidemiology of OA, literature update. *Curr Opin Rheumatol.* 30: 160–167.

Vormann J., C. Forster, U. Zippel, E. Lozo, T. Gunther, H. Merker, and R. Stahlmann. 1997. Effects of magnesium deficiency on magnesium and calcium content in bone and cartilage in developing rats in correlation to chondrotoxicity. *Calcif Tissue Int.* 61: 230–238.

Wu Y., Y. Shen, X. Wu, et al. 2018. Hydrolysis before stir-frying increases the isothiocyanate content of broccoli. *J Agric Food Chem.* 66: 1509–1515.

Xie L., H. Xie, C. Chen, Z. Tao, et al. 2019. Inhibiting the PI3K/AKT/NF-κB signal pathway with nobiletin for attenuating the development of osteoarthritis: in vitro and in vivo studies. *Food Funct.* 10: 2161–2175.

Xu, G.H., J.C. Chen, D.H. Liu, et al. 2008. Minerals, phenolic compounds and antioxidant capacity of citrus peel extract by hot water. *J Food Sci.* 73(1): C11–C18.

Yoshimura N., S. Muraki, H. Oka, S. Tanaka, H. Kawaguchi, K. Nakamura, and T. Akune. 2012. Accumulation of metabolic risk factors such as overweight, hypertension, dyslipidaemia, and impaired glucose tolerance raises the risk of occurrence and progression of knee osteoarthritis: a 3-year follow-up of the ROAD study. *Osteoarthr Cartil.* 20(11): 1217–1226.

Yuan G-F., B. Sun, J. Yuan, and Q.M. Wang. 2009. Effects of different cooking methods on health promoting compounds of broccoli. *J Zhejuang Univ Sci B.* 10: 580–588.

Zeng C., J. Wei, H. Li, et al. 2015. Relationship between serum magnesium concentration and radiographic knee osteoarthritis. *J Rheumatol.* 42: 1231–1236.

Zhang C., Z.Y. Su, T.O. Khor, and A.N. Kong. 2013. Sulforaphane enhances Nrf2 expression in prostate cancer TRAMP C1 cells through epigenetic regulation. *Biochem Pharmacol.* 85: 1398–1404.

Zhao Q., et al. 2016. A specialized flavone biosynthetic pathway has evolved in the medicinal plant Scutellaria baicalensis. *Sci Adv.* 2: e1501780.

Zhuo Q., W. Yang, J. Chen, and Y. Wang. 2012. Metabolic syndrome meets osteoarthritis. *Nat Rev Rheumatol.* 8(12): 729–737. doi: 10.1038/nrrheum.2012.135.

9 Providing Community-Centered Culinary Medicine-Based Patient Education

Kofi Essel
Children's National Hospital
The George Washington University School
of Medicine & Health Sciences

Graciela Caraballo
The George Washington University School
of Medicine & Health Sciences

CONTENTS

The residents of the District of Columbia often witness what has become far too common across the country, what we often describe as a "tale of two cities" (District of Columbia Behavioral Risk Factor Surveillance System, 2017). We see populations affected and marginalized by social injustices. We see the role of racism in concentrated poverty, housing instability, and increased unemployment (Health Equity Report for the District of Columbia 2018). But at the same time, we see a city ranked in the top three for most fit cities in the country every year (2020 Summary Report ACSM American Fitness Index). We see a city that harbors the most influential political powerhouses along with an incredible amount of wealth. The disparities that exist are reflected in the gravity of diet-related chronic diseases that disproportionately affect the most marginalized. The effects of food apartheid leave some sections in the city with 2–3 grocery stores for ~150,000 people, while other areas in the city with half the population experience more than double the number of full-service grocery stores (Health Equity Report for the District of Columbia, 2018). As clinicians, we find it crucial to advocate for our patients in and outside of the four walls of our clinic. We use culinary medicine as a powerful tool to support our patients and families struggling with food insecurity and diet-related chronic diseases. We have come to recognize that without considering systems of disenfranchisement and patients' contexts – cultural, family, household, and community – any such efforts around health and nutrition may quickly become futile. We are encouraged and influenced by frameworks that highlight families' lived experiences, social determinants of health, and health equity (Davison et al., 2013; Kumanyika, 2019; Dietz et al., 2017). Culinary medicine has improved the self-efficacy of our families and has allowed them to feel empowered and more adept to take control of their own health.

PHYSICIAN PERSPECTIVE: EXPERIENTIAL LEARNING IN CULINARY EDUCATION

I have always had an interest in the role food and nutrition plays in the health of people. Over a decade ago, I began working with families around nutrition education and behavioral change and initially focused on a simplified approach of community lectures. I believed that if my families had the "knowledge," then everything might be solved. I now know that my misdirected and yet passionate approach as a young medical student was important but limited in its ability to sustainably impact the care of my families. Over the course of several years, I conducted multiple community lectures, cooking demonstrations and workshops, incorporated motivational interviewing practices and set Specific, Measurable, Attainable, Realistic, and Timely (S.M.A.R.T.) goals with families. As a medical student and trainee, I found these experiences to be life-changing in helping me understand the assets and challenges of the communities I worked alongside; however, my families continued to struggle with generalizing these short tangible experiences into real-world settings.

David Kolb, an educational theorist, is famous for his descriptions and framework known as Experiential Learning (Murphy, 2007). In this advanced learning technique, the learner is thrust into real-world settings, allowing for an in-depth understanding of the subject. This experience may be transferable to future, relevant experiences. This experiential learning was a critical piece often missing from my understanding and approach to nutrition education. As I came across the cooking class model through community partnerships with family-centered organizations (i.e., Common Threads, YMCA), I noticed a level of engagement and sustained buy-in from my families that I had not noticed in years of community programming. I became convinced that having children and adults in an actual kitchen preparing meals and practicing the new skills we were teaching them allowed them to truly develop a level of self-agency to change behavior and ideally impact their health (Jarpe-Ratner et al., 2016; Trubek et al., 2017).

MEDICAL STUDENT PERSPECTIVE: OPTIMIZING HOLISTIC CARE THROUGH CULINARY EDUCATION

Historically, the practice of medicine has been reduced from healthcare to sick care, reacting to chronic disease that has existed untreated and undiagnosed long before its acute presentation to the emergency room as a disabling stroke. I left my first night of shadowing in a low-income emergency department with one clear thought… "Health begins outside the hospital, and healthcare must do the same." Fortunately, I began my training as medicine was experiencing a renaissance of holism and prevention, expanding its approach to consider many social, economic, and political conditions that influence health. In stride, I conducted research that explored the high burden of chronic disease in historically underserved neighborhoods and increasingly became interested in the relationship between eating behaviors and health.

Shortly after beginning medical school, I began teaching hands-on community cooking classes and leading table discussions (through George Washington University Culinary Medicine Program & Health Meets Food Culinary Medicine Program) surrounding the impact that food choices can have in the prevention of disease. After some time working with this model, I realized its massive potential as a public health intervention. First of all, it was practical. Culinary medicine fills an important and often overlooked gap in the current care model by moving beyond simply recommending dietary change to helping individuals actually incorporate these changes into their everyday life. Hands-on learning in the kitchen is complemented by a discussion that includes pragmatic concepts like how to best store and cross-utilize the day's left-overs. My students were leaving each class with new skills but more importantly, with the confidence and knowledge required to put those skills to use.

Besides its practicality, the cooking class model is unique in that it is also personal. Spending time gathering around a table to share a meal and discuss the lesson proved effective in helping me engage my students' concerns and individualize my approach. In order to combat the recurring idea that a fast-food establishment's breakfast sandwich was the quickest and cheapest solution to a busy morning, my team created comparison tables for our next lesson. These tables juxtaposed our participants' favorite fast-food breakfast options with our similar home-made breakfast recipes, including side-by-side comparisons of price, preparation time, and nutrition facts. Adapting our curriculum to address the concerns of our participants proved successful in directly combating the stigma that home-made meals are expensive and time consuming, which had previously been a significant misconception.

The flexibility of the curriculum extends beyond individual lessons, allowing us to adjust courseware across a variety of socioeconomic and cultural contexts. Recently, I adapted our community courseware for Hispanic populations, tailored our recipes to feature traditional ingredients predominant in the Latino diet, and launched our curriculum in Spanish. While the core lessons remained the same, modifying the courseware to make it more culturally sensitive allowed me to better engage the audience I was targeting. Ameliorating community health requires us to move away from one-size-fits-all healthcare. Culinary medicine education provides an exciting avenue through which this may be accomplished, allowing providers to work directly with individuals to find personalized solutions to health problems.

ADVANCING COMMUNITY HEALTH

Western medicine has failed in giving the next generation of clinicians sound, applicable tools to improve the lifestyles of the families they serve. We have done a phenomenal job industrializing health but have stigmatized lifestyle medicine as an alternative and ineffective approach to optimizing health. We have encouraged clinicians to rely on their strong clinical acumen to manage chronic diseases. We have highlighted lifestyle as a core means of managing and preventing every diet-related chronic disease but have struggled with its incorporation into clinical practice and lack of confidence in its effectiveness (Danaei, Ding and Mozaffarrian, 2011; Kolasa and Rickett, 2010). As a result of limited training, providers unfortunately lean on their personal experiences and common misunderstandings about nutrition (Crowley, Ball and Hiddink, 2019). We know that the majority of medical schools do not meet the minimum number of hours of nutrition education for their students (Adams, Butsch and Kohlmeir, 2015). A combination of limited training and implicit unawareness of root contributors to these same diseases creates clinicians that have unreal expectations about behavior change and leads to frustration and worsening stigma toward patients (Pont et al., 2017).

Effective interventions around nutrition take time, especially because the foods we eat are far more than nutrients, but incorporate our culture, emotions, taste, and finances, among other factors. Deep relationships are required to unwind these layers, and the limited time given in clinical encounters may hinder the ability for physicians to intervene. Although the clinician is burdened with the responsibility of dynamically changing the patient's lifestyle, the more realistic approach will lean heavily on clinical-community partnerships with the family and health equity being at the center. Culinary medicine approaches that create a pipeline between clinical settings to community settings allow for interventions that meet families where they are and allow for more sustainable change.

CULINARY MEDICINE

As discussed in previous chapters, over time, the culture of cooking has diminished and stabilized throughout the country (Smith, Ng and Popkin, 2013). In fact, it now seems like cooking is a sign of privilege. While poverty is synonymous with preparation of your own foods in many cultures around the world, Western culture seems quite the opposite. Poverty is expensive, and the weight of poverty and marginalization limits one's ability to effectively plan, think ahead, and access a culture of cooking in one's household (a term known as "temporal discounting") (Bickel et al., 2012).

To counteract these tangible challenges, we created community-clinical partnerships with local organizations to address areas of food insecurity and diet-related chronic disease through culinary interventions. Our partnerships allowed us to rent teaching kitchen space and create easy-to-follow recipes based on a Supplemental Nutrition Assistance Program (formerly food stamp program) budget. Recognizing the malleability of the palate, we challenge families to try new foods, flavors, and methods of making cuisines that they know and love. Clinicians use food insecurity screening tools (i.e., Hunger Vital Sign™) and clinical and laboratory risk factors to determine if families are eligible (Council, on Community Pediatrics, and on Nutrition Committee, 2015; Hager et al., 2010). Motivated families who meet our inclusion criteria are invited to attend our 6-week course (1 session per week) where they can learn methods of bulk cooking, buying on a budget, improving the nutritional value of their foods, or just advancing the health of their families.

Our classes primarily focus on family-centered approaches to cooking, even allowing children to take part in the preparation of the meal to increase their self-efficacy and empower whole households to learn skills they can easily apply in the home together. Our programs often bring a chef or community partner to teach classes, while local student volunteers help families and clean the kitchen space. In addition, because many families lack some of the basic cooking appliances, our grants and partnerships provide cooking instruments to many of our families to start building their own collection at home. Lastly, after working hard to make delicious meals, our families take a moment to sit together, talk, and reflect on their experiences and how they would apply them at home. Through our qualitative measures, our families have returned to the clinic and shared their feedback. They share amazement with seeing their children participate in preparing home meals, emphasize the health lessons learned in balancing their meals, and even celebrate health goals their family has been able to set and achieve.

Our culinary medicine programs provide a safe space while at the same time giving families the freedom and time to be immersed in the training. The combination of hands-on training with specific feedback and lessons fuels their learning. We are able to build rapport with families, revisit lessons from past classes, and reflect on home experiences in order to challenge our families to continue to succeed.

VIRTUAL SPACES

Following the global pandemic of COVID-19, teaching kitchens have had to rapidly respond to meet the needs of families in a virtual space. We have taken advantage of video platforms and food delivery services to counteract areas of food apartheid and create a flexible venue for reaching families worldwide. Online courses provide an opportunity to overcome many logistical barriers to access, including time constraints, lack of childcare, and transportation (Adam et al., 2015). The comfort of receiving a home-based education made the commitment less intimidating for participants, helped reduce the perceived inconvenience of attending traditional in-person classes, and better accommodated variations in personal and professional schedules, contributing to low attrition rates. We also found that our home-based education encouraged other family members to participate in the lessons, providing opportunities for entire households to learn together.

However, transitioning experiential courseware to a virtual space does not come without its challenges. Initially, we were concerned that the constraints of the marginalized areas we were targeting may impact community members' ability to meaningfully engage in the culinary experience. In the traditional teaching kitchen setting, participants are not tasked with accessing a local grocery store, purchasing fresh ingredients, or owning their own kitchen equipment. While these obstacles could be mitigated by providing households with common appliances and organizing food delivery services, limited funding does not always allow for these measures to be taken. Instead, we used this opportunity as a teaching tool and encouraged individuals to learn within the conditions of their local communities. In response, participants actually gained a better understanding of the assets around them and learned how to prepare and store food utilizing the equipment they had at their disposal. Instructors also benefited from observing individuals' behaviors and obstacles in their natural environments and were available to provide personalized assistance and real-time substitutions when participants could not find an ingredient or lacked a necessary appliance. Participants became more flexible and dynamic as they learned how to substitute one acid for another in their salad dressing or realized that a fork mixed batter just as effectively as a whisk. The resilience gained from these experiences improved the self-efficacy of our families, giving them the confidence to not only continue to practice healthful behaviors in their everyday lives but also translate their knowledge and skills into new settings. By shifting our focus away from external obstacles and instead emphasizing individuals' abilities to overcome those obstacles, we can empower diverse communities to take a more active and intentional role in their health.

The emergence of virtual learning platforms presents an exciting, scalable opportunity to meet the needs of a diverse, global audience. Free of geographic constraints, communities no longer require local teaching kitchens or local instructors as prerequisites for participation. The ability to log on from any location allows for class discussions that feature a broader range of perspectives, including instructors with diverse, interdisciplinary backgrounds. This increases participants' access to nutritional expertise while simultaneously improving collaboration among providers. In a time of rapid healthcare innovation, leveraging technologies will become increasingly vital to improving access and optimizing the health of our communities. Virtual culinary education has the potential to improve technology literacy among community members and contribute to a more inclusive and diverse healthcare system.

TAKE-HOME LESSONS IN FAMILY-CENTERED COMMUNITY-BASED CULINARY EDUCATION

Our experiences conducting family-centered cooking classes have yielded several insights about creating effective community-centered culinary education programs.

1. **First, meet families where they are**: It is essential that we work with staff to ensure messaging is consistent, evidence-based, and takes into account families' lived experiences. Team members must meet families where they are and walk alongside them on their journey, allowing them to be the authors of their own story. Families often differ in their priorities and face unique barriers to healthy eating. Adapting the lessons to directly respond to what matters most to them is a more effective way to challenge misconceptions and encourage long-lasting behavioral change. The same holds true in the kitchen, make sure participants know that recipes are guidelines, not rulebooks, and empower them to be flexible and use the resources at their disposal.

2. **Find the right time**: One of the most frustrating challenges with community programming is fighting attrition and improving retention. It is important to find times for cooking classes that work well for families and staff. Sometimes these programs may need to be considered on weekends to accommodate family extracurricular activities and cultural moments.

3. **Make sure families are invested**: A commitment to a weekly cooking course is a large investment for busy families. It is important to attempt to ensure that families are able to commit to the entirety of the program. But at the same time, remember to be flexible, and if every lesson builds off of the past lesson, recognize how that may limit the family's experience.

4. **Include the entire family**: Children can play a very important role in preparing meals for families. Also, when they are assisting with the preparation of food, they are more likely to eat the foods. Even if the clinician identifies the child with obesity, it is important that we focus on the health of the whole family and do not isolate the child and worsen stigma toward them.

5. **Appreciate the process**: Having a captive audience does not require you to bombard your families with didactic lessons. Recognize that you have multiple weeks with the family and make sure to praise their successes as you continue to build rapport and spend time working alongside them.

6. **Create a safe space for your families**: In the years of doing work in obesity, we have recognized the importance of using "person-first" language. It is important to recognize obesity as a disease a person has versus them being synonymous with the word. When the person is the disease, they are then associated with all the incredible societal biases tied to obesity, such as being lazy, tired, unmotivated, etc. In order to create a safe space, all volunteers and staff must use person-first language, so that families feel the freedom to ask any and all questions and make mistakes – even many – in the kitchen.

7. **Consistency and rapport are beneficial**: Many of my patients are used to groups swooping into their communities and using "savior" language and departing after funding ends. Children may experience this from a variety of traditional anchors in their lives including teachers, family members, community members, etc. Children who experience toxic stress need reliable relationships and connections. Establishing consistency among volunteers and staff helps build rapport with children and families, allowing for increased transparency and counteracting attrition.

8. **Clinical-community partnerships are beneficial**: Clinics have patients and communities have infrastructures in place. Having a champion who can help create pivotal partnerships with key informants and community organizations allows for strong relationships, shared goals, consistent messaging, and ultimately the improved health of families.

9. **Collect metrics**: The effectiveness of culinary medicine as a teaching tool continues to be debated. Our feedback through qualitative measures has been outstanding; however, creating a more structured methodology to study and measure these interventions is necessary to move the intervention forward.

10. **Think about next steps**: After the cooking classes end, families return to obesogenic environments full of stressors and challenges. It is important for programs and partners to consider secondary programs that can further support families' health behavior changes. Secondary programs can strengthen families' commitment to healthy lifestyles by providing them opportunities to be health ambassadors and influencing others.

REFERENCES

2020 Summary Report ACSM American Fitness Index. https://americanfitnessindex.org/wp-content/uploads/2020/07/2020-American-Fitness-Index-Summary-Report.pdf.

Adam M, Young-Wolff KC, Konar E., et al. (2015). Massive open online nutrition and cooking course for improved eating behaviors and meal composition. *International Journal of Behavioral Nutrition and Physical Activity*, 12(143). doi: 10.1186/s12966-015-0305-2.

Adams KM, Butsch WS, & Kohlmeier M. (2015). The state of nutrition education at US Medical Schools. *Journal of Biomedical Education*: 1–7. doi: 10.1155/2015/357627.

Bickel WK, Jarmolowicz DP, Mueller ET, Koffarnus MN, Gatchalian KM. (2012 Jun). Excessive discounting of delayed reinforcers as a trans-disease process contributing to addiction and other disease-related vulnerabilities: emerging evidence. *Pharmacology & Therapeutics*, 134(3): 287–297.

Council, on Community Pediatrics, and on Nutrition Committee. (2015). Promoting food security for all children. *Pediatrics*, 136(5): e1431.

Crowley J, Ball L, & Hiddink GJ. (2019). Nutrition in medical education: a systematic review. *The Lancet Planetary Health*, 3(9): e379–e389.

Danaei G, Ding EL, Mozaffarian D, et al. (2011 Jan). The preventable causes of death in the United States: comparative risk assessment of dietary, lifestyle, and metabolic risk factors [published correction appears in *PLoS Med*, 8(1). doi: 10.1371/annotation/0ef47acd-9dcc-4296-a897-872d182cde57]. *PLoS Med*. 2009;6(4):e1000058. doi:10.1371/journal.pmed.1000058.

Davison KK, Jurkowski JM, & Lawson HA. (2013 Oct). Reframing family-centred obesity prevention using the Family Ecological Model. *Public Health Nutrition*. 16(10): 1861–1869. doi: 10.1017/S1368980012004533. Epub 2012 Oct 22. PMID: 23089267; PMCID: PMC5500251.

Dietz WH, Belay B, Bradley D, Kahan S, Muth ND, Sanchez E, & Solomon L. (2017). A Model Framework that Integrates Community and Clinical Systems for the Prevention and Management of Obesity and Other Chronic Diseases. NAM Perspectives. Discussion Paper, National Academy of Medicine, Washington, DC. doi: 10.31478/201701b.

District of Columbia Behavioral Risk Factor Surveillance System (BRFSS). 2017. https://dchealth.dc.gov/sites/default/files/dc/sites/doh/publication/attachments/BRFSS%20 2017%20Annual%20Report%20Final.pdf.

Hager ER, Quigg AM, Black MM, Coleman SM, Heeren T, Rose-Jacobs R, Cook JT, Ettinger de Cuba SA, Casey PH, Chilton M., et al. (2010). Development and validity of a 2-item screen to identify families at risk for food insecurity. *Pediatrics*, 126: e26–e32.

Health Equity Report for the District of Columbia. 2018. https://app.box.com/s/yspij8v8 1cxqyebl7gj3uifjumb7ufsw.

Jarpe-Ratner E, Folkens S, Sharma S, Daro D, & Edens, N. (2016). An experiential cooking and nutrition education program increases cooking self-efficacy and vegetable consumption in children in grades 3–8. *Journal of Nutrition Education and Behavior*, 48(10): 697–705.e1. doi: 10.1016/j.jneb.2016.07.021.

Kolasa KM, & Rickett K. (2010). Barriers to providing nutrition counseling cited by physicians: a survey of primary care practitioners. *Nutrition in Clinical Practice*, 25: 502–509.

Kumanyika SK. (October 1, 2019). A framework for increasing equity impact in obesity prevention. *American Journal of Public Health* 109(10): 1350–1357. doi: 10.2105/AJPH.2019.305221.

Murphy E. (2007). Prior Learning Assessment: a review of Bloom's taxonomy and Kolb's theory of experiential learning: practical uses for prior learning assessment. *The Journal of Continuing Higher Education*, 55(3): 64–66. doi: 10.1080/07377366.2007.10400135.

Pont S, Puhl R, Cook S, & Slusser W. (2017). Stigma experienced by children and adolescents with obesity. *Pediatrics*, 140(6). doi:10.1542/peds.2017-3034.

Smith LP, Ng SW, & Popkin BM. (2013). Trends in US home food preparation and consumption: analysis of national nutrition surveys and time use studies from 1965–1966 to 2007–2008. *Nutrition Journal*, 12: 45. Published 2013 Apr 11. doi:10.1186/1475-2891-12-45.

Trubek A, Carabello M, Morgan C, & Lahne J. (2017). Empowered to cook: the crucial role of "food agency" in making meals. *Appetite*, 116: 297–305. doi: 10.1016/j.appet.2017.05.017.

10 Healthy Cooking Techniques

Joel J. Schaefer and Mary Schaefer
Your Allergy Chefs

CONTENTS

DOI: 10.1201/b22377-10

Cooking becomes healthier when focusing on real, whole foods along with healthy cooking techniques. Whole foods are foods that are as close to their natural form such as fruits and vegetables.

Most deaths in the United States are preventable and are related to diet. Diet is the number one cause of premature death and the number one cause of disability (Lenders et al., 2013). According to Dr. Michael Greger, whatever genes may be inherited, diet can affect how those genes affect health. The power is on the plate.

Many of the foods consumed today in modern diets are not real whole foods but foods processed to various degrees that contain antibiotics, pesticides, preservatives, trans fats, high-fructose corn syrup, monosodium glutamate (MSG), artificial sweeteners and colors, additives, man-made proteins, and genetically modified foods (GMOs). Food choices play a great role in our health from helping maintain a healthy weight to preventing the onset or progression of many chronic conditions.

Food selection and preparation must take into account our individual needs. For instance, foods that may prevent the onset of chronic diseases for one person may harm or even kill someone with a severe allergy. Walnuts are a healthy nut, containing a large amount of polyunsaturated fats, which includes omega-3 fatty acids that reduce inflammation. While they are healthy for some, they are also high in phosphorus which doesn't make them a good choice for someone with chronic kidney disease, and they can be fatally harmful to someone with a severe tree nut allergy.

There is no one perfect eating plan or lifestyle that fits all. It's about each individual person. What particular health challenges does one live with or want to prevent? It's important to know what foods heal and those that harm.

The reality is, in dealing with a health challenge, cutting back on certain foods can help. However, it doesn't have to be a sacrifice. Eating more of the good foods makes it easier to cut back on the bad foods.

This chapter is about education – the basic knowledge, skills, and confidence – to select and cook real foods.

Without the confidence that comes from knowing how to prepare healthy foods, people are left vulnerable to the aggressive marketing tactics of the food industry. The industry is all too eager to promote highly refined and processed foods that cause obesity and countless other health issues (Hyman, 2018).

Whole foods are as close to their natural form as possible. They are minimally processed or refined, if at all and are free from additives and artificial substances. Some examples of whole foods are vegetables, fruits, nuts, seeds, whole grains, beans, baked chicken breast, baked potato, and brown rice. Just a few examples of what's not a whole food are fruit rollups, fruit drinks, chicken nuggets, potato chips, and brown rice syrup.

READING FOOD LABELS

Food labels are a crucial tool in building a healthy diet. Understanding what's in food is helpful in making healthier choices. Food labels are also helpful in avoiding certain ingredients for those who have a food allergy or intolerance or are following a diet that excludes certain ingredients, such as dairy or soy.

Reading labels can also help in limiting the amount of fat, sodium, sugar, and cholesterol in the diet by making it easy to compare one food item with another to determine the brand with lower amounts. For someone with a chronic condition, such as high blood pressure, it's crucial to pay attention to the sodium content. Moreover, food labels are an important tool to gather information regarding the amount of each nutrient as well as its quality. Whereas knowing the fat content in a food product is important, learning about the relative content of saturated vs. unsaturated fats is equally important.

The nutritional information found on a food label is based on one serving of that particular food. The information on serving size is particularly important since the nutrient information listed is often for more than one serving. Always look at what makes one serving and how many servings the package contains.

Food labels also include exactly what's in the package. The first ingredient on the list represents the ingredient with the largest amount. The second ingredient is the second highest amount and so on.

Sodium is present in foods as part of a wide variety of many ingredients and has many names other than salt. MSG is a flavor enhancer. Many other sources of sodium start with the word sodium, so be aware of these products. Sodium benzoate is a preservative. Sodium nitrite is a source of sodium found in hot dogs and lunch meats and is also used as a preservative in many foods. Another example is sodium phosphate, which is a generic term for a variety of salts and sodium and phosphate. (Figure 10.1).

Hidden Sodium Names	Foods High in Sodium
Disodium guanylate (GMP)	Breads and Rolls
Disodium inosinate (IMP)	Pizza
Fleur de sel	Sandwiches
Himalayan pink salt	Colds Cuts & Cured Meats
Kosher salt	Canned Soups & Vegetables
Monosodium glutamate (MSG)	Burritos & Tacos
Rock salt	All savory snacks
Salt	Chicken, whole pieces
Sea Salt	Cheese
Sodim chloride	Eggs and omelets
Sodium bicarbonate	Pasta dishes like Macaroni and Cheese
Sodium citrate	Bacon, Hot dogs, Sausages
Sodium diacetate	Tomato-based condiments
Sodium erythorbate	Salad dressings
Sodium glutamate	Microwave meals i.e. frozen dinners
Sodium lactate	Cakes & Pies
Sodium lauryle sulfate	Ready-to-eat cereals
Sodium metabisulfite	
Sodium nitrate	
Sodium phosphate	
Trisodium phospate	
Source: American Heart Association: February 2017	Source: American Heart Association: February 2018

FIGURE 10.1   Chart with "hidden" sodium names and with foods high in sodium.

The Dietary Guidelines for Americans recommend no more than 2.3 g of sodium a day (https://health.gov/our-work/food-nutrition/2015-2020-dietary-guidelines/guidelines/appendix-7/). That is one teaspoon of salt and prepared foods can be high in sodium. When shopping for ingredients that are generally high in sodium, such as soy sauce, canned soups, prepared broths or stocks, and condiments, look for low- or reduced-sodium versions.

Added sugar can also be listed on food labels as corn syrup, high-fructose corn syrup, dehydrated cane juice, and agave nectar just to name a few. It may be listed as the fifth ingredient in a product, so thought not to be bad. However, other sugars such as high-fructose corn syrup may also be listed as an ingredient in the same product, adding more sugar and making it not so good (Figure 10.2).

CREATING A "HEALTHY COOKING ZONE"

Creating a "healthy cooking zone" is important for general food safety. The following information helps to ensure safe and enjoyable dining experiences at home.

HAND WASHING

Keeping food safe from bacteria, viruses, and food allergens takes a lot of work. The first step in prevention is hand washing. Many diseases and conditions are spread by not washing hands properly. Follow these safe steps:

1. Rinse hands with water as warm as can be tolerated.
2. Add soap and rub hands together to create suds, and continue to do this for 10–15 seconds.
3. Rinse hands under warm water.
4. Dry hands with a single-use paper towel. Avoid using a kitchen towel, unless changed daily, as it can be one of the most bacteria laden items in your kitchen.

PROPER REFRIGERATION OF FOODS

It is critical that raw foods, cooked foods, and ready-to-eat foods are stored away from each other. Raw foods include uncooked poultry, beef, pork, seafood, fish, and eggs. Cooked foods include rice, potatoes, vegetables, and eggs that have been cooked. Examples of ready-to-eat foods are deli meats, breads, cereals, dried fruits and nuts, or any food item ready for immediate consumption (Figure 10.3).

When storing food in the refrigerator, it is best to keep ready-to-eat foods above cooked foods and cooked foods above raw foods. This keeps any unwanted food drippings from spilling onto other foods that may not be cooked before eating.

Raw foods that will be cooked should always be stored in the bottom of the refrigerator. When storing multiple raw meats on the bottom shelf or drawer, it's important that they are separated. The final internal cooking temperature varies from

Sugar Names - Sugars with Sucrose & Fructose	Sugar Names - Sugars with Glucose
High-Fructose Corn Syrup (HFCS)	Barley Malt
Agave Nectar	Brown Rice Syrup
Beet Sugar	Corn Syrup
Blackstrap Molasses	Corn Syrup Solids
Brown Sugar	Dextrin
Buttered Syrup	Dextrose
Cane Juice Crystals	Diastatic Malt
Cane Sugar	Ethyl Maltol
Caramel	Glucose
Carbo Syrup	Glucose Solids
Castor Sugar	Lactose
Coconut Sugar	Malt Syrup
Confectioner's Sugar	Maltodextrin
Date Sugar	Maltose
Demerara Sugar	Rice Syrup
Evaported Cane Sugar	
Florida Crystals	Common Foods High in Sugar
Fruit Juice	Low-fat Yogurt
Fruit Juice Concentrate	BBQ Sauce
Golden Sugar	Ketchup
Golden Syrup	Fruit Juice
Grape Sugar	Spaghetti Sauce
Honey	Sports Drinks
Icing Sugar	Chocolate Milk
Invert Sugar	Granola
Maple Syrup	Flavored Coffees
Molasses	Protein Bars
muscovado Sugar	Premade Soups
Panela Sugar	Canned Fruits
Raw Sugar	Canned Baked Beans
Refiner's Syrup	Breakfast Cereal
Sorghum Syrup	
Sucanat	
Treacle Sugar	
Turbinado Sugar	
Yellow Sugar	
Source: Healthline.com June 2017	Source: Healthline.com June 2017

FIGURE 10.2 Chart with different types of sugar and foods with high sugar content.

meat to meat. When storing multiple raw meats, here is the order they should be stored, from top to bottom:

- Fish and whole cuts of beef, veal, lamb, and pork
- Ground meats (beef, veal, lamb, and pork)
- Poultry (chicken, turkey, Cornish game hens), ground chicken, and ground turkey

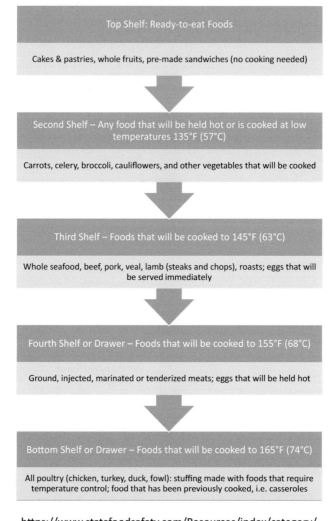

Refrigerator Food Storage Chart

Food should be stored based on the internal cooking temperature of the food, starting with highest cooking temperature on the bottom shelf

Top Shelf: Ready-to-eat Foods

Cakes & pastries, whole fruits, pre-made sandwiches (no cooking needed)

Second Shelf – Any food that will be held hot or is cooked at low temperatures 135°F (57°C)

Carrots, celery, broccoli, cauliflowers, and other vegetables that will be cooked

Third Shelf – Foods that will be cooked to 145°F (63°C)

Whole seafood, beef, pork, veal, lamb (steaks and chops), roasts; eggs that will be served immediately

Fourth Shelf or Drawer – Foods that will be cooked to 155°F (68°C)

Ground, injected, marinated or tenderized meats; eggs that will be held hot

Bottom Shelf or Drawer – Foods that will be cooked to 165°F (74°C)

All poultry (chicken, turkey, duck, fowl): stuffing made with foods that require temperature control; food that has been previously cooked, i.e. casseroles

https://www.statefoodsafety.com/Resources/index/category/Posters

FIGURE 10.3   Chart on proper storage of foods in the refrigerator.

A hypothetical example of what could happen with improper storage of raw meats is presented as follows. If raw chicken, which is often contaminated with salmonella and campylobacter, is stored above salmon fillets, juices from the raw chicken can drip onto the raw salmon. The salmon is cooked to 145°F, never reaching the temperature of 165°F, which is required to kill the pathogens in the chicken. Serious complications could occur, including bacteremia, typhoid fever, Guillain-Barré syndrome, and reactive arthritis (Healthline). This can be serious for even a healthy individual but worse for someone with a weak immune system or other health issues.

CHILLING COOKED FOODS

After food is cooked (see Figure 10.4 for proper cooking temperatures), it needs to be cooled quickly to keep bacteria from multiplying. It only takes 4 hours for a food stored between the temperatures of 41°F–135°F to contain an unhealthy level of bacteria. The rule of thumb is to reduce the internal temperature of the food from 135°F to 70°F within the first 2 hours and then below 41°F within the next 4 hours. This can be done by placing hot liquids such as soup in a stainless-steel container and then placing the container over an ice bath. The liquid should be stirred often to

Category	Food	Temperature (°F)	Rest Time
Ground Meat & Meat Mixtures	Beef, Pork, Veal, Lamb	160	None
	Turkey, Chicken	165	None
Fresh Beef, Veal, Lamb	Steaks, Roasts, Chops	145	3 minutes
Poultry	Chicken & Turkey, whole	165	None
	Poultry breasts, roasts	165	None
	Poultry thighs, legs, wings	165	None
	Duck & Goose	165	None
	Stuffing, (cooked alone or in bird)	165	None
Pork & Ham	Fresh Pork	145	3 minutes
	Fresh Ham (raw)	145	3 minutes
	Precooked Ham (to reheat)	140	None
Eggs & Egg Dishes	Eggs	Cook until yolk and white are firm	None
	Egg dishes	160	None
Leftovers & Casseroles	Leftovers	165	None
	Casseroles	165	None
Seafood	Fin Fish	145 or cook until flesh is opaque and seperates easily with fork	None
	Shrimp, Lobster, & Crab	Cook until flesh is pearly and opaque	None
	Clams, Oysters, and Mussels	Cook until shells open during cooking	None
	Scallops	Cook until flesh is milky white or opaque and firm	None

Source: https://www.foodsafety.gov/keep/charts/mintemp.html

FIGURE 10.4 Diagram of cooking temperatures.

speed the cooling process before it is placed in the refrigerator. Other foods such as large cuts of meat should be cut into smaller pieces, placed in a shallow container, uncovered and stored in the refrigerator. Once cooled, all food should be wrapped, labeled, and dated.

REHEATING FOODS

When reheating food, the internal temperature of all precooked foods should reach 165°F for 15 seconds. When using a microwave, foods should be stirred halfway through the cooking process to distribute the heat and assure that any bacteria will be killed. When reheating soups or sauces, bring to a complete boil and simmer for 1 minute before serving.

CROSS-CONTAMINATION VERSUS CROSS-CONTACT

Cross-contamination: Cross-contamination is the transference of bacteria and is a common factor in the cause of foodborne illness. Microorganisms such as bacteria and viruses from different sources can contaminate foods during preparation and storage. However, proper cooking of the contaminated food in most cases will reduce or eliminate the chances of a foodborne illness (Figure 10.5).

Cross-contact: Cross-contact is the transference of proteins. This occurs when an allergen is inadvertently transferred from a food containing an allergen to a food that does not contain the allergen.

The truth is cooking does not reduce or eliminate the chances of a person with a food allergy having a reaction to the food eaten. This can happen when utensils, pots, pans, or hands are not properly washed and sanitized between food preparations (Figure 10.6).

To put it simply, cross-contamination can lead to food poisoning, and cross-contact can lead to allergic reactions.

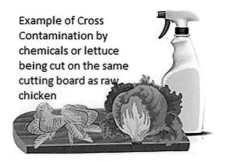

Example of Cross
Contamination by
chemicals or lettuce
being cut on the same
cutting board as raw
chicken

FIGURE 10.5   Picture of cross-contamination.

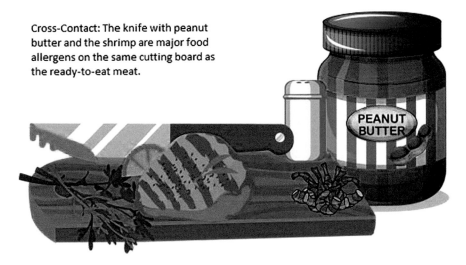

Cross-Contact: The knife with peanut butter and the shrimp are major food allergens on the same cutting board as the ready-to-eat meat.

FIGURE 10.6   Picture of cross-contact.

SETTING UP YOUR KITCHEN

A healthy kitchen is a safe and clean kitchen with an organized pantry.

- Review all food products. Look over ingredient labels to identify foods that need to be avoided, and discard these food items. Give to a neighbor or donate to a local food bank.
- Check condiment labels. Throw out any that have gone bad and get rid of any that are laden with sugar and/or salt.
- Look for canned goods and plastic containers that are BPA (bisphenol A)-free.
- Replace unused spices and herbs every 6 months.
- Organize the fridge weekly. Every 3–4 months, take everything out and give it a deep cleaning.
- Use a sticker or marker to date all foods placed in the refrigerator. Date any products after opening. Leftovers should be held no more than 5–7 days after cooking.
- To control portions, use small plates to trick the brain into seeing an over-flowing, full plate.
- Buy local and organic produce when possible, especially those fruits and vegetables laden with the highest amounts of pesticides. https://www.ewg.org/foodnews/dirty-dozen.php

MISE EN PLACE

Mise en place is the French term meaning "everything in its place." It's all the preparation and organization that takes place before actual cooking begins and the most important technique practiced in the kitchen. Mise en place is the first thing every culinary student learns in school. However, mise en place is more than just a technique. It's a frame of mind that gives confidence in the kitchen.

The steps of mise en place include studying the recipe. It's important to read through the recipe at least three times before beginning to cook. This will help to understand ingredients, procedures, and timing. It's important to gather mixing bowls, measuring cups, tools, and equipment before starting to cook. Understand the equipment needed. For example, if making a gravy and the recipe says to strain through a chinois, do research on a chinois if unsure of what it is. A chinois is a fine mesh conical-shaped strainer. If you don't have a chinois, find an alternative method such as straining through cheesecloth, which can be purchased online or at kitchen specialty shops.

Good knife skills are critical because the knife is the most commonly used tool in the kitchen.

- Keep knives sharp; a dull knife is more dangerous than a sharp one.
- Always cut on a cutting board, not on glass, marble, or metal. Place a damp towel underneath the cutting board to keep the board from sliding while cutting.
- When carrying a knife, hold it pointing down, parallel and close to the leg while walking.
- A falling knife has no handle, so don't attempt to catch a falling knife; step back and allow it to fall.
- Never leave a knife in a sink of water. Anyone reaching into the sink could be injured, or the knife could be dented by pots or other utensils (Labensky, Hause, & Martel, 2011).

Look for tasks that can be done before beginning to cook. Meat may need to be marinated for 4 hours, or time may need to be allotted for proofing dough or for defrosting frozen vegetables. Having these tasks done ahead of time will make the cooking process much easier and less stressful.

Oftentimes, cooks make the mistake of not fully understanding the recipe. An example is blanching tomatoes and realizing an ice bath (bowl of ice water) to stop the cooking process is not set up. What happens? The tomatoes are overcooked by the time they are plunged into cold water.

Measure each ingredient according to the recipe and organize them in order of preparation, storing conveniently at proper temperatures. Ovens and cooking surfaces should be preheated as necessary.

Mise en place or being organized in the kitchen saves time and frustration, especially in the middle of the cooking process.

HEALTHY COOKING METHODS DEFINED

Sautéing/Dry Sautéing: To cook quickly in little or no fat in a pan on the stovetop.

Stir-Frying: Similar to sautéing, in which items are cooked in a wok over very high heat, using little fat and kept moving constantly. Stir-fried dishes can be great choices for healthy meals because they are usually loaded with vegetables and grains, with smaller amounts of fish or meats.

Baking: To cook foods by surrounding them with hot, dry air, usually in an oven.

Simmering: To cook in a liquid that is bubbling gently at a temperature of about 185°F–205°F. Most foods cooked in a liquid are simmered as boiling can be detrimental to foods.

Poaching: To cook in a small amount of liquid that is hot but not actually bubbling. Poaching is ideal for fragile foods such as fish, eggs, and fruit.

Steaming: To cook items in direct steam created by boiling water or other liquids. Steaming is most often used for fish and vegetables.

Braising or Stewing: To cook covered in a small amount of liquid, usually after preliminary browning. Stewing is most often associated with smaller pieces of food.

Sous Vide: To cook a food item that is vacuum-packed in a special water bath at a constant low temperature.

Pan Steam: To cook foods in a very small amount of liquid in a covered pan over direct heat.

En Papillote: A moist-heat cooking method similar to steaming, in which items are enclosed in parchment or foil and cooked in the oven.

GRILLING AND DEEP FRYING

All high-temperature cooking methods, including grilling, broiling, roasting, and frying, can result in potentially carcinogenic substances forming on foods.

Scientists at the Lawrence Livermore National Laboratory in California found that marinating foods for as little as 5 minutes before grilling can dramatically reduce the presence of some carcinogens (Salmon, Knize, and Felton, 1997).

Deep frying at home can be made better by the type of oil and how it is used. The ideal temperature of the oil for frying is 350°F–375°F. When breaded or battered food is cooked in oil at this temperature, its surface cooks almost instantly and forms a type of "seal" that the oil cannot penetrate. If the temperature is too low, the oil will seep into the food, making it greasy. Also, crowding the skillet or overloading the fryer basket greatly lowers the temperature of the oil. On the other hand, if the temperature is too high, the oil can oxidize, posing serious health risks. High temperatures can also burn the exterior of the food while not fully cooking the interior.

Some oils can withstand much higher temperatures than others. Fry with an oil that has a high smoke point. Heating oil to the point where the oil begins to smoke produces toxic fumes and harmful free radicals, unstable atoms that can cause oxidative damage in the body, contributing to a number of different diseases including dementia, cancer, and cardiovascular disease (Figure 10.7).

COOKING WITHOUT OILS

Many oils are advertised as good oils and healthy foods. But not all oils are healthy. Oils are highly processed and pure fat with all nutrients stripped away. Replacing bad fats (saturated and trans) with healthier fats (monounsaturated and polyunsaturated) is better for the heart, according to the American Heart Association. Here's an

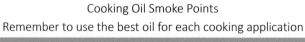

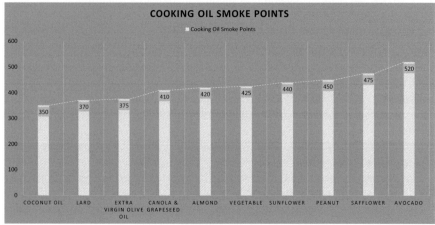

FIGURE 10.7   Chart of smoke points of oils.

alphabetical list of common cooking oils that contain more of the "better-for-you" fats and less saturated fat.

- Avocado
- Canola
- Corn
- Olive
- Peanut
- Safflower
- Soybean
- Sunflower

http://www.heart.org/HEARTORG/HealthyLiving/HealthyEating/Simple CookingandRecipes/Healthy-Cooking-Oils_UCM_445179_Article.jsp#.W2N Ejy2ZP6Y

However, for one on a diet which restricts oil, here are a few simple techniques that can be used in cooking without using added fats such as oil or butter.

As simple as it sounds, when sautéing or stir-frying, all that's needed is a good pan and a little water. If choosing to avoid Teflon, use a good-quality, heavy-bottomed stainless-steel pan. Enamel-coated cast iron and ceramic titanium pans are also good options.

Sautéing and Stir-Frying: Replace the oil in sautéing with a small amount of water or vegetable broth. Heat the pan first, and then add a tablespoon or two of liquid to start with, depending on how much you are cooking. When the liquid sizzles, add the food and stir. Keep the food moving so it doesn't burn. If too dry, add an additional tablespoon of water. Do this as often as needed to cook and brown the food, without steaming it.

Steaming: Steaming is the easiest way to cook vegetables without oil, while retaining nutrients, color, and flavor. Use an electric steamer or a steamer basket in a pot with a small amount of simmering water.

Browning and Caramelizing: Oil is not needed for browning or caramelizing. Start with a heated nonstick pan, and add a tablespoon of water, allowing it to evaporate while lightly browning the vegetables. If you are caramelizing onions, add a pinch of salt, which draws out the moisture of the onion which then evaporates, providing a sweet, caramelized effect.

Baking or Roasting: To bake or roast without adding oil, line a baking sheet with a good-quality nonstick baking sheet or parchment paper to prevent sticking. Toss vegetables with enough vegetable broth to coat. This will add moisture and flavor while allowing the vegetables to cook evenly. In baking, applesauce, mashed bananas, and date paste are great substitutions for oil.

HEALTHY ALTERNATIVES TO REPLACE SALT

Garlic: Add raw or cooked garlic, garlic powder or flakes to chicken, fish, lean red meat, and vegetables.

Onions: Raw or cooked, onions complement nearly any savory dish from soups and stews to burgers, pizza, and pasta sauces.

Lemon juice: Lemon juice adds a bright taste and is a great replacement for salt. Add a squeeze of lemon to salads, steamed or roasted vegetables, grilled fish or chicken, soups, and sauces.

Vinegar: Balsamic, white balsamic, apple cider, red wine, white wine, and champagne vinegars are the ultimate flavor enhancers. They are the perfect condiment to salads and perfect to splash over poultry, seafood, and vegetables.

Salsas and chutneys: Homemade salsas and chutneys are easy to make and a great accompaniment to grilled meats, appetizers, chips, omelets, fish, and tacos.

Mushrooms: Mushrooms bring natural umami flavors. Ditch the soy sauce, Worcestershire sauce, and other high-sodium condiments for mushrooms. Caramelize onions with mushrooms and add a dash of balsamic vinegar.

Herbs and spices: Pick up some fresh rosemary, thyme, chives, or basil at the market. Cayenne can be used in a variety of dishes including meats, grains, soups, and vegetables. Cumin adds a distinct smoky and earthy flavor to food and works well with lean meats like chicken, beef, and lamb. Add Herbs de Provence, coriander, lemon pepper, and no-salt seasonings to your pantry.

https://www.nhlbi.nih.gov/health/educational/healthdisp/pdf/tipsheets/Use-Herbs-and-Spices-Instead-of-Salt.pdf

GRAINS

Grains are the edible seeds of various members of the grass family. Each seed consists of four parts:

- The husk – an inedible fibrous outer layer that is removed during processing
- The endosperm – the starchy mass that forms most of the kernel

- The bran – a tough but edible layer covering the endosperm
- The germ – the tiny embryo that forms the new plant when the seed sprouts

There are two types of grains: whole grains and refined grains. To qualify as a whole grain, the cereal kernel must have the endosperm, bran, and germ, while refined grains do not include the bran or germ.

Whole grains such as whole wheat flour contain nutrients and fiber. Refined grains, such as white flour and white rice, are milled, a process that strips out both the bran and germ to give them a finer texture and longer shelf life. The refining process also removes many nutrients, including fiber (Whole Grains Council).

Eat whole grains rather than refined grains as often as possible. Examples of whole grains include the following:

Amaranth – gluten-free
Barley
Brown rice – gluten-free
Buckwheat – gluten-free
Bulgur (cracked wheat)
Corn – gluten-free
Farro
Millet – gluten-free
Oats
Quinoa – gluten-free
Sorghum – gluten-free
Triticale
Wheat berry
Wild rice – gluten-free

COOKING GRAINS

Most grains are cooked by one of three cooking methods: the simmering method, the pilaf method, and the risotto method.

Simmering Method (Table 10.1)

1. For whole grains, wash the grain in cold water as necessary. Drain.
2. Combine the grain with the proper amount of water or other liquid in a heavy saucepot. Bring to a boil. Stir.
3. Cover and cook over very low heat for the proper cooking time, depending on the grain.
4. Test for doneness; cook for a few additional minutes if necessary.
5. Remove from heat. Drain excess liquid if necessary. Let stand, covered, to allow moisture to be absorbed uniformly by the grain.
6. For rice and any grains that stick together, fluff with a fork and turn out into a pan to let steam escape and stop the cooking.

Pilaf Method (Table 10.1)

1. Heat the desired fat (such as butter or olive oil) in a heavy pan. Add chopped onion or other aromatic vegetable, if desired, and sauté until soft but not browned.

2. Add the grain. Stir to coat the grains with fat.
3. Cook the grain in the fat, stirring, to toast the grain lightly.
4. Add the proper amount of hot liquid.
5. Bring to a simmer, stirring occasionally.
6. Cover tightly. Cook on the stovetop or in an oven for the correct length of time, depending on the grain.
7. Remove from the heat and let stand, covered, to allow the moisture to be absorbed uniformly by the grain.

Risotto Method

1. Heat the desired fat (such as butter or olive oil) in a heavy pan. Add chopped onion or other aromatic vegetable, if desired, and sauté until soft but not browned.
2. Add the grain. Stir to coat the grains with fat.
3. Cook the grain in the fat, stirring, to toast the grain lightly.
4. Add a small amount of hot liquid. Cook slowly, stirring, until the liquid is absorbed by the grain.
5. Add a second small amount of liquid, and repeat the procedure.
6. Continue adding a small quantity of liquid at a time, stirring constantly and waiting until the liquid is absorbed before adding more.
7. Stop adding liquid when the grain is tender but still firm. It should be moist and creamy but not runny.

TABLE 10.1

Cook Times (in Minutes) for Various Grains Using the Simmering or Pilaf Methods[a]

Grain (1 Cup)	Simmering Method		Pilaf Method	
	Liquid (Cups)	Cook Time (minutes)	Liquid (Cups)	Cook Time (minutes)
Amaranth	2	20–25	25–30	2.5
Barley, pearled	2	35	35	2
Buckwheat	2	20	25–35	2
Bulgur	2	10–15	20–30	2
Kamut[b]	4	45–60	45–60	2
Millet	2.5	20–25	25–30	2.5
Quinoa	2	20–25	25–30	2
Rice, brown	2.5	40–50	45–60	2.5
Rye berries[b]	4	45–60	45–60	3
Sorghum	4	25–40	30–40	3
Spelt berries[b]	4	40–50	45–60	3
Teff	3	20–25	25–30	2.5
Wheat berries	4	45–60	45–60	2.5
Wild rice	3	40–50	45–60	2

[a] Some simmering method cook times and liquid requirements were obtained from The Whole Grains Council.
[b] Requires overnight soak.

THE SWEETENING POWER OF FRUIT

The best sources for sugar alternatives are whole foods, such as dates, bananas, applesauce, and pureed and dried fruit. Dates are an effective sweetener; they contain fiber, and their flavor can sweeten breads, cakes, smoothies, and desserts.

When substituting sugar for fruits, their moisture content has to be taken into account, which may change the proportion of liquids and other ingredients added to the mix. A second consideration is the sugar composition of several fruits, which is primarily glucose and fructose. These simple sugars (monosaccharides) promote nonenzymatic browning (Maillard reaction) because they are reducing sugars. In contrast, table sugar (sucrose) is not a reducing sugar and thus, may not promote Maillard browning to the same extent as that of reducing sugars. However, most fruits have a pH level in a range from 2.5 to 4.5, which helps decrease the rate of nonenzymatic browning, which increases greatly in alkaline (pH > 7.0) conditions.

IN CONCLUSION

Cooking at home is cheaper and healthier than eating out. Teach yourself to cook healthy things you love that are easy to prepare. Everyone's ideal diet is different. Talk to your physician about your specific needs. The best way to maintain health is through a healthful lifestyle. It's not always possible to avoid disease completely, but protecting our health through diet and exercise and by doing as much as we can to develop resilience is a step we can all take.

REFERENCES

https://health.gov/our-work/food-nutrition/2015-2020-dietary-guidelines/guidelines/appendix–7/.
https://wholegrainscouncil.org.
https://www.ewg.org/foodnews/dirty-dozen.php.
https://www.healthline.com/health/what-happens-if-you-eat-raw-chicken#symptoms.
http://www.heart.org/HEARTORG/HealthyLiving/HealthyEating/SimpleCookingand Recipes/Healthy-Cooking-Oils_UCM_445179_Article.jsp#.W2NEjy2ZP6Y.
https://www.nhlbi.nih.gov/health/educational/healthdisp/pdf/tipsheets/Use-Herbs-and-Spices-Instead-of-Salt.pdf.
Labensky, Hause, & Martel. *On Cooking*, (New York: Pearson, 2011) p. 78.
Lenders C, Gorman K, Milch H, Decker A, Harvey N, Stanfield L, Lim-Miller A, Salge-Blake J, Judd L, Levine S. A novel nutrition medicine education model: the Boston University experience. *Adv Nutr*. 2013 Jan 1;4(1):1–7.
Mark Hyman, MD. *Food, What the Heck Should I Eat?* (New York, Boston: Little, Brown and Company, 2018) pp. 17–18.
NutritionFacts.org. https://nutritionfacts.org/2019/07/11/dialing-down-the-grim-reaper-gene/.
Salmon CP, Knize MG, Felton JS. Effects of marinating on heterocyclic amine carcinogen formation in grilled chicken. *Food Chem Toxicol*. 1997 May;35(5):433–41. doi: 10.1016/s0278-6915(97)00020-3. PMID: 9216741.

APPENDIX: HEALTHY RECIPES

SPAGHETTI SQUASH WITH SPINACH, ARTICHOKES, AND MEATBALLS

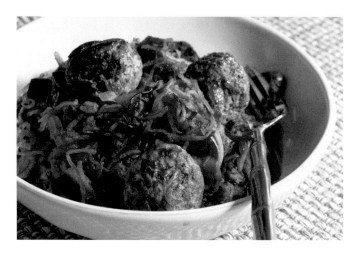

Free of added salt, oil, and sugar, this dish is loaded with flavor. If you've never prepared spaghetti squash before, it's much easier than you might think.

Makes: 4 servings

Spaghetti Squash
    1 medium spaghetti squash

Meatballs
    1–2 tbsp water
    1 cup finely chopped red onion
    1 pound lean ground dark turkey
    2 tsp minced garlic
    1 tbsp Dijon or whole grain mustard
    1 tsp dried Italian seasoning
    ¼ tsp black pepper

Sauce
    ¼ cup water, divided
    1 cup chopped onion
    1 cup chopped red bell pepper
    1 tsp Italian dried seasoning
    ¼ tsp crushed red pepper flakes
    1 (14.5-ounce) can diced tomatoes
    1 (14.5-ounce) can artichoke hearts, quartered, rinsed, and drained
    4 cups fresh baby spinach, firmly packed
    ¼ cup fresh chopped parsley

Method

1. **For the spaghetti squash,** preheat oven to 400°F. Cut spaghetti squash in half, lengthwise. Scoop out seeds and discard. Place squash cut side down on a baking pan lined with parchment paper or foil. Bake for 35–40 minutes until tender but not overcooked. Cooking time may vary depending on oven and size of squash.

2. Remove from oven and allow to cool slightly. Flip squash over, and use a fork to shred into "spaghetti," and transfer to a bowl. Set aside. The spaghetti squash can be prepared a day in advance.

3. **For the meatballs,** preheat oven to 400°F.

4. Heat a small sauté pan over medium heat. Add 1 tablespoon water. It should sizzle. Add the onions, and cook for 3 minutes, adding an additional tablespoon of water as needed.

5. Transfer onions to a bowl. Add turkey, garlic, mustard, Italian seasoning, and pepper. Mix well.

6. Portion into meatballs, about two tablespoons per meatball. Place on a parchment- or foil-lined baking pan. The yield is about 16 meatballs.

7. Heat a large nonstick sauté pan over medium heat. Add the meatballs, working in batches so not to overcrowd the pan. Sear, turning with tongs, until all sides are browned, about 5–7 minutes. Return the seared meatballs to the baking pan.

8. Set aside while preparing the sauce. When the sauce is almost ready, place meatballs in oven and bake for 8–10 minutes, until meatballs are cooked through and thermometer registers 165°F.

9. **For the sauce,** heat a deep skillet over medium-high heat. Add 1 tablespoon of water. It should sizzle. Add the onions and reduce heat to medium. Cook for 3 minutes, adding a tablespoon of water at a time, as needed. Add bell pepper and cook another minute.

10. Add Italian seasoning and red pepper flakes and cook for 1 minute. Add undrained tomatoes and cook for 4 minutes.

11. Add artichokes and spinach. Cover and cook until spinach is wilted, about 3 minutes.

12. Measure out 3 cups of spaghetti squash. Add squash and parsley to skillet, and gently stir to heat through.

13. Portion into bowls, and top with turkey meatballs.

CREAMY VEGETABLE SOUP

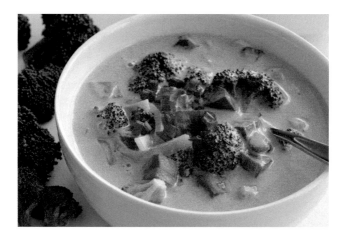

A delicious easy-to-make soup packed with veggies in a creamy broth.

Makes: 6 (1 ¼ cup) servings

Cashew Cream
   1 cup whole raw cashews
   3 ½ cups water, divided (2 cups + 1 ½ cups)
   2 tbsp nutritional yeast

Soup
   1 tbsp water
   1 cup sliced onions
   ½ cup thinly sliced celery
   2 tsp minced garlic
   4 cups low-sodium vegetable broth
   1/8 tsp black pepper
   1 ½ cups half-inch diced carrots
   3 cups broccoli, cut into small florets
   2 tbsp sliced green onions, optional garnish

Method
   1. **For the cashew cream,** place the cashews in a medium bowl and cover with two cups of water. Set aside uncovered at room temperature for 3–4 hours. Drain and rinse. Place the drained cashews, 1 ½ cups water, and nutritional yeast in a high-speed blender. Blend until completely smooth, about 1 minute. Transfer to an airtight container, and refrigerate until ready to use. Cashew cream holds for up to 5 days in the refrigerator.

2. **For the soup,** heat a large saucepan over medium-high heat. Add water. When water starts to sputter, add onions and celery and cook, stirring frequently for 3 minutes, adding an additional tablespoon of water as needed. Add garlic, and cook for an additional 30 seconds.
3. Add vegetable broth and pepper and bring to a boil. Lower heat to medium. Add carrots and gently simmer for 5 minutes.
4. Add broccoli and simmer for 2 minutes. Add cashew cream, and increase heat to medium-high. Once it comes to a boil, reduce heat to medium and simmer for about 3 minutes, until broccoli is crisp tender.
5. Garnish with green onions, if desired.

BROCCOLI RISOTTO

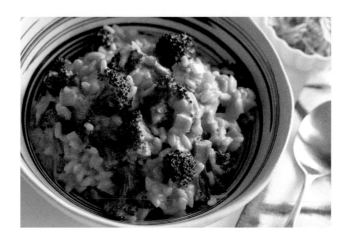

We've taken out the butter, heavy cream, and cheese, and this risotto still rivals that of any restaurant.

Makes: 4 servings

Ingredients
   4 cups broccoli florets
   1 quart low-sodium vegetable broth
   1 cup water
   1 tbsp grapeseed oil or olive oil
   1 cup diced onion
   1/8 tsp sea salt
   1 ½ cups Arborio rice
   ½ cup dry white wine, such as Sauvignon Blanc
   1 tbsp lemon juice

Method

1. Bring 2 inches of water to a boil in a large pot. Place a steamer basket in the pot. Place broccoli florets in the steamer basket and reduce heat to medium. Cover and steam for approximately 5 minutes, until crisp tender. Remove from heat and rinse under cold running water to stop the cooking process and drain. Chop the broccoli. Set aside.
2. In a medium saucepan, heat the broth and 1 cup water just until hot. Turn heat to low to keep the broth warm.
3. Heat oil in a large saucepan. Add onion and a pinch of salt and sauté over medium-low heat for 5 minutes until onions begin to soften, being careful not to brown them.
4. Add Arborio and stir with a wooden spoon for 2 minutes until all the grains are well coated with oil. Set your timer for 18 minutes. This is the approximate time it takes to make risotto. Add wine. Stir until completely absorbed. Begin to add hot broth, ½ cup at a time, stirring frequently. Wait until each addition is almost completely absorbed before adding the next half cup, stirring frequently to prevent sticking.
5. Since stoves and sizes of pots vary, check risotto for doneness after 17 and 18 minutes of cooking.
6. When the rice is tender but still firm, add ¼ cup broth and broccoli, stirring briefly until broccoli is heated through. You may have a little broth leftover. Remove from heat and stir in lemon juice. Let sit for 5 minutes before serving.

TERIYAKI STIR-FRIED VEGGIES

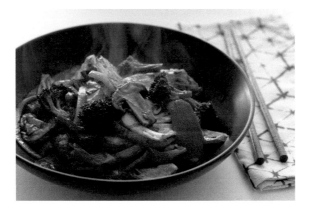

Dive into deliciousness as we replace soy sauce in this teriyaki sauce with coconut aminos, a healthy replacement that contains 73% less sodium.

Makes: 4 servings

Sauce

    6 tbsp coconut aminos
    6 tbsp pineapple juice
    3 tbsp water
    2 ¼ tsp minced garlic
    2 ¼ tsp minced ginger
    4 tsp cornstarch

Stir-fry

    2 tsp grapeseed or olive oil
    2 cups sliced yellow onions
    4 cups chopped green cabbage (about ¼ head)
    2 cups sliced mushrooms (about 4 ounces)
    2 cups broccoli florets, steamed or blanched
    2 cups carrots, cut on the diagonal/bias, steamed or blanched

Method

1. **For the sauce,** whisk together coconut aminos, pineapple juice, water, garlic, and ginger in a small bowl. Whisk in cornstarch and set aside.
2. **For the stir-fry,** heat a wok or sauté pan over high heat. Add oil. Add onions and stir-fry for 1 ½ minutes.
3. Add cabbage and stir-fry for another 1 ½ minutes.
4. Add mushrooms and cook for 1 ½ minutes.
5. Add broccoli and carrots. Stir sauce and pour over vegetables. Stir-fry 1 minute.

SORGHUM PILAF, 4-BEAN SALAD & ROASTED TOMATO VINAIGRETTE

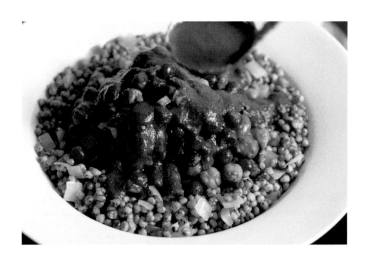

This healthy grain retains the majority of its nutrients since it doesn't have an inedible hull like many other grains.

Makes: 6 servings

4-Bean Salad

3 cups precooked green beans, cut into 1-inch pieces (see recipe notes)
1 (15-ounce) can black beans (no added salt), drained and rinsed
1 (15.5-ounce) can pinto beans (no added salt), drained and rinsed
1 (15.5-ounce) can garbanzo beans (no added salt), drained and rinsed
1 ½ cups frozen peas, thawed
1 ½ cups frozen corn, thawed (optional)
½ cup diced red onion, soaked in ice water for 10–15 minutes & drained (see recipe notes)
¾ cup chopped tomato (approximately 1 medium tomato)
¼ cup apple cider vinegar
2 tbsp fresh lemon juice
2 tbsp Dijon style mustard
1 tbsp honey
1 tsp ground cumin
1 tsp chopped garlic

Spicy Tomato Vinaigrette

1 (14.5-ounce) can diced tomatoes, no salt added
2 tbsp olive oil
2 tbsp fresh oregano, stems removed
2 tbsp fresh Italian parsley, stems removed
4 tsp Balsamic vinegar
1 tsp harissa
1/8 tsp white pepper

Sorghum Pilaf

2 cups uncooked whole grain sorghum
2 quarts low-sodium vegetable broth
1 ½ cups chopped white or yellow onion

Method

1. **For the 4-bean salad,** place green beans, black beans, pinto beans, garbanzo beans, peas, corn, and onion in a large bowl. Set aside.
2. Place tomato, vinegar, lemon juice, mustard, honey, cumin, and garlic into a blender; blend until smooth. Pour over the bean mixture and stir to combine. Set aside in refrigerator.
3. **For the spicy tomato vinaigrette,** place undrained tomatoes, oil, oregano, parsley, vinegar, harissa, and pepper in a blender; blend until smooth.
4. Transfer to a container and place in the refrigerator.

5. **For the pilaf,** rinse the sorghum and place in a medium saucepan with the broth and heat over medium-high heat. When it comes to a boil, reduce heat to medium-low and cover. Simmer for 1 hour, or until grains are tender, but still chewy. Remove from heat and drain through a strainer.
6. In a nonstick pan, sauté the onions over medium heat using 1–2 tablespoons of water or broth at a time as needed to cook the onions, without steaming them. Sauté for approximately 8–10 minutes, stirring periodically so they don't burn.
7. Add the cooked sorghum to the pan and stir until heated through.
8. **To assemble,** place ¾ cup of sorghum pilaf in each bowl. Top with one cup of 4-bean salad, and drizzle with spicy tomato vinaigrette.

Recipe Notes:
- To cook green beans, trim the ends. You can steam them or cook in boiling water, covered. This will take about 4–6 minutes. Cook until the beans are tender, but not mushy. Quickly transfer the beans to a large bowl of ice water. Placing the beans in ice water stops the cooking process and helps set the vibrant green color. When cool, remove beans from water and pat dry.
- Soaking onions in ice water for 10–15 minutes mellows their flavor. The cold water keeps the onion super crunchy, while the sulfur compounds that give onion its pungent, harsh flavor dissipate in the water.

GRILLED SALMON WITH BLACK RICE AND MANGO SALSA

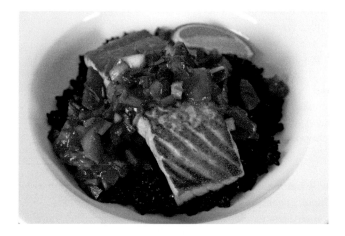

Legend has it that this forbidden rice was once reserved for emperors of China. Black rice is a natural source of antioxidants called anthocyanins.

Makes: 4 servings
Ingredients
   2 cups chopped mango
   ½ cup chopped red bell pepper
   2 tbsp chopped red onion, soaked in ice water for 10–15 minutes and drained
   2 tbsp chopped cilantro
   1 jalapeño pepper, seeded and minced (about 2 tbsp)
   1 tbsp fresh lime juice
   1 cup raw forbidden (black) rice, cooked according to package directions
   4 (4-ounce) salmon fillets

Method
   1. For the salsa, in a small bowl, combine the mango, bell pepper, onion, cilan-
      tro, jalapeño, and lime juice. Set aside in the refrigerator.
   2. Prepare the rice according to package instructions.
   3. When the rice is almost done, grill or broil the salmon until just cooked
      through.
   4. To assemble, divide the rice between 4 plates. Top each with a piece of
      salmon and salsa.

Recipe Notes:
   • Soaking onions in ice water for 10–15 minutes mellows their flavor. The cold
     water keeps the onion super crunchy, while the sulfur compounds that give
     onion its pungent, harsh flavor dissipate in the water.

VEGETABLE BROTH

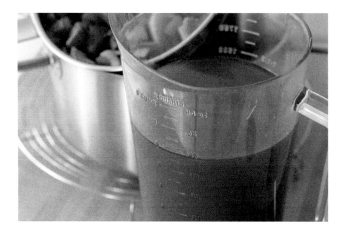

*This healthy broth makes the perfect base for soups, sauces, gravy, and all kinds of
recipes, without the sodium packed in most store-bought brands. You'll never want
to buy the boxed broth again.*

Makes: 4 ½ cups
Ingredients
  2 quarts plus 1 tbsp water, divided
  2 ½ cups chopped onions (about 2 medium onions)
  2 cups carrots, peeled and chopped (about 4 medium carrots)
  2 cups celery stalks, sliced (about 4 medium stalks)
  4 cloves garlic, peeled
  2 quarts water
  ¼ cup fresh Italian parsley
  1 tsp black peppercorns
  ½ tsp dried thyme
  2 bay leaves

Method
  1. In a large saucepan, heat 1 tablespoon water over medium heat. When the water starts to sputter, add onions, carrots, celery, and garlic. Cook for about 5 minutes, stirring occasionally. Add a tablespoon of water as needed to prevent sticking.
  2. Add 2 quarts water, parsley, peppercorns, thyme, and bay leaves. Increase heat to high. When it comes to a boil, stir and reduce heat to medium-low. Simmer, uncovered, for about an hour.
  3. Place a fine mesh strainer over a large pot. Carefully pour contents into the strainer. Reserve broth and discard solids. If freezing, allow broth to cool completely before transferring to freezer-safe storage containers.

LEMONY CHICKEN SOUP

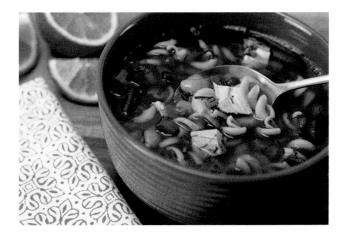

This comfort food classic will have everyone thinking you spent all day cooking it from scratch. Brimming with vegetables, chicken and pasta, this soup is hearty and comforting for the whole family. Soups on!

Makes: 4 servings

Ingredients
  4 ounces uncooked shell pasta, fusilli, or other short pasta
  1 tbsp water
  1 cup diced onions
  ½ cup diced celery
  6 cups low-sodium chicken or vegetable broth
  1 bay leaf
  12 ounces chicken breasts, skinless and boneless
  1 cup diced carrots
  1 cup frozen peas, thawed
  2 tbsp lemon juice
  1 tbsp finely chopped dill
  1 tbsp finely chopped Italian parsley

Method

1. Cook pasta according to package directions. Drain in a colander, and rinse under cold water. Set aside.
2. Heat a medium saucepan over medium heat. Add water. When it starts to sputter, add onions and celery. Cover pan and sweat for 6 minutes, stirring occasionally.
3. Add broth and bay leaf. Increase heat and bring to a boil.
4. Add chicken breasts. Cover and reduce heat to medium-low and simmer for 7 minutes.
5. Add carrots and simmer another 5–7 minutes, until carrots are tender and chicken is cooked. Turn off heat and remove pan from stove.
6. Remove bay leaf and discard. Remove chicken breasts and allow to cool slightly. When cool enough to handle, chop into bite-size pieces.
7. Return the pan to the stove over medium heat. Bring to a gentle simmer and add peas, diced chicken, and pasta and gently simmer approximately 3 minutes, until peas, chicken, and pasta are heated through.
8. Remove from heat and stir in lemon juice, dill, and parsley.

Recipe Notes:
- Sweating is the gentle heating of vegetables. By keeping the lid on, you use their own liquid to sweat or steam them.
- For a veggie version, replace chicken broth with vegetable broth and chicken with one (15-ounce) can white beans, drained and rinsed.

ROASTED TOMATO WHITE BEAN DIP

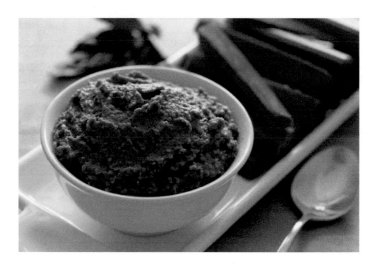

This tomato white bean dip is wonderful with veggies, crackers or crostini, and even wrapped up in kale or romaine leaves.

Makes: 2 ½ cups
Ingredients
   1 garlic bulb (see recipe notes)
   1 tsp olive oil
   2 (15-ounce) cans great northern white beans, drained and rinsed
   2 tbsp fresh lemon juice (about 1 lemon)
   1/3 cup oven roasted tomatoes (or 6–8 sun dried)
   2 tbsp fresh basil, chopped (about 6 large leaves)
   ½ tsp sea salt
   1/8 tsp ground white pepper
   ¼ cup low-sodium vegetable broth, or more as needed

Method
   1. Preheat oven to 400°F.
   2. To roast the garlic, peel and discard the loose layer of the bulb, leaving cloves intact. With a sharp knife, cut ¼ to ½-inch from the top to expose cloves. Rub a little oil over the exposed cloves. Tightly wrap the bulb in foil, and bake for about 30–40 minutes, until the cloves are soft. Do not over-bake and brown the garlic bulb; the flavor will be too strong for this dip. Keeping in foil, set garlic aside to cool slightly.
   3. Place beans in a food processor.
   4. When cool enough to handle, squeeze roasted garlic flesh from the bulb. Measure out 1 tablespoon of roasted garlic and add to the beans, reserving remaining garlic for another use.

5. Add lemon juice, tomatoes, basil, salt, pepper, and vegetable broth to food processor. Process until smooth. If the dip is too thick, add an additional tablespoon of broth as needed, and process for an additional 30 seconds.

6. Transfer to an appropriate container and store in the refrigerator for up to 3 days.

Recipe Notes:

You can substitute 2 teaspoons of raw minced garlic for the roasted garlic. We prefer roasted garlic, as raw garlic has a strong, pungent, and heated taste. Garlic mellows and sweetens considerably when cooking. Roasted garlic offers a well-balanced, delicate, sweet, and nutty flavor.

Roasting garlic also changes the chemical makeup of the garlic, so it's easier to digest.

CINNAMON SCENTED QUINOA PILAF

This quinoa pilaf is dressed up with sautéed onions, raisins, and cinnamon sticks. A healthy and easy side dish!

Makes: 4 cups

Ingredients

1 tbsp water
1 ½ cups sliced yellow onions
3 tbsp fresh lime juice
2 cups low-sodium vegetable broth
1 cup white quinoa
¼ cup golden raisins
¼ cup dark raisins
2 each cinnamon sticks
¼ tsp sea salt

Method

1. Heat a 2-quart saucepan over medium heat. Add water. When water starts to sputter, add onions. Cook, stirring occasionally for 6 minutes to slightly caramelize onions. Add an additional tablespoon of water as needed.

2. Add lime juice to deglaze pan, cooking for 1 minute.

3. Add broth, quinoa, golden and dark raisins, cinnamon sticks, and salt. Stir to combine. Increase heat to medium-high and bring to a boil. Cover and reduce heat to medium-low. Cook for 20 minutes.

4. When quinoa is done, remove from heat. Let rest for 5 minutes. Then fluff with a fork and remove cinnamon sticks.

BREAKFAST HASH BROWNS

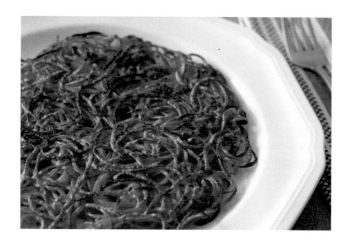

Crispy hash browns without the salt and oil, the perfect breakfast side!

Makes: 2 servings

Ingredients
   2 small Yukon Gold potatoes (8 ounces), peeled
   1/8 tsp ground black pepper
   1 cup unsweetened applesauce, optional

Method
   1. Slice the potatoes using the coarse blade of a vegetable spiralizer. You can also grate the potatoes using the larger holes on a box grater.
   2. Pat the potatoes dry between paper towels.
   3. Preheat a large nonstick frying pan over medium heat. Place the shredded potatoes into the hot pan, spreading to an even 1-inch layer.
   4. Cook for 5–7 minutes with the lid partially off. When the hash browns are a medium brown, flip them, and cook partially covered for another 5–7 minutes.
   5. Serve immediately, seasoned with a little black pepper and a side of applesauce, if desired.

CITRUS GUACAMOLE

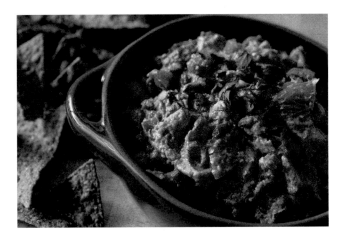

Citrus guacamole brings a burst of sunshine to your palate. Great with tortilla chips, toast, bell peppers, radishes, carrots, or added to your favorite veggie wrap.

Makes: 6 servings

Ingredients

1 poblano pepper
1 tsp olive oil
1 cup firmly packed kale, stems removed (about 1 ounce)
3 large ripe avocados or 4 medium
1 tbsp fresh lime juice
1 pink grapefruit, segmented and chopped
1 orange, segmented and chopped
¼ cup diced red onion, soaked in ice water for 10–15 minutes and drained (see recipe notes)
2 tbsp chopped cilantro
½ tsp ground cumin

Method

1. Preheat oven to 400°F. Rub pepper with olive oil. Place on a small baking pan lined with foil and roast until soft and a bit charred, about 15–20 minutes, turning pepper halfway through. Remove from oven and place in a small bowl. Cover bowl tightly with plastic wrap and allow to cool for 10–15 minutes. This process will help to loosen the skin, making it easier to remove. Remove the stem, seeds, and outer skin. Dice pepper. You will have approximately 1/3 cup.

2. Wash and clean the kale to remove any grit. Remove the stems by grabbing the leaves with your hand and pulling the stem away in the opposite direction.

3. Place kale in a steaming basket and set in a large saucepan with about 2-inches of boiling water. Cover and steam kale until wilted, about 2–3 minutes. Remove from heat, and when cool, squeeze out excess moisture, chop, and set aside.

4. Slice the avocados in half, around the pit. Remove the pit. Slice the avocados while still in the shell but not cutting through the skin. Scoop the avocado with a spoon into a medium bowl.

5. Add lime juice, and lightly smash avocados with a potato masher or fork until coarsely mashed.

6. Add kale, grapefruit, orange, chile, onion, cilantro, and cumin. Gently mix to combine ingredients.

Recipe Notes

• Soaking onions in ice water for 10–15 minutes mellows their flavor. The cold water keeps the onion super crunchy, while the sulfur compounds that give onion its pungent, harsh flavor dissipate in the water.

Index

Note: **Bold** page numbers refer to tables and *italic* page numbers refer to figures.

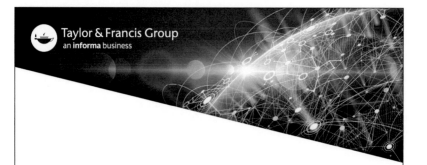